LAST MINUTE REVISION
FOR
NBE/DNB/NEET/PGMEE/FMGE

Fourth Edition

Mathew R John MBBS MD
Psychiatry (NIMHANS)
Consultant Psychiatrist
Community Mental Health Programme
Kottayam, Kerala, India

Simi Babu MBBS DMRD
Consultant Radiologist
Govt. Medical College Kottayam
Kottayam, Kerala, India

Sanish Babu MBBS
Postgraduate Trainee in Pathology
Regional Cancer Centre (RCC)
Thiruvananthapuram, Kerala, India

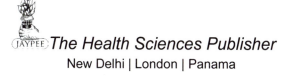

The Health Sciences Publisher
New Delhi | London | Panama

Jaypee Brothers Medical Publishers (P) Ltd

Headquarters

Jaypee Brothers Medical Publishers (P) Ltd
4838/24, Ansari Road, Daryaganj
New Delhi 110 002, India
Phone: +91-11-43574357
Fax: +91-11-43574314
Email: jaypee@jaypeebrothers.com

Overseas Offices

J.P. Medical Ltd
83 Victoria Street, London
SW1H 0HW (UK)
Phone: +44 20 3170 8910
Fax: +44 (0)20 3008 6180
Email: info@jpmedpub.com

Jaypee-Highlights Medical Publishers Inc
City of Knowledge, Bld. 235, 2nd Floor, Clayton
Panama City, Panama
Phone: +1 507-301-0496
Fax: +1 507-301-0499
Email: cservice@jphmedical.com

Jaypee Brothers Medical Publishers (P) Ltd
Bhotahity, Kathmandu, Nepal
Phone +977-9741283608
Email: kathmandu@jaypeebrothers.com

Jaypee Brothers Medical Publishers (P) Ltd
17/1-B Babar Road, Block-B, Shaymali
Mohammadpur, Dhaka-1207
Bangladesh
Mobile: +08801912003485
Email: jaypeedhaka@gmail.com

Website: www.jaypeebrothers.com
Website: www.jaypeedigital.com

© 2018, Jaypee Brothers Medical Publishers

The views and opinions expressed in this book are solely those of the original contributor(s)/author(s) and do not necessarily represent those of editor(s) of the book.

All rights reserved. No part of this publication may be reproduced, stored or transmitted in any form or by any means, electronic, mechanical, photocopying, recording or otherwise, without the prior permission in writing of the publishers.

All brand names and product names used in this book are trade names, service marks, trademarks or registered trademarks of their respective owners. The publisher is not associated with any product or vendor mentioned in this book.

Medical knowledge and practice change constantly. This book is designed to provide accurate, authoritative information about the subject matter in question. However, readers are advised to check the most current information available on procedures included and check information from the manufacturer of each product to be administered, to verify the recommended dose, formula, method and duration of administration, adverse effects and contraindications. It is the responsibility of the practitioner to take all appropriate safety precautions. Neither the publisher nor the author(s)/editor(s) assume any liability for any injury and/or damage to persons or property arising from or related to use of material in this book.

This book is sold on the understanding that the publisher is not engaged in providing professional medical services. If such advice or services are required, the services of a competent medical professional should be sought.

Every effort has been made where necessary to contact holders of copyright to obtain permission to reproduce copyright material. If any have been inadvertently overlooked, the publisher will be pleased to make the necessary arrangements at the first opportunity. The **CD/DVD-ROM** (if any) provided in the sealed envelope with this book is complimentary and free of cost. **Not meant for sale.**

Inquiries for bulk sales may be solicited at: jaypee@jaypeebrothers.com

Last Minute Revision

First Edition: 2014
Second Edition: 2015
Third Edition: 2017
Fourth Edition: **2018**
ISBN: 978-93-5270-432-3
Printed at Nutech Print Services - India

Dedicated to the great teachers in
NIMHANS
and
BMCRI

Preface to the Fourth Edition

Another year of competitive learning......our new edition comes with newer question patterns as well as some fuel to keep you going. During long and dry study hours, it is important to rediscover motivation, remember purpose and renew energy stores. We have added some quotes by men of history, both medical and others, to keep your spirits up.

Otherwise, it is business as usual. Needless to say, the importance of image based questions is increasing as is evident from NEET 2018. Still it is also important to familiarize oneself with the regular stock of often repeated questions. And to use whole brain thinking—not memory alone, but logical reasoning, common sense, thinking outside the box and multiple choice skills to get to maximum probability of getting a correct answer.

Wishing everyone a rocking 2018........claim your dreams!!!

Mathew R John
Simi Babu
Sanish Babu

From the Publisher's Desk
We request all the readers to provide us their valuable suggestions/errors (if any)
at: *jaypeemcqproduction@gmail.com*
so as to help us in further improvement of this book in the subsequent edition.

Preface to the First Edition

There are books and more books than one can imagine in the Medical PG Entrance field. As candidates who have successfully overcome the entrance barrier, we feel that it is not the sheer volume of facts that one skims through, but the retention of facts which matter ultimately in the entrance challenge.

As neuroscience tells us, consolidation of short term memories into lasting long term memories occurs in the hippocampus and this requires a constant revision of facts. Especially on the last week of the entrance days, there is a great requirement of revision of factoids with the maximum probability of being asked in the test.

With this aim in mind, we have designed a book which will give you maximum yield in the entrance exams with a focus on the new pattern of All India Exams. Hope you will benefit greatly from the book.

Mathew R John
Simi Babu
Sanish Babu

Acknowledgments

The authors of this book wish to convey their sincere and heartfelt gratitude to Shri. Jitendar P Vij (Group Chairman) and Mr Ankit Vij (Group President) M/s Jaypee Brothers Medical Publishing (P) Ltd, New Delhi India for providing the opportunity to see this book in print.

The authors wish to convey their gratitude to Ms Chetna Malhotra Vohra (Associate Director–Content Strategy) and Ms. Payal Bharti (Senior Manager- Publishing) for the great support and enthusiasm extended throughout the process of creating this book.

Special thanks to Sam Mathew and Steven Mathew for continuing to be sources of great love and inspiration.

Some Tales, Less Told..........

We have always thought that the students who qualify for MBBS are above average students. So the Postgraduate Medical Entrance test is a competition among very good students. In all sense, a battle royale!

Everybody wants to perform well, a lot of them actually perform well, and few end up in courses or specialities of their original choice – specialities to which their talents can make a lasting contribution.

So what is decisive is the extra edge. There is not much margin for error, both in the profession as well as the exam. Even less so in the exam. The edge, friends, is only with those people who actually perform a little extra, a little more than the norm, not necessarily with:

Those who study more, cram in as much information as possible

Those who take more stress for the exam

Those who sacrifice a lot of things

Those who invest the maximum hours.

The edge is with those students who can retain a lot of information, who can put their logic on the best bet even if they do not know the real answer, those who are familiar with the real art of multiple choice questions.

So, study smart, make learning fun because it is a long road out there……

Just for information sake, we are presenting two factoids which are not very popular, little known among most students but strangely true……..which I think will be of good use to you….

- Most students learn more from summaries than whole chapters.
- Most students benefit significantly on an average, by changing their answers, not relying on their first impressions.

Both these facts are proven with the help of years of extensive research……..now it is up to you to decide what to do……..

Contents

Image Based Questions

1. Anatomy — 1-20
2. Physiology — 21-40
3. Biochemistry — 41-53
4. Pathology — 54-79
5. Microbiology — 80-100
6. Pharmacology — 101-117
7. Preventive and Social Medicine — 118-133
8. Forensic Medicine — 134-150
9. ENT — 151-164
10. Ophthalmology — 165-183
11. Orthopaedics — 184-199
12. Medicine — 200-227
13. Surgery — 228-252
14. Obstetrics and Gynecology — 253-267
15. Pediatrics — 268-284
16. Dermatology — 285-300
17. Anesthesia — 301-311
18. Psychiatry — 312-325
19. Radiology — 326-342

Image Based Questions

1. The type of muscle present in the image shown is:

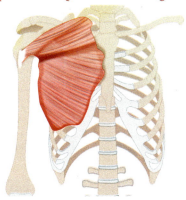

Ans. Cruciate/Convergent Muscle. (Pectoralis major is an example for convergent/cruciate muscle.)

(NEET PATTERN 2018)

2. Which nerve palsy causes Winging of Scapula ?

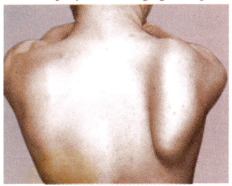

Ans. Long Thoracic Nerve.[Q]

3. The commonest anatomical position of the appendix is:

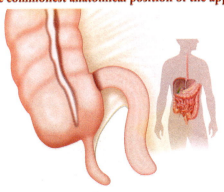

Ans. Retrocaecal position.[Q]

4. Muscle which is NOT a part of this muscle complex:

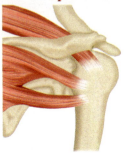

Ans. Teres Major[Q]

Rotator Cuff Muscles: Supraspinatus/Infraspinatus/Teres Minor/Subscapularis.

5. Function of the muscle shown in the picture:

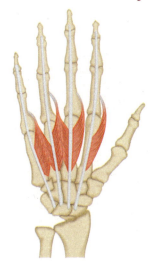

Ans. Flexion.[Q] *(NEET PATTERN 2018)*

Action of lumbricals: Flexion at MCP joint and extension at interphalangeal joints.

6. Ishihara charts are used to detect:

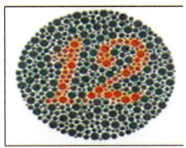

Ans. Colour Blindness.[Q]

7. 'A' wave in JVP is due to:

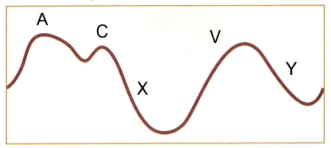

Ans. Atrial Contraction.^Q

8. Blood Testes barrier is formed by:

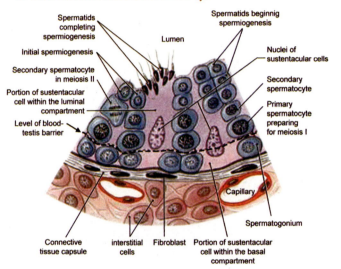

Ans. Basal lamina and adjacent sertoli cells.^Q

9. Name this structure thematically represented in the figure:

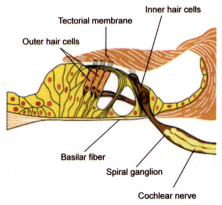

Ans. Organ of corti.^Q

10. This test can be used to measure:

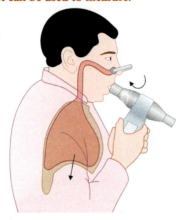

Ans. Tidal Volume. (Spirometry)[Q]

11. Casal's Necklace is due to deficiency of:

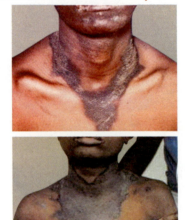

Ans. Niacin.[Q]

12. Which vitamin deficiency can cause glossitis?

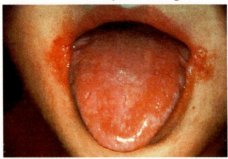

Ans. Riboflavin.[Q]

13. **This is known as:**

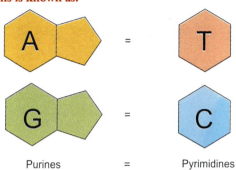

Ans. Chargaff's Rule.

14. **Organic compound seen in picture is formed by:**

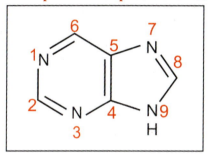

Ans. Aspartate, Glycine, Glutamine.[Q] (Structure shown: Purine)

15. **Pigmentation of Ear Cartilage is due to deficiency of:**

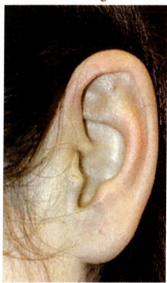

Ans. Homogenetisic Acid Oxidase.[Q]
This is seen in Ochronosis or Alkaptonuria.

16. The following histopathological slide from an orbital mass is indicative of:

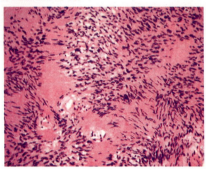

Ans. Schwannoma.^Q

17. The following peripheral smear is indicative of:

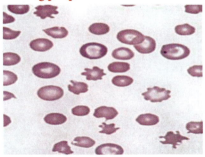

Ans. Acanthocytes.^Q

18. Identify the following histopathology specimens^Q:

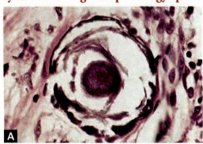

A
Psammoma bodies

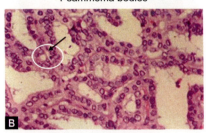

B
Orphan annie eye nuclei

Ans. Papillary Carcinoma thyroid

19. **Multinucleate Giant Cells seen in Measles:**

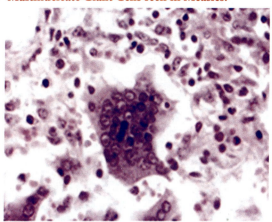

Ans. Warthin Finkledy Cells

20. **Identify the haematological abnormality:**

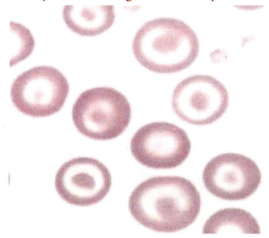

Ans. Target Cells.[Q]

21. **Name the virus in the figure which causes epidemics.**

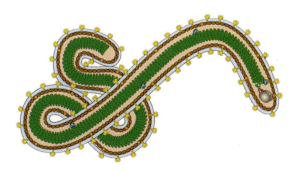

Ans. Ebola Virus[Q]

22. Name the virus shown in the picture which causes microcephaly:

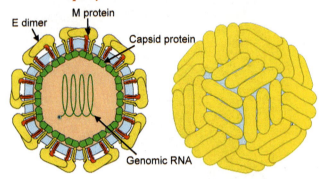

T=3-like organization of surface dimers

Ans. Zika Virus[Q]

23. The term Vaccine was introduced by: Louis Pasteur[Q]

Rabies and Anthrax vaccine were invented by Pasteur[Q]

Father of Modern Microbiology: Louis Pasteur[Q]

Father of microbiology: Antoni Van Leewenhoek

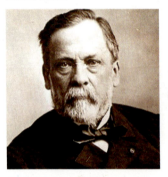
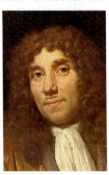

24. The following smear is indicative of:

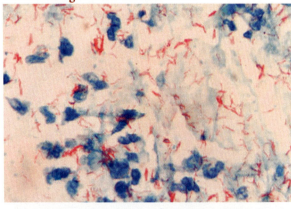

Ans. Mycobacterium Tuberculosis.[Q] *(AIIMS PATTERN 2017)*

25. Identify the organism in the picture:

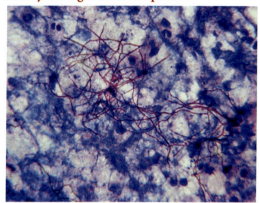

Ans. Nocardia[Q] (AIIMS PATTERN 2017)

26. Which organism is this image of endoflagella about?

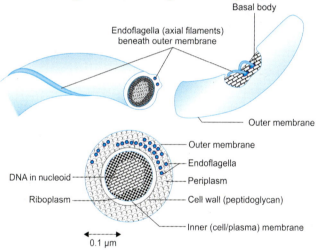

Ans. Leptospira icterohemorrhagica.[Q]

(AIIMS PATTERN 2017)

27. Hyphae branching in acute angulation is a feature of:

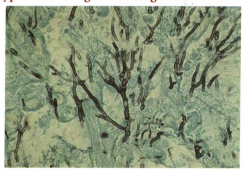

Ans. Aspergillus[Q]

28. The following image is the life cycle of:

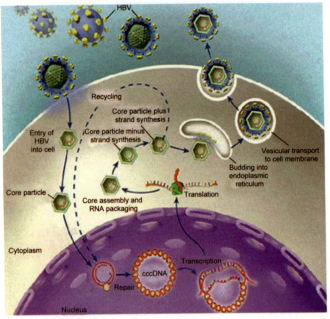

Ans. Hepatitis B Virus.^Q.   *(AIIMS PATTERN 2017)*

29. The organism shown in the image is:

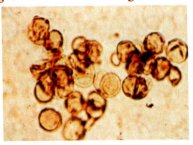

Ans. Chromoblastomycosis.^Q

30. Molar Tooth Colonies are seen in agar in:

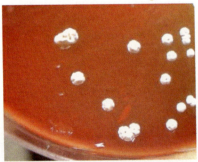

Ans. Actinomyces/Nocardia.
Typically described for Actinomyces israelii.

31. **Patient having HIV presented with fever and diarrhoea for 3 weeks. He was started on Sulphamethoxazole-Trimethoprim. His diarrhoea responded but his fever persisted. Bone marrow aspirate showed the following picture.**

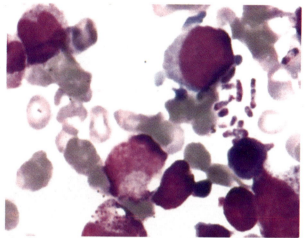

Ans. NOT correct about the pathogenetic organism:
(AIIMS PATTERN 2017)

It does NOT grow on SDA medium.[Q]

(The pathogenetic organism is Pencillium marneiffei which typically grows on Sabouraoud's Dextrose Agar-SDA- medium.)

32. **The classification system seen below is called:**

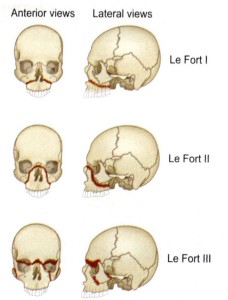

Ans. Lefort Classification.[Q]

33. Identify the cyst shown in the picture below:

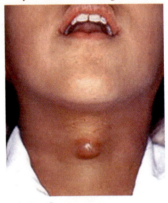

Ans. Thyroglossal Cyst[Q]

34. Identify the lesion:

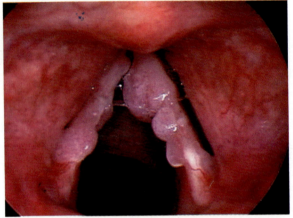

Ans. Respiratory Papillomatosis[Q] *(AIIMS PATTERN 2017)*

35. Condition shown in picture is due to hyperplasia of:

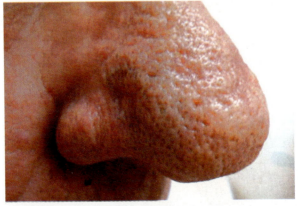

Ans. Sebaceous Glands.[Q]

Rhinophyma is also called Potato Nose/Tapir Nose[Q]

36. This ear ossicle develops from:

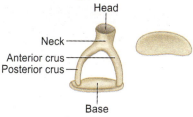

Ans. 2nd Branchial Arch.[Q]

37. The Tympanogram is indicative of:

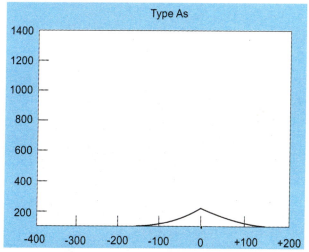

Ans. Otosclerosis.[Q]

38. The following picture is suggestive of:

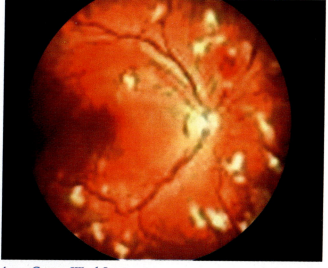

Ans. Cotton Wool Spot

39. The picture depicted below is indicative of:

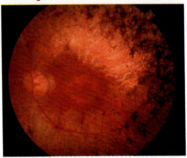

Ans. Retinitis Pigmentosa.^Q

40. Red Bag is used for:

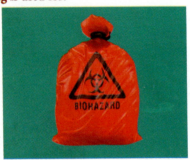

Ans. Biohazardous Waste.^Q   *(AIIMS PATTERN 2017)*

41. Identify the following X-ray:

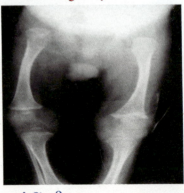

Ans. Wimberger's Sign^Q

- The **Wimberger's sign**, also called Wimberger's corner sign, refers to localized bilateral metaphyseal destruction of the medial proximal tibias. It is a pathognomonic sign for congenital syphilis.
- **Wimberger's Ring Sign**: Wimberger's ring sign refers to a circular calcification surrounding the osteoporotic epiphyseal center of ossification in scurvy, which may result from bleeding.

42. Identify the radiographic sign:

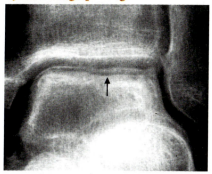

Ans. Hawkins Sign[Q]
- Hawkins sign
- In healing talar fractures
- Indicates good prognosis
- Indicates less chance for AVN talus

43. The following X-ray is suggestive of:

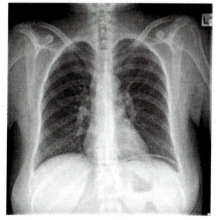

Ans. Gas under the Diaphragm.[Q]

44. The following X-ray image is suggestive of:

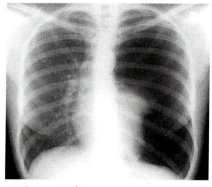

Ans. Pneumothorax Left Lung.

45. Identify the neurological syndrome given below:

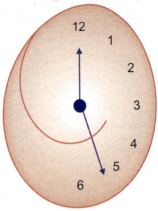

Ans. Hemineglect[Q]

46. Identify this condition:

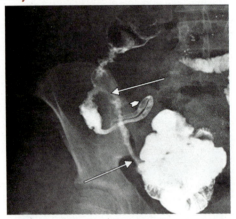

Ans. String Sign of Kantor in Crohn's Disease.

47. The following X-ray image is suggestive of:

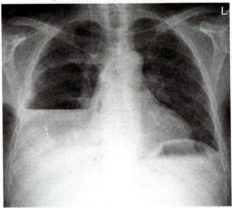

Ans. Empyema Thoracis.[Q]

48. The following X-ray is suggestive of:

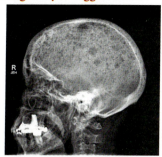

Ans. Punched Out Skull seen in Multiple Myeloma.^{Q}

49. The following X-ray is indicative of:

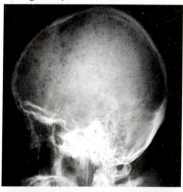

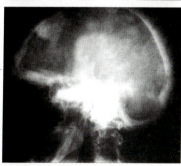

Ans. Paget's Disease.

50. Identify the following ECG:

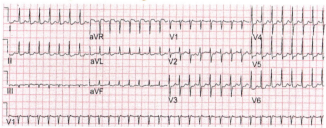

Ans. Supraventricular Tachycardia.

51. Identify the following ECGs.

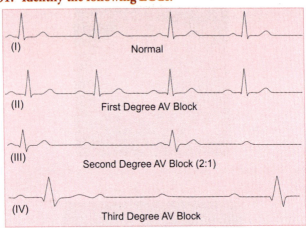

Ans. (I) Normal
(II) First Degree AV block
(III) Second Degree AV block (2:1)
(IV) third Degree AV block

52. Identify the following ECG:

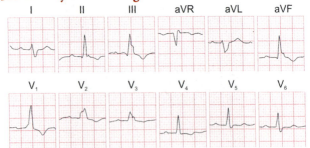

Ans. Right Bundle Branch Block.

53. Identify the instrument:

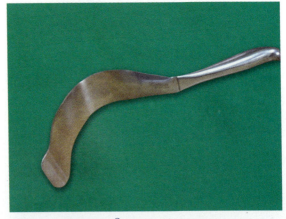

Ans. Deawer's Retractor[Q]

54. **Identify the instrument:**

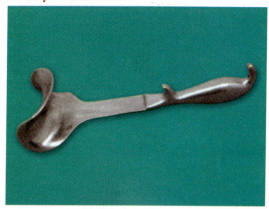

Ans. Doyen's Retractor[Q]

55. **Identify the instrument:**

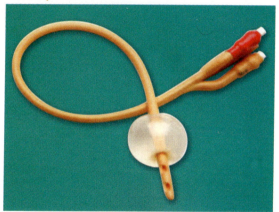

Ans. Foley's Catheter

Diameter of the Foley's Catheter is indicated by French size (Fr)

56. **Identify the instrument:**

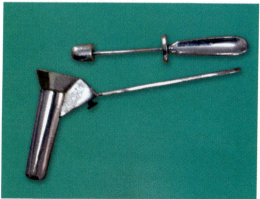

Ans. Proctoscope[Q]

57. **Identify the instrument:**

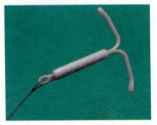

Ans. Mirena^Q

58. **Identify this logo:**

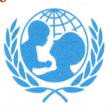

Ans. UNICEF

59. **Identify this picture:**

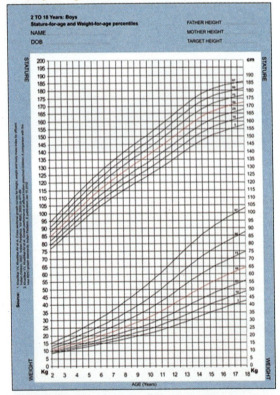

Ans. Growth Chart^Q

Growth Charts were developed by: David Morley

60. **Identify this clinical sign**

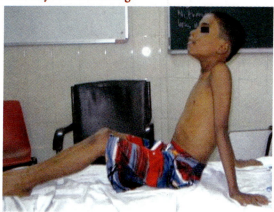

Ans. Tripod Sign[Q]

Tripod sign is seen usually in Poliomyelitis and meningitis'

61. **The skin lesion seen below is indicative of:**

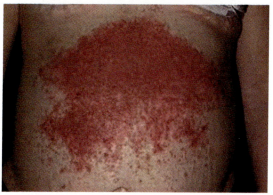

Ans. Dermatitis Herpetiformis[Q]

62. **The bullous lesion seen below is indicative of:**

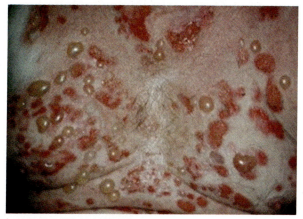

Ans. Bullous Pemphigoid[Q]

63. What is this dermatological lesion ?

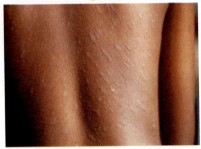

Ans. Christmas Tree Pattern in Pityriasis Rosea.
Other findings. Hanging Curtains Sign/Herald Patch/Mother Patch.

64. Identify the dermatological lesion:

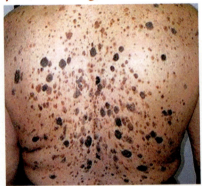

Ans. Leser Trelat Sign
The Leser-Trélat sign is the explosive onset of multiple seborrheic keratoses (many pigmented skin lesions) often with an inflammatory base. This can be an ominous sign of internal malignancy as part of a paraneoplastic syndrome.

65. Identify the dermatological lesion given below:

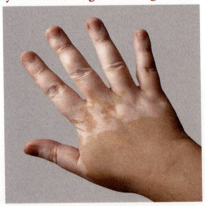

Ans. Vitiligo.[Q]

66. Identify the dermatological lesion given below:

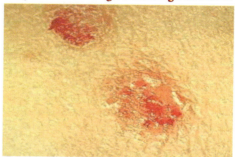

Ans. Ausptiz Sign in Psoriasis.^Q

67. Identify the dermatological lesion shown below:

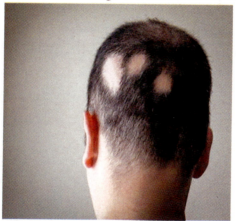

Ans. Alopecia Areata

68. The following picture is indicative of a key finding in a syndrome characterised by Seizures, Mental Retardation and angiofibromas on face. It is:

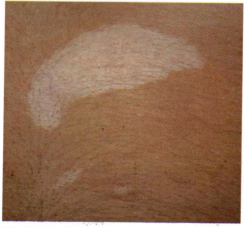

Ans. Ashleaf Macule^q

69. This skin lesion is pathognomonic of this viral disease:

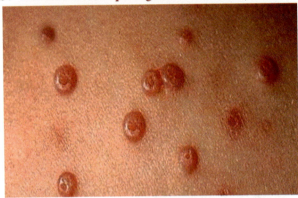

Ans. Molluscum Contagiosum. (Target lesions)

70. Identify this mucosal white lesions:

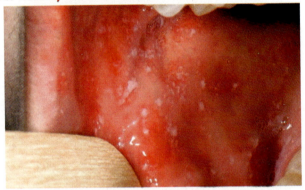

Ans. Koplik's Spots.[Q]

71. Name this Apparatus:

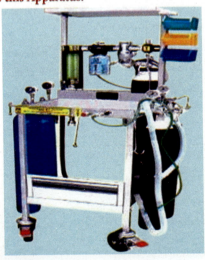

Ans. Boyle's Apparatus.[Q]

72. **Identify these cylinders:**

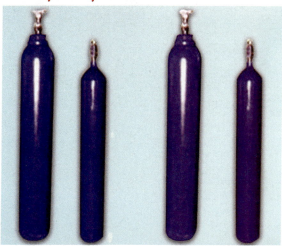

Ans. Nitrous Oxide.[Q]

73. **Identify the Instrument.**

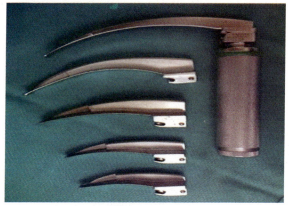

Ans. Laryngoscope.

74. **What historical incident does this picture depict?**

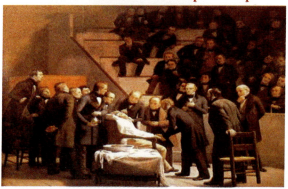

Ans. The first use of Anaesthesia by William Morton.

75. Identify this Mapleson Circuit

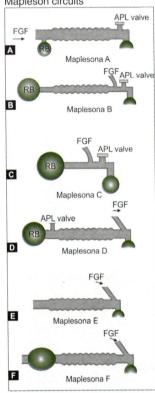
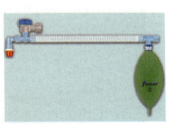

Ans. Magill Circuit. (Mapleson's)[Q]

76. Identify this scientist who discovered Nitrous Oxide:

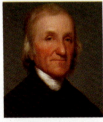

Ans. Joseph Priestley.[Q]

77. Identify this instrument:

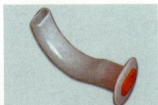

Ans. Guedel's Airway

78. Identify this instrument:

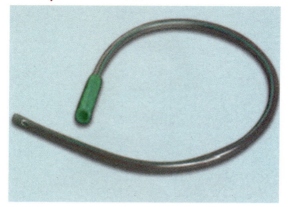

Ans. Nasal Cannula

79. Identify this instrument:

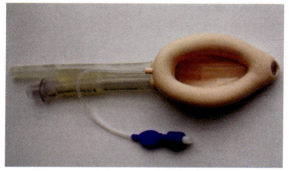

Ans. Laryngeal Mask.(Brain Mask)

80. This person was the first to introduce Obstetric Anaesthesia:

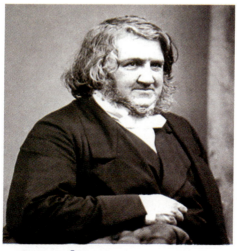

Ans. James Simpson.[Q]   *(NEET 2016 PATTERN)*

81. **This person is known as the Father of Anaesthesia:**

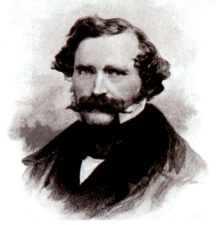

Ans. **William Morton.**[Q]

82. **Mallampatti Classification is used to assess:**

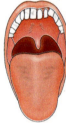 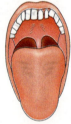 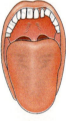 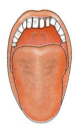

Class I	**Class II**	**Class III**	**Class IV**
Full visibility of tonsils, uvula and soft palate	Visibility of hard and soft palate, upper portion of tonsils and uvula	Soft and hard palate and base of the uvula are visible	Only hard palate visible

Ans. **Oral Cavity before Intubation.**[Q]

83. **Identify this instrument:**

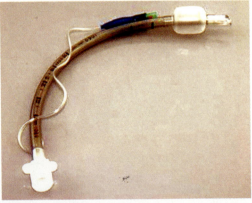

Ans. **Armoured Endotracheal Tube.**

84. Following image is indicative of:

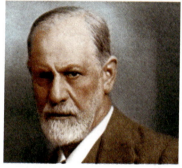

Ans. **Guedel's Stages of Anaesthesia.**

85. Identify the person.

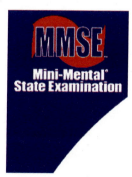

Ans. **Sigmund Freud[Q]**

Founder of Psychoanalysis[Q]
Wrote 'The Interpretation of Dreams'
Proposed Oedipus Complex[Q]

86.

Minimum Score[Q] – 24/30
Maximum Score[Q] – 30
Another name for MMSE Folstein's Test[Q]

87. Psychiatric Disorders belong to which category[Q]?

TENTH REVISION

ICD-10

INTERNATIONAL CLASSIFICATION OF DISEASES

ICD-10 is a new code set for reporting medical diagnoses & inpatient procedures.

Ans. F

Total number of chapters[Q] 21

Symptoms and signs of unknown etiology are classified under: R category[Q]

88. Name of this Test.

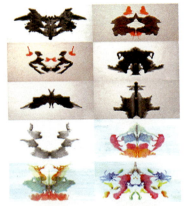

Rorschasch Ink Blot Test.
RIBT is an example of: Projective Test.[Q]

89. Identify the Psychological Test shown below:

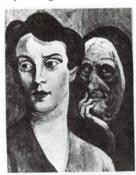

Ans. Thematic Apperception Test[Q]

TAT is a type of Projective Test[Q]

In this test, a person's responses reveal underlying motives, concerns, and the way they see the social world through the stories they make up about ambiguous pictures of people.

90. What is the name of this test?

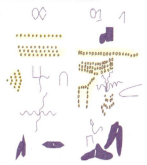

Ans. Bender Gestalt Test.

The Bender Visual Motor Gestalt Test is a psychological test first developed by child neuropsychiatrist Lauretta Bender. The test is used to evaluate "visual-motor maturity to screen for developmental disorders, or to assess neurological function or brain damage".

91. Which disorder does this ribbon represent?

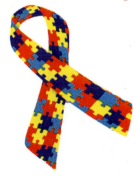

Ans. Autism.

92. Name this person regarded as a pioneer of Psychosomatic Medicine:

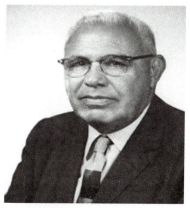

Ans. Franz Alexander

93. Who coined the word 'Schizophrenia'?

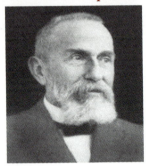

Ans. Eugene Bleuler.^Q

- Bleuler proposed the 4 As of Schizophrenia.^Q
  Ambivalence
  Autistic Thinking
  Abnormal affect
  Abnormal Associations.

94. This psychiatrist coined the term Dementia Precox. He is:

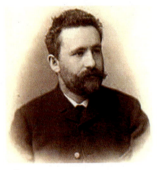

Ans. Emil Kraepelin

Dementia Precox was initially another name for Schizophrenia^Q

95. This Gallium-67 Citrate Scan image is indicative of:

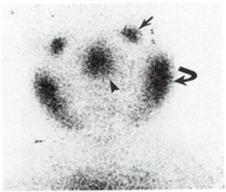

Ans. Panda Sign in Sarcoidosis.^Q

96. The MRI image of FACE OF THE GIANT PANDA Sign on MRI is indicative of:

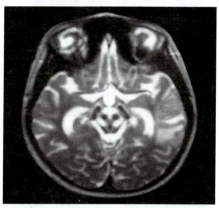

Ans. Wilson's Disease.[Q]

97. The following MRI image is indicative of:

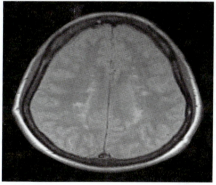

Ans. Dawson's Fingers in Multiple Sclerosis.[Q]

98. The following CT Scan image is indicative of:

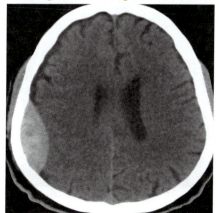

Ans. Extradural Hematoma[Q] (Lentiform/Lens Shaped/Biconvex)

99. The following CT scan image is indicative of:

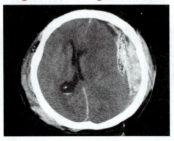

Ans. Subdural Hematoma.^Q (Crescentic/Banana shaped/Concave)

100. The following image of THE EYE OF THE TIGER Sign is seen in:

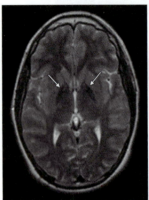
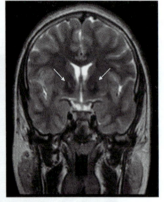

Ans. Hallevorden Spatz Disease.

101. MRI picture is indicative of:

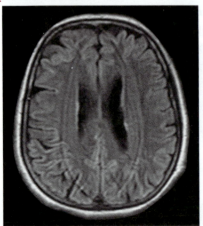

Ans. Prion Disease.
Sporadic Cruetzfeldt Jakob Disease.
Cortical Ribboning in MRI.

102 Type of Neurotransmitter involved in this condition:

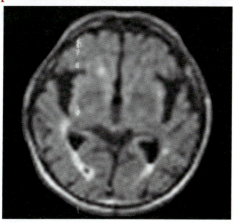

Ans. Acetyl Choline

Scan suggestive of Alzheimer's Disease.^Q

103. Identify the following CT scan image:

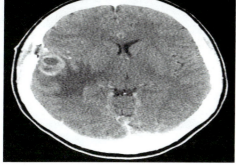

Ans. Temporal Abscess Rt Side.

104. Identify the following CT scan image:

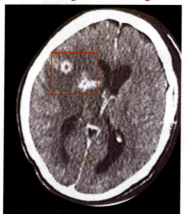

Ans. Toxoplasmosis.

105. In which disease is the following condition seen?

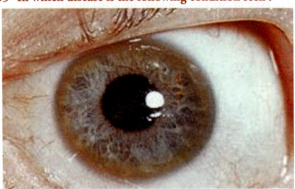

Ans. Wilson's Disease. (Kayser Fleischer Ring)

106. The following picture is indicative of:

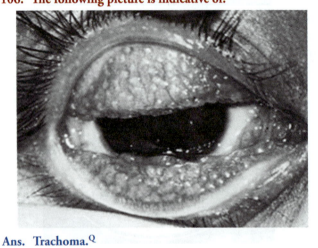

Ans. Trachoma.[Q]

107. Picture depicted here is a logo of:

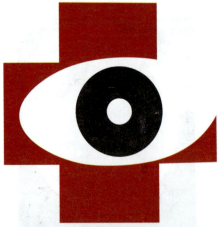

Ans. National Programme for Control of Blindness (NPCB)[Q]

108. The following image is indicative of:

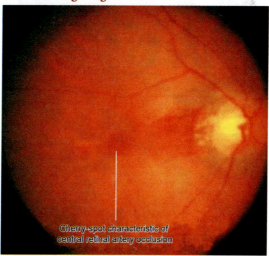

Cherry-spot characteristic of central retinal artery occlusion

Ans. Cherry Red Spot.

109. Identify the ocular lesion:

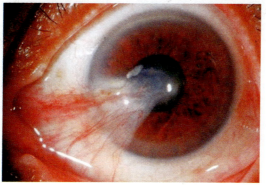

Ans. Pterygium.^Q

110. Name the systemic disease presenting with drooping of one eye:

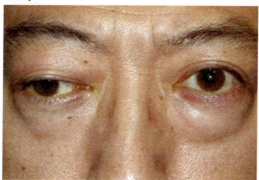

Ans. Myasthenia Gravis.

111. Which nerve palsy presents with such a lesion ?

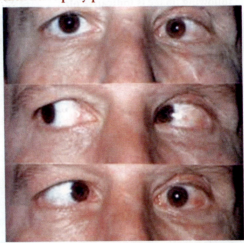

Ans. Abducens (6th nerve) palsy.

112. Name the following visual test:

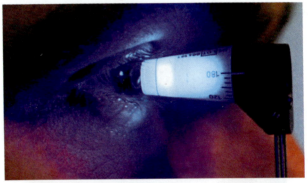

Ans. Tonometry[Q]

113. Identify the following ocular lesion:

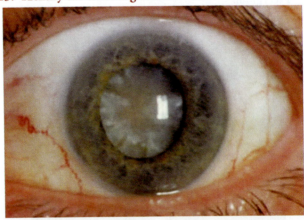

Ans. After Cataract.[Q]

114. Picture depicted here is the logo of:

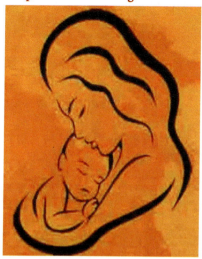

Ans. Janani Suraksha Yojana (JSY)^Q

115. This is a logo of:

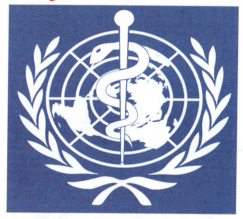

Ans. World Health Organisation (WHO)^Q

116. This is a logo of:

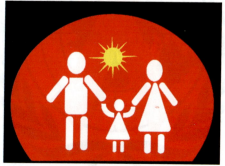

Ans. National Health Mission. (NHM)^Q

117. This is a logo of:

Asn. National Leprosy Eradication Programme (NLEP)^Q

118. The following picture depicts:

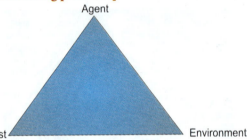

Ans. Epidemiological Triad.^Q

119. This is a logo of:

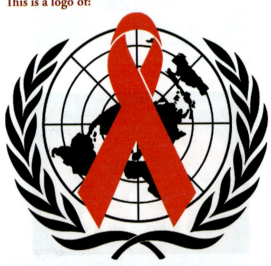

Ans. UNAIDS^Q

120. **Identify the insect:**

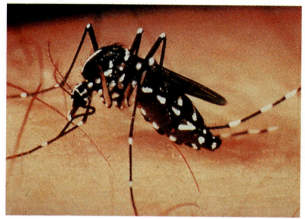

Ans. Aedes Mosquito.[Q]

121. **Identify the insect shown below:**

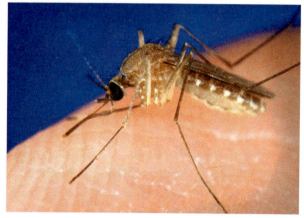

Ans. Culex Mosquito.[Q]

122. **Identify the insect shown below:**

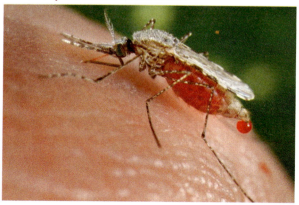

Ans. Anopheles Mosquito[Q]

123. Identify the insect shown below:

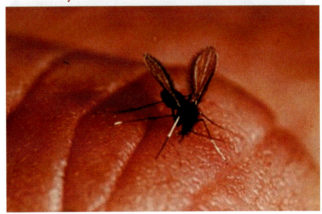

Ans. Sandfly.[Q]

1 ANATOMY

*"If you can't fly, run.
If you can't run, walk.
If you can't walk, crawl.
But, by all means, keep moving."*
—*Martin Luther King Jr.*

REFERENCES
- *Gray's Anatomy, 41st ed.*
- *Last Anatomy, 12th ed.*

LEVEL I: BASIC REPEATS

EMBRYOLOGY

- Muscles of Mastication arises from the: mesoderm of first pharyngeal arch.
  (DNB PATTERN 2003, 2008, NEET PATTERN 2013)
- Stapes is a derivative of: 2nd branchial arch.
  (DNB PATTERN 2003, NEET PATTERN 2014, 2015)
- NOT developing from 2nd branchial arch: Anterior belly of digastric.
  (DNB PATTERN DEC 2009, FMGE PATTERN 2008)
- FAQ ON Pharyngeal Pouches/Arches.

1st pouch	TongUe [U for uni (1)]
2nd pouch	TonSil (S for second)
3rd pouch (THIrd)	TH*ymus, I*nferior Parathyroid gland
4th pouch	Superior parathyroid gland

1st arch	M list (Mandibular nerve, Maxillary artery, meckels cartilage, mastication muscles)
Second arch	S list (Seventh nerve, stapedial artery, stapes*, stapedius and stylohyoid muscle) and posterior belly of digastrics
3rd arch	9th (3*3) nerve and anterior belly of digastrics
4th arch	Cricothyroid* muscle and SLN (Superior laryngeal nerve)
6th arch	Recurrent laryngeal nerve

- Styloid process is derived from—2nd arch.
  (NEET PATTERN 2015)
- Artery of 2nd pharyngeal arch is—stapedial artery
  (NEET PATTERN 2013)

- Artery of 3rd arch—common carotid artery
  (DNB PATTERN NOV 2015)
- The muscle of 3rd pharyngeal arch is: Stylopharyngeus
  (DNB PATTERN NOV 2013, NOV 2014)
- Double aortic arch is persistent right 4th aortic arch.
  (DNB PATTERN 2000, JUNE 2015)
- Nerve of 6th pharyngeal arch—vagus.
  (NEET PATTERN 2013)
- Epiglottis is derived from—4th arch.
  (NEET PATTERN 2013)
- Parathyroid glands develop from the: Branchial pouches.
  (DNB PATTERN DEC 2011, 2014).
- Tonsils are derived from the: 2nd branchial pouch.
  (DNB PATTERN 2003, 2014, FMGE PATTERN 2009).
- Inferior parathyroid gland is derivative of: 3rd pharyngeal pouch.
  (DNB PATTERN 2009, FMGE PATTERN PATTERN 2008, 2010, NEET PATTERN 2013, 2015).
- Branchial cyst is derived from—2nd branchial cleft.
  (NEET PATTERN 2016)

EMBRYOLOGY OF GENITALIA (REFER TABLES 1.1 TO 1.3)

- Ureter develops from Mesonephric duct
  (DNB PATTERN 2009, DNB PATTERN JUNE 2016)
- Gartner's cyst arises from remnant of Mesonephric duct.
  (DNB PATTERN DEC 2009)
- Prostatic utricle is NOT derived from Mesonephric duct.
  (DNB PATTERN 2002, 2008)
- Excretory portion of kidney is formed by: Mesonephric duct
  (DNB PATTERN NOV 2013, AIPG 2014)
- Lower one third of vagina is developed from Sinovaginal bulb. *(DNB PATTERN JUNE 2011, AIPG)*
- Vestibule of the vagina develops from Urogenital sinus.
  (DNB PATTERN JUNE 2010, FMGE PATTERN 2013)
- Appendix of testis is derived from Paramesonephric duct.
  (DNB PATTERN DEC 2011)
- In males mullerian duct forms: Appendix of testis.
  (DNB PATTERN NOV 2013)
- Ovary develops from Genital ridge.
  (DNB PATTERN JUNE 2011)
- Testes are developed from: Genital Ridge.
  (DNB PATTERN NOV 2013, NOV 2014)

Anatomy

- Genitals are developed from which part of mesoderm: Somatic mesoderm. *(DNB PATTERN NOV 2013)*
- Clitoris develops from: Genital tubercle. *(FMGE PATTERN SEP 2011)*
- Primordial germ cell develops from: Epiblast *(DNB PATTERN DEC 2009, AIPGME 2015)*
- Ureteric Bud develops from: Mesonephros. *(NEET PATTERN 2018)*

SPERMATOGENESIS AND OOGENESIS

- Spermatogenesis begins at—birth. *(NEET PATTERN 2016)*
- Development of sperm from spermatogonium takes how much time—70-75 days. *(DNB PATTERN NOV 2014)*
- Primary spermatocyte chromosome number is—46XY. *(DNB PATTERN NOV 2014)*
- In early phase division of spermatogonia by—Mitosis. *(DNB PATTERN NOV 2014)*
- True about spermatid—derived from secondary spermatocyte. *(DNB PATTERN JULY 2015)*
- Sperm acquire motility in Epididymis. *(NEET PATTERN 2014, 2015)*
- Sperm maturation takes place in female genital tract. *(NEET PATTERN 2013, 2016)*
- Acrosome cap of sperm is derived from—Golgi body. *(DNB PATTERN NOV 2014)*
- Middle piece of sperm contain Mitochondria. *(DNB PATTERN JULY 2015)*
- Primary oocyte is formed after Mitotic division. *(NEET PATTERN 2013)*
- First polar body is formed after First meiosis. *(NEET PATTERN 2014)*
- Diplotene and zygotene stages are seen in—Prophase. *(DNB PATTERN JULY 2015)*
- Cells which surround the oocyst in graafian folicle are called—Cumulus oophorcus. *(NEET PATTERN 2014)*
- Nerves of the Branchial Arch are derived from: Neural Crest. *(NEET PATTERN 2018)*

GENERAL EMBRYOLOGY

- Kerckring's center for ossification is associated with Occipital bone. *(DNB PATTERN 2006)*
- Persistent primitive streak leads to—sacrococcygeal teratoma. *(DNB PATTERN JUNE 2008)*

- Nucleus pulposus arises from the Notochord. *(DNB PATTERN 2005)*
- Meckel's diverticulum arises from Ileum. *(DNB PATTERN 2006)*
- NOT a derivative of midgut: Descending colon. *(DNB PATTERN JUNE 2010)*
- Gastrosplenic ligament is derived from Dorsal mesogastrium. *(DNB PATTERN JUNE 2010)*
- Umbilical vein becomes Ligamentum teres. *(DNB PATTERN 2001, DEC 2009)*

HISTOLOGY

CELLS

- Pericytes are pluripotent cells lining the capillaries. *(DNB PATTERN JUNE 2012)*
- The supporting cells of the testes are the Sertoli cells. *(DNB PATTERN 2000)*
- Cells NOT present in cerebellum: Pyramidal cells. *(DNB PATTERN DEC 2009)*
- Goblet cells are NOT present in Stomach. *(DNB PATTERN 2007, DEC 2009)*
- Germinal cells do NOT form coverings of Graafian follicle. *(DNB PATTERN JUNE 2011)*
- In CNS, Myelin sheath of neurons are formed by oligodendroglial cells. *(DNB PATTERN DEC 2010)*
- Stem cells are located from which region of hair follicle? Bulge of follicle. *(DNB PATTERN DEC 2010)*
- Bipolar cells are NOT seen in Cerebellar cortex. *(DNB PATTERN 2009)*
- Strongest layer of Oesophagus is: Submucosa. *(NEET 2016 PATTERN)*
- Hard Palate is: Keratinised, dense submucosa with accessory salivary glands. *(NEET PATTERN 2018)*
- Hard Palate is: Keratinised, dense submucosa with accessory salivary glands. *(NEET PATTERN 2018)*

CARTILAGES

- Which is formed of Elastic cartilage? Auditory tube. *(DNB PATTERN DEC 2010)*
- Microscopic examination of Articular surface of a synovial joint demonstrates Hyaline cartilage. *(DNB PATTERN DEC 2010)*
- Which is an example of hyaline cartilage? Thyroid cartilage *(DNB PATTERN JUNE 2011)*

- Pinna is NOT White fibrocartilage.
  (DNB PATTERN DEC 2011)
- Intervertebral disc is an example of fibrocartilage.
  (DNB PATTERN JUNE 2011)
- Pseudounipolar neurons are seen in dorsal root ganglion.
  (DNB PATTERN DEC 2010)
- Submucosal glands are present in Duodenum.
  (DNB PATTERN 2000)
- Mitochondria of a sperm is located in the Body.
  (DNB PATTERN 2005)
- Von Braun's nest is seen in Normal Urothelium.
  (DNB PATTERN 2009)
- Implantation occurs after how many days of ovulation— 7-9 days. *(DNB PATTERN JUNE 2009)*
- Centromere near the end of chromosome: Acrocentric.
  (DNB PATTERN DEC 2010)
- Chromatin condensation occurs in Prophase.
  (DNB PATTERN DEC 2010)
- Epithelial lining of lingual surface of epiglottis is Stratified squamous epithelium. *(DNB PATTERN JUNE 2012)*
- Epithelial lining of Vagina is Stratified squamous non-keratinized. *(DNB PATTERN JUNE 2010)*
- Not a type of epiphysis: Friction epiphysis
  (DNB PATTERN DEC 2011)
- Which gland has fibromuscular stroma? Prostate.
  (DNB PATTERN DEC 2010)
- Temporomandibular joint is a Condyloid joint.
  (DNB PATTERN DEC 2009)
- Incudomalleal joint is a saddle joint.
  (DNB PATTERN JUNE 2011)

HEAD AND NECK

- Intrinsic laryngeal muscles are supplied by Recurrent laryngeal nerve. *(DNB PATTERN JUNE 2011)*
- Taste sensation of anterior two thirds of tongue are carried by facial nerve. *(DNB PATTERN JUNE 2011)*
- Sphenopalatine foramen opens in which wall of pterygopalatine fossa? Medial wall. *(DNB PATTERN JUNE 2011)*
- Sphenopalatine foramen opens in which wall of pterygopalatine fossa? Medial wall. *(DNB PATTERN JUNE 2009)*
- Structure seen in lateral wall of tonsillar fossa is superior constrictor muscle. *(DNB PATTERN JUNE 2009)*
- Muscle not attached to apex of orbit: Inferior oblique.
  (DNB PATTERN JUNE 2009)

- Which bone does not contribute to medial wall of orbit? Zygoma. *(DNB PATTERN JUNE 2009)*
- Structure in close proximity to lower third molar is Inferior alveolar nerve. *(DNB PATTERN JUNE 2009)*
- Skin over the angle of mandible is supplied by C2/C3. *(DNB PATTERN DEC 2011)*
- Ridge of Passavant is found in Palatopharyngeus. *(DNB PATTERN 2000)*
- Which artery can be felt at anterior border of masseter against the mandible? Facial artery. *(DNB PATTERN DEC 2009)*
- Taste sensation of anterior two thirds of tongue is facial nerve. *(DNB PATTERN DEC 2009)*
- The triangular interval between the medial border of scalenus anterior and longus colli does NOT contain internal carotid artery. *(DNB PATTERN DEC 2010)*
- Anterior ethmoidal artery closely relates to Nasociliary nerve. *(DNB PATTERN JUNE 2010)*
- Which layer of scalp is vascular? Subcutaneous tissue. *(DNB PATTERN DEC 2009)*
- Mandibular nerve is NOT a terminal branch of facial nerve. *(DNB PATTERN JUNE 2010)*
- Maximum contribution to the floor of orbit is by Maxillary bone. *(DNB PATTERN DEC 2010)*
- Diploic bone—Frontal bone. *(DNB PATTERN JUNE 2008)*
- Not true about Scalenus anterior—Subclavian artery lies anteriorly. *(DNB PATTERN JUNE 2008)*
- Whitnall's Ligament refers to: Superior Transverse ligament of the eye. *(NEET 2016 PATTERN)*
- Position of the Thyroid isthmus: C6 -C7 level. *(NEET 2016 PATTERN)*
- Lateral Atlanto Axial Joint belongs to the variety of: Plane Synovial Joint. *(NEET 2016 PATTERN)*
- NOT a muscle of Tongue: Palatoglossus. *(NEET 2016 PATTERN)*
- Acute Tonsillitis affects which nerve? – Glossopharyngeal Nerve. *(NEET 2018 PATTERN)*
- Newly erupted teeth is covered by: Nasmyth's Membrane. *(NEET 2018 PATTERN)*
- Tensor of Vocal Cord: Cricothyroid. *(NEET 2018 PATTERN)*

NEUROANATOMY

- CSF pressure depends primarily on rate of CSF absorption. *(DNB PATTERN 2008)*

Anatomy

- Magendie foramen drains CSF from 4th ventricle. *(DNB PATTERN JUNE 2011)*
- Endolymphatic duct drains into subarachnoid space. *(DNB PATTERN DEC 2010)*
- Cells NOT present in cerebral cortex are Bipolar cells. *(DNB PATTERN 2008)*
- Closure of neural tube begins at Cervical end. *(DNB PATTERN 2008)*
- NOT a part of Epithalamus: Geniculate Bodies. *(DNB PATTERN 2008)*
- Nucleus in brain common to 9, 10, 11 cranial nerves: Nucleus ambiguus. *(DNB PATTERN 2008)*
- NOT a tract of Inferior cerebellar peduncle: Pontocerebellar fibers. *(DNB PATTERN 2008)*
- Dorsal nucleus of Vagus belongs to the general visceral efferent column. *(DNB PATTERN 2008)*
- Not a part of Internal Capsule–Optic radiation. *(DNB PATTERN JUNE 2008)*
- Edinger-Westphal nucleus—is part of General visceral efferents. *(DNB PATTERN JUNE 2008)*
- Junction of anterior and posterior horn of lateral ventricle is called as Trigone of lateral ventricle. *(DNB PATTERN JUNE 2009)*
- Infection of CNS spreads in inner ear through Cochlear aqueduct. *(DNB PATTERN DEC 2011)*
- Striae of Gennari seen in—Layer 4C of the primary visual cortex from the Lateral geniculate nucleus. *(DNB PATTERN JUNE 2008)*
- Posterior communicating artery is a branch of the Middle cerebral artery. *(DNB PATTERN 2005)*
- The chorda tympani nerve arises from the facial nerve. *(DNB PATTERN 2003)*
- NOT at risk in anterior cranial fossa fracture: Sphenoid sinus. *(DNB PATTERN 2003)*
- Taste fibers are relayed in tractus solitarius. *(DNB PATTERN 2003)*
- Craniosacral outflow is mediated by parasympathetic preganglionic fibers. *(DNB PATTERN DEC 2011)*
- Most lateral deep cerebellar nucleus is dentate nucleus. *(DNB PATTERN DEC 2009, JUNE 2011)*
- Broca's area is located in inferior frontal gyrus. *(DNB PATTERN DEC 2009)*
- This structure gets decussated in superior medullary velum-4th nerve. *(DNB PATTERN DEC 2009)*

- NOT a structure present in the lateral wall of cavernous sinus—Optic nerve. *(DNB PATTERN JUNE 2009)*
- Ophthalmic artery is a branch of—Intracranial internal carotid artery. *(DNB PATTERN JUNE 2008)*
- Vital point is found in Medulla oblongata. *(DNB PATTERN 2007)*
- Broca's Area is located in: Inferior Frontal Gyrus. *(NEET 2018 PATTERN)*

UPPER LIMB AND BREAST

- Protractor of Scapula is serratus anterior. *(DNB PATTERN JUNE 2011)*
- Which does not form posterior wall of axilla? Supraspinatus. *(DNB PATTERN DEC 2010)*
- Which is present in posterior axillary wall? Subscapular artery. *(DNB PATTERN DEC 2010)*
- Axillary artery occlusion does NOT affect Suprascapular artery. *(DNB PATTERN JUNE 2010)*
- Winging of scapula is due to injury to nerve to Serratus anterior. *(DNB PATTERN 2000, 2006)*
- Serratus anterior does NOT form a boundary of the triangle of auscultation. *(DNB PATTERN 2008)*
- Winging of scapula is due to injury to nerve to serratus anterior. *(DNB PATTERN 2000)*
- Winging of scapula is due to damage to nerve supply of trapezius. *(DNB PATTERN JUNE 2009, JUNE 2010)*
- Lower angle of scapula lies at the level of T7. *(DNB PATTERN 2001, JUNE 2012)*
- Lateral border of cubital fossa is bounded by the Brachioradialis. *(DNB PATTERN 2000)*
- Musculocutaneous nerve does NOT supply brachioradialis. *(DNB PATTERN JUNE 2010)*
- Fascia around the nerve bundle of brachial plexus is derived from prevertebral fascia. *(DNB PATTERN 2007)*
- Porter's tip deformity is seen in Erb's paralysis. *(DNB PATTERN 2000)*
- Erb's point is C5-C6. *(DNB PATTERN 2004)*
- Klumpke's paralysis involves C8/T1. *(DNB PATTERN DEC 2011)*
- Carcinoma of upper and outer quadrant of breast will NOT metastasize to parasternal nodes. *(DNB PATTERN 2001)*
- Pain along medial aspect of arm in Carcinoma breast is mediated through Intercostobrachial nerve. *(DNB PATTERN JUNE 2008)*

Anatomy

- True about Level 3 nodes in axilla is they are superomedial and above the pectoralis minor.

  (DNB PATTERN DEC 2010)

- Delphic Nodes are: Pretracheal Nodes.

  (DNB PATTERN 2008)

> Easy Mnemonic: Dolphin squashes water through Tracheostomy Hole (Delphi-Pretracheal)

- Epiphysis at the tip of coracoids process is atavistic epiphysis.

  (DNB PATTERN 2001)

- Which of the following is an atavistic epiphysis? Coracoid process. *(DNB PATTERN JUNE 2011)*

- Superior radioulnar joint is Pivot joint.

  (DNB PATTERN 2002, 2005)

- Latissimus dorsi is NOT an elevator of the scapula.

  (DNB PATTERN 2006)

- Paralysis of opponens muscle leads to loss of pinching action of the hand. *(DNB PATTERN 2007)*

- First bone to ossify in the body is the Clavicle.

  (DNB PATTERN 2007)

- Wrist drop is seen in damage of radial nerve.

  (DNB PATTERN JUNE 2009)

> w[R]ist drop – [R]adial nerve injury

- Median nerve supplies all except adductor pollicis.

  (DNB PATTERN DEC 2010)

- Ape hand deformity is due to damage of median nerve.

  (DNB PATTERN JUNE 2009)

- Median nerve injury above the elbow does NOT cause flexion at 4th and 5th DIP joints. *(DNB PATTERN DEC 2010)*

- Carpal tunnel syndrome involves the Median nerve.

  (DNB PATTERN JUNE 2008)

- Carpal tunnel does NOT contain Palmaris longus.

  (DNB PATTERN JUNE 2009)

- Which of the following is a subcutaneous muscle? Palmaris brevis. *(DNB PATTERN JUNE 2011)*

- Superficial palmar arch is at the level of distal border of extended thumb. *(DNB PATTERN DEC 2011)*

- Clavipectoral fascia is NOT pierced by Medial pectoral nerve.

  (DNB PATTERN DEC 2011)

- Maximum area of representation in cerebral cortex is for first metacarpophalangeal joint. *(DNB PATTERN JUNE 2010)*

- Pectoralis major is a: Multipennate Muscle.

  (NEET PATTERN 2018)

- Function of Lumbricals: Flexion of Metacarpophalangeal joints and extension of Interphalangeal Joints.
  (NEET 2018 PATTERN)
- Muscles which contributes to two triangles in the back: Latissimus dorsi. *(NEET 2016 PATTERN)*

THORAX

- Sympathetic supply to the Heart is from T1–T5.
  (DNB PATTERN 2001)
- Structure related to the arch of aorta is: Pulmonary trunk.
  (DNB PATTERN 2002)
- Structure which passes through the Aortic Hiatus: Azygos vein. *(DNB PATTERN 2000, NEET PATTERN 2016)*
- NOT a branch of arch of aorta? Right common carotid.
  (DNB PATTERN DEC 2010)
- Membranous part of interventricular septum is situated in between left ventricle and right atrium.
  (DNB PATTERN 2003)
- Left gonadal vein is NOT a tributary of inferior vena cava.
  (DNB PATTERN 2003)
- Anterior cardiac veins open into right atrium.
  (DNB PATTERN 2004)
- All veins open into the coronary sinus except anterior cardiac vein. *(DNB PATTERN DEC 2009)*
- The thoracic duct terminates into the left brachiocephalic vein at the junction of Internal jugular vein and subclavian vein. *(DNB PATTERN 2003)*
- Ectopia cordis is associated with the organ—heart.
  (DNB PATTERN 2006)
- Foramen of Morgagni refers to an opening in the diaphragm.
  (DNB PATTERN 2006)
- Diaphragm is at the lowest level during standing.
  (DNB PATTERN 2004)
- Oesophagus crosses diaphragm at the level of T10.
  (DNB PATTERN 2004)
- Constrictions of the esophagus are all except at the level of left atrium. *(DNB PATTERN JUNE 2010)*
- Pleura extends to which rib in mid axillary line? 10th rib.
  (DNB PATTERN 2001)
- Pleural reflection on left mid axillary line is at 10th intercostal space. *(DNB PATTERN 2004)*
- Sequestration of lung is most commonly seen in posterior part of left lung. *(DNB PATTERN 2006)*

- Which is a typical intercostal nerve? Third.
(DNB PATTERN DEC 2009)
- Root value of phrenic nerve is C3–C5.
(DNB PATTERN DEC 2011)
- Structure NOT passing through the Esophageal Hiatus of the Diaphragm: Thoracic Duct. *(NEET 2016 PATTERN)*
- Structure NOT passing through Aortic opening: Vagus Nerve. *(NEET 2018 PATTERN)*
- Incorrect about Sibson's Fascia: Attached to 2nd Rib.
(NEET PATTERN 2018)

ABDOMEN

- Transpyloric plane separates—Hypochondrium from lumbar region. *(NEET PATTERN 2015)*
- Transtubercular plane lies at—L5 vertebral level.
(NEET PATTERN 2013)
- Highest point of iliac crest is at—L4 vertebral level.
(NEET PATTERN 2014)
- Fundus of gallbladder at–L1 vertebral level.
(DNB PATTERN NOV 2015)
- Supracristal plane is above—highest point of iliac crest.
(DNB PATTERN JULY 2016)
- True about scarpas fascia—forms suspensory ligament of penis. *(NEET PATTERN 2015)*
- Function of external oblique—active expiration.
(NEET PATTERN 2016)
- Pyramidalis is supplied by—subcostal nerve.
(NEET PATTERN 2015)
- The efferent limb of Cremasteric Reflex is provided by—genital branch of genitofemoral nerve.
(DNB PATTERN NOV 2014)
- Cremasteric muscle is supplied by—genital branch of genitofemoral nerve. *(NEET PATTERN 2016)*
- Floor of petit triangle is formed by—internal oblique.
(DNB PATTERN JULY 2016)
- Not forming boundary of petit triangle—inguinal ligament.
(NEET PATTERN 2016)
- Ovarian artery is a branch of—abdominal aorta.
(NEET PATTERN 2013)
- Superior pancreaticoduodenal artery is a branch of—gastroduodenal artery. *(NEET PATTERN 2013)*
- The vein which drain directly into IVC—hepatic vein.
(NEET PATTERN 2013)
- The cisterna chili are situated in the abdomen.
(NEET PATTERN 2014)

- ➢ (Cisterna chili is in front of L1 and L2 vertebra, immediately to right of abdominal wall)
- ❑ Which is derived from thoracolumbar fascia? Lateral arcuate ligament. *(DNB PATTERN JULY 2016)*
- ❑ Right suprarenal vein drains into IVC. *(DNB PATTERN JUNE 2009)*
- ❑ Foramen of winslow is between the Greater sac and the Lesser sac. *(DNB PATTERN 2000)*
- ❑ The portal vein is formed from the superior mesenteric vein and the splenic vein at the second lumbar vertebra. *(DNB PATTERN 2000, DEC 2010)*
- ❑ Pectinate line is an important landmark because it marks a divide in nerve supply/it marks a location in change in type of epithelium/it represents a lymphatic and venous divide. *(DNB PATTERN 2000)*
- ❑ Superior border of epiploic foramen is formed by caudate lobe of liver. *(DNB PATTERN JUNE 2009)*
- ❑ Renal angle is the angle between 12th rib and erector spinae. *(DNB PATTERN DEC 2010)*
- ❑ Superior border of epiploic foramen is formed by caudate lobe of liver. *(DNB PATTERN JUNE 2011)*
- ❑ The tympanic note on percussion in traube's space on chest wall is due to fundus of stomach. *(DNB PATTERN DEC 2010)*
- ❑ True statement regarding portal venous system is whole system is valveless. *(DNB PATTERN JUNE 2011)*
- ❑ Midgut is supplied by superior mesenteric artery. *(DNB PATTERN JUNE 2011)*
- ❑ Which is a flexor of abdomen? External oblique. *(DNB PATTERN DEC 2011)*
- ❑ PECTEN of anal canal is lined by: Non keratinised stratified squamous epithelium. *(NEET 2016 PATTERN)*

INGUINAL CANAL

- ❑ Length of inguinal canal—4 cm. *(NEET PATTERN 2013)*
- ❑ Deep inguinal ring is a deficiency in the—Transversalis fascia. *(NEET PATTERN 2013, 2015)*
- ❑ Content of deep inguinal ring—spermatic cord. *(NEET PATTERN 2016)*
- ❑ Nerve of inguinal canal—ilioinguinal nerve. *(DNB PATTERN NOV 2015)*
- ❑ Inguinal ligament forms the boundaries of–femoral triangle and hesselbach's triangle *(NEET PATTERN 2013)*

- Inferior epigastric artery forms the boundary of—hesselbachs triangle. *(NEET PATTERN 2013)*
- Protective mechanisms of inguinal canal-obliquity of inguinal canal, contraction of cremasteric muscle, contraction of conjoint tendon. *(DNB PATTERN JULY 2016)*
- Inguinal ligament is derived from—external oblique. *(NEET PATTERN 2016)*

UROGENITAL SYSTEM

- Left testicular vein drains into left renal vein. *(DNB PATTERN JUNE 2011)*
- Testicular volume at prepubertal age is 5 mL. *(DNB PATTERN JUNE 2010)*
- Testes completely descend into scrotum by the age of end of 9th month of intrauterine life. *(DNB PATTERN JUNE 2009)*
- Normal constrictions of ureter are at all of the following sites except crossing iliac artery. *(DNB PATTERN DEC 2010)*
- Ureter in ureteric tunnel is inferior to uterine artery. *(DNB PATTERN JUNE 2012)*
- Relations of left ureter are all except quadratus lumborum. *(DNB PATTERN JUNE 2010)*
- Urinary bladder is supplied by L1 and L2 branches of the Lumbar plexus. *(DNB PATTERN JUNE 2012)*
- Uterine artery is a branch of internal iliac artery. *(DNB PATTERN DEC 2011)*
- Lymphatic drainage of cervix is into internal iliac nodes. *(DNB PATTERN DEC, JUNE 2010)*
- Denonvillier's fascia is between Prostate and Rectum. *(DNB PATTERN DEC 2011)*
- During ejaculation, sperms are released from epididymis. *(DNB PATTERN DEC 2011)*
- True regarding prostate gland is that it has glandular tissue and fibromuscular stroma. *(DNB PATTERN DEC 2011)*
- Ilioinguinal nerve is NOT a content of spermatic cord. *(DNB PATTERN JUNE 2010)*
- Weakest support of uterus is broad ligament. *(DNB PATTERN JUNE 2011)*
- Which is not a true support of uterus? Infundibulopelvic ligament. *(DNB PATTERN DEC 2010)*
- Lymphatic drainage of cervix drains into which nodes? internal iliac nodes. *(DNB PATTERN DEC 2010)*
- Uterine epithelium develops from—Fusion of paramesonephric ducts. *(DNB PATTERN JUNE 2008)*
- Muscle in deep perineal pouch—Sphincter urethrae. *(DNB PATTERN JUNE 2008)*

- Pudendal nerve–root value S2, S3, S4.
  (DNB PATTERN JUNE 2008)
- Pudendal canal is bounded between Obturator membrane and Fascia lunata. *(DNB PATTERN JUNE 2008)*
- Uvula seen in bladder is median lobe of prostate.
  (DNB PATTERN 2005)

LOWER LIMB

- Upper border of pubic ramus forms—Arcuate line.
  (DNB PATTERN JUNE 2014)

  Upper border of pubic ramus (pectineal line/pectin pubis) forms arcuate line.
- Lower border of pubic ramus forms upper margin of obturator foramen
- True about attachment of ischial tuberosity—origin of semimembranosus from superolateral area.
  (DNB PATTERN JULY 2015)
- Blood supply to femoral head is mostly by—Profunda femoris. *(NEET PATTERN DEC 2013)*
- Medial circumflex artery, branch of profunda femoris is the major vessel supplying blood to femoral head.
- True about linea aspera—Continue as gluteal tuberosity.
  (NEET PATTERN DEC 2013)
- Muscle attached to medial lip of linea aspera of femur—vastus medialis. *(DNB PATTERN JULY 2015)*
- Lower end of femur is ossified from—1 ossification center.
  (NEET PATTERN 2013)
- Secondary ossification center for lower femur—present at birth.
- Secondary ossification center of lower end of femur appears at 9th month of IUL (present at birth).
- Ligament below head of talus is—spring ligament.
  (NEET PATTERN 2013)
- Ligament supporting the talus is—spring ligament.
  (NEET PATTERN 2013)
- Ligament not attached to talus—spring ligament.
  (NEET PATTERN 2013, 2015)
- Spring ligament (plantar calcaneonavicular ligament) connects the calcaneum with navicular bone. It is not attached to talus, but related to (supports) talus.
- Strongest flexor of hip—iliopsoas muscle.
  (NEET PATTERN 2015)
- Trendelenburg sign is due to paralysis of—gluteus medius.
  (NEET PATTERN 2013, DNB PATTERN 2015)
- Positive Trendelenburg sign: Superior gluteal nerve injury leads to paralysis of hip abductors (gluteus medius and minimus).

- Positive Trendelenburg's test is NOT seen with Paralysis of gluteus maximus.
  (DNB PATTERN JUNE 2009, NEET PATTERN 2014, 2016)
- Defect in Gluteus maximus does NOT lead to positive Trendelenburg test. *(DNB PATTERN JUNE 2010)*
- Tibial collateral ligament is the degenerated part of—Adductor magnus. *(DNB PATTERN JULY 2016)*
- Origin of PCL—posterior part of intercondylar area of tibia. *(DNB PATTERN JULY 2015)*
- ACL originates from—anterior part of intercondylar area of tibia. *(DNB PATTERN JULY 2015)*
- ACL prevents—anterior dislocation of tibia.
  (NEET PATTERN 2014, 2016)
- Oblique popliteal ligament is pierced by—middle genicular branch of popliteal artery.
  (NEET PATTERN 2013, 2015)
- Blood supply of anterior cruciate ligament is middle genicular artery. *(NEET PATTERN 2013;2015;2016)*
- Locking of knee joint occurs due to—medial rotation of femur during last degree of extension.
  (DNB PATTERN JULY 2015, NEET PATTERN 2016)
- Physiological unlocking is caused by popliteus.
  (NEET PATTERN 2015)
- Most common ligament damaged in knee injuries—MCL.
  (NEET PATTERN 2016)
- Dorsiflexion of ankle joint—Tibialis anterior.
  (NEET PATTERN 2015)
- Abduction and adduction of foot occurs at which joint? Subtalar. *(NEET PATTERN 2016)*
- Inversion is sole of foot inward. *(NEET PATTERN 2013)*
- Medial aspect of great toe supplied by deep peroneal nerve
  (NEET PATTERN 2013;2015;2016)
- Ossification center which appears first is Lower end of femur.
  (DNB PATTERN JUNE 2009)
- Medial border of Hesselbach's triangle is formed by Linea semilunaris. *(DNB PATTERN JUNE 2011)*
- Nerve to obturator externus is NOT a structure passing through lesser sciatic foramen.
  (DNB PATTERN JUNE 2011)
- Popliteal artery is NOT a content of Adductor canal.
  (DNB PATTERN JUNE 2010)
- Evertor of ankle inserted into the medial cuneiform is Peroneus longus. *(DNB PATTERN DEC 2009)*

- A sesamoid bone is present in the tendon of flexor hallucis brevis. *(DNB PATTERN DEC 2010)*
- Structure which does NOT pass under extensor retinaculum—Anterior interosseous artery. *(DNB PATTERN JUNE 2008)*
- Sectioning of fibular nerve leads to Foot drop. *(DNB PATTERN JUNE 2008)*
- Abduction of toes is by—Dorsal interossei. *(DNB PATTERN JUNE 2008)*
- Muscle which pulls the base of 5th metatarsal in a case of 5th metatarsal fracture—Peroneus brevis. *(DNB PATTERN JUNE 2008)*
- Ligament NOT involved in external rotation in semi flexed knee—Fibular collateral ligament. *(DNB PATTERN JUNE 2008)*
- In walking, gravity tends to tilt the pelvis and trunk to unsupported side, major factor preventing this unwanted movement is: Gluteus medius and minimus. *(DNB PATTERN 2000)*
- Main action of muscle gemellus is: Lateral rotation of thigh. *(DNB PATTERN 2000)*
- Common segmental joint innervation for the movements of Knee and Ankle joints is: L4, L5, S1. *(NEET 2016 PATTERN)*

LEVEL II: HIGH YIELD FACTORS

Table 1.1: Derivatives of mesonephric ducts (Wolffian ducts)

Male	Female
Ureteric bud	Broad ligament
Trigone of urinary bladder	Paraovarian cyst
Urethra	Gartner duct and cysts
Seminal vesicle + Ejaculatory duct	Mesonephric tubules
Vas deferens and epididymis	Organ of rosenmuller
Paradidymis	
Appendix of epididymis	

Table 1.2: Derivatives of paramesonephric ducts (Mullerian ducts)

Hydatid of Morgagni
Appendix of testis
Prostatic utricle
Upper 4/5th of vagina
Uterovaginal canal
Uterus and cervix
Fallopian tubes

Anatomy

Table 1.3: Derivatives of three germ layers

Endoderm	Ectoderm	Mesoderm
Pharyngeal pouches	Pharyngeal clefts	Pharyngeal arches
Urethra	Membranous labyrinth	Dura mater
Liver and Gall bladder	Lens	Trigone of urinary bladder
Urinary bladder	Adrenal medulla	Adrenal cortex
		Ciliary body
		Sclera, choroid, vitreous

Table 1.4: Derivatives of urogenital sinus

	Male	Female
Ventral and Pelvic part	Urinary bladder, Prostatic urethra (supra montanal region)	Urinary bladder urethra
Phallic/urethral region	Inframontanal prostatic urethra	Vaginal vestibule
Sinovaginal bulb	Part of prostatic utricle	Lower 1/5th of vagina

Table 1.5: Derivatives of branchial arches

Arch	Nerve	Muscles	Structures
1st	**M**andibular	**M**uscles of mastication [**MATT**] • Mylohyoid • **Anterior belly of digastric** • Tensor tympani and tensor palati	**M**eckel's cartilage **M**alleus/Incus
2nd	Facial	Muscles of facial expression Occipitofrontalis platysma **Posterior belly of Digastric** Stapedius	**R**eichert's cartilage **S**tapes **S**tyloid process **S**tylohyoid ligament **S**maller cornu of Hyoid **S**uperior part of body of Hyoid
3rd	**G**losso-pharyngeal	Stylopharyngeus	Greater cornu of Hyoid Lower part of body of Hyoid
4th	Superior laryngeal nerve	Muscles of pharynx and larynx	Cartilages of larynx

Contd...

Contd...

5th	Disappears	
6th	Recurrent laryngeal nerve	Muscles of larynx and pharynx

Table 1.6: Important vertebral levels

Bifurcation of common carotid artery	C3
Thyroid cartilage	C5
Cricoid cartilage	C6
Arch of aorta	T4
Tracheal bifurcation (Standing)	T6
Xiphoid process	T9
Transpyloric plane	L1
Subcostal plane	L3
Bifurcation of abdominal aorta	L4
Transtubercular plane	L5

Table 1.7: Important foramina and their contents

Mandibular foramen	Inferior alveolar nerve and vessels
Foramen rotundum	Maxillary nerve
Foramen spinosum	Middle meningeal artery and vein Meningeal branch of Mandibular Nerve.
Foramen lacerum	Internal carotid artery
Jugular foramen	9, 10, 11 nerves
Foramen ovale	Mandibular nerve, Emissary vein, Lesser petrosal nerve, Accessory meningeal artery
Carotid sheath	Common carotid artery, Internal jugular vein, Vagus nerve
Cavernous sinus	3, 4, 6, Ophthalmic and Maxillary Branch of 5th nerve, Internal Carotid Artery

Table 1.8: Named structures

Hassall's corpuscles	Thymus
Malpighian bodies	Spleen
Kupffer cells	Liver
Purkinje cells	Only output axons from cerebellar cortex
Reticular cells	Lymph node
Jacobsen's nerve	Tympanic branch of 9th nerve
Arnold's nerve	Auricular branch of 10th nerve
Nerve of latarjet	Branch of vagus in the stomach
Vidian nerve	Nerve of pterygoid canal
Rivinus duct	Duct of sublingual salivary gland

Contd...

Contd...

Wharton's duct	Duct of submandibular salivary gland
Waldeyer's fascia	Condensation of pelvic fascia behind rectum.
Kugel's artery	Branch of left coronary
Valve of gerlach	Guards the opening of appendix into caecum
Dentate line	Mucocutaneous junction located 1.5 cm above the anal verge
Valves of Kerckring	Circular fold of mucus membrane present in 2nd part of duodenum/jejunum/proximal ileum
Peyer's patches	Present in ileum
Paneth cells	Seen in base of crypts in small intestine, secrete lysozyme
Meibomian glands	Modified sebaceous glands
Brunner's glands	Mucus secreting glands in the submucosa of Duodenum.

Table 1.9: Joints

Largest joint in the body	Knee joint
Gomphosis or tooth socket joint is	Fibrous joint
Interosseous membrane between Radius and Ulna is example of	Syndesmosis
Vomer sphenoidal rostrum junction is example of	Schindylesis
Atlanto axial joint is an example of	Pivot joint
Incudo malleolar joint is	Saddle type of Synovial joint
Incudo stapedial joint is an example of	Ball and socket type of Synovial joint
Meta carpo phalangeal joint is an example of	Bicondylar Joint

EMBRYOLOGY

Rule of 2 FOR 2ND wk of IUL	2 Germ layers–Epiblast and Hypoblast 2 Cavities–Amniotic cavity, yolk sac 2 Components to placenta–syncytiotrophoblast/cytotrophoblast
Rule of 3 for 3rd wk of IUL	3 Germ Layers–Ectoderm/Endoderm/Mesoderm
Rule of 4 for 4TH wk of IUL	4 heart chambers/4 limb buds
Sonic hedgehog gene	Involved in patterning along Anteroposterior Axis
Homeobox genes (HOX)	Involved in organisation of the embryo in a craniocaudal direction
Morula stage	Day 3
Blastocyst occurs by	Day 5
Implantation occurs by	Day 6

Gastrulation occurs by	3rd week.
Neural Tube is formed by	3–8 weeks
Heart begins to beat by	4th week
Fetal movements occur by	8th week
Genitalia show male/female characteristics by	10th week
Fetal erythropoiesis occurs by	
Yolk Sac	3–8 weeks
Liver	6–30 weeks
Spleen	9–28 weeks
Bone Marrow	28 weeks onward

2. Physiology

"I am not the richest, smartest or the most talented person in the world, but I succeed because I keep going and going and going."
—**Sylvester Stallone**

REFERENCE
- *Ganong's Review of Physiology, 25th ed.*

LEVEL I: BASIC REPEATS

NERVOUS SYSTEM AND MUSCULAR SYSTEM

- Peripheral and central chemoreceptors respond to increased arterial CO_2. *(DNB PATTERN DEC 2011)*
- TRUE statement about Oligodendrocytes: They form myelin sheath. *(DNB PATTERN DEC 2011)*
- Hormone which decreases appetite: LEPTIN. *(DNB PATTERN DEC 2011)*

  ➤ Leptos means thin. Leptin is primarily secreted by White Adipose Tissue.
  ➤ Leptin counter acts the effects of Neuropeptide Y/Anandamide.
  ➤ Ghrelin increases Appetite.

- Orexins are NOT implicated in sexual behavior. *(DNB PATTERN DEC 2011)*
- Time duration required to generate an action potential is Rheobase. *(DNB PATTERN DEC 2011)*
- Satiety centre is located at ventromedial nucleus of thalamus. *(DNB PATTERN DEC 2011)*
- Nucleus ambiguus true is—9th and 10th nerve arise from it. *(DNB PATTERN JUNE 2008)*
- Serotonin secreting cell in brain is raphe nucleus. *(DNB PATTERN DEC 2011)*
- Achromatopsia is due to lesion in which area of occipital cortex? Area V4. *(DNB PATTERN JUNE 2011)*
- Band not covered by actin filament is H band. *(DNB PATTERN DEC 2011)*
- ADH is secreted by supraoptic nucleus. *(DNB PATTERN JUNE 2012)*

- Oxytocin is NOT involved in milk production. *(DNB PATTERN JUNE 2012)*
- Photoreceptors on stimulation release–Glutamate. *(DNB PATTERN JUNE 2008)*
- Tract which controls skilled voluntary movements is lateral corticospinal tract. *(DNB PATTERN JUNE 2011)*
- Seen in REM Sleep: Brain is very active but muscles are virtually paralysed. *(DNB PATTERN JUNE 2011)*
- Insulin increases glucose uptake in skeletal muscle. *(DNB PATTERN JUNE 2012)*
- During denervation of smooth muscle, there is increased sensitivity to chemical mediators. *(DNB PATTERN DEC 2010)*
- Nerve fibre with slowest conduction velocity – C fibre. *(DNB PATTERN DEC 2010)*
- Nerve fibre most susceptible to local anaesthetic: C fibre. *(DNB PATTERN DEC 2010)*
- RMP of cell is dependent on the permeability of the cell membrane to K^+ being greater to Na^+. *(DNB PATTERN DEC 2010)*
- During repolarisation phase of action potential of a neuron, there is increased permeability to Potassium. *(DNB PATTERN DEC 2010)*
- No of Golgi tendon organs for every 100 muscle fibres—0–10. *(DNB PATTERN DEC 2010)*
- Hemiplegia is most commonly due to occlusion of Middle Cerebral Artery. *(DNB PATTERN DEC 2010)*
- Prolactin secretion is Not increased by Dopamine. *(DNB PATTERN DEC 2010)*
- Renshaw cells are inhibitory interneurons found in grey matter of spinal cord. *(DNB PATTERN JUNE 2010)*
- Volume receptors are low pressure receptors, provide afferents for taste control and mediate vasopressin release. *(DNB PATTERN JUNE 2010)*
- Bruxism is NOT a feature of REM sleep. *(DNB PATTERN JUNE 2010)*
- Contractile unit of muscle is Sarcomere. *(DNB PATTERN DEC 2009)*
- Medial Geniculate Body is related to Hearing. *(DNB PATTERN DEC 2009)*
- Specific gravity of CSF 1.006–1.009. *(DNB PATTERN JUNE 2009)*
- Pretectal area is responsible for light reflex. *(DNB PATTERN JUNE 2009)*

- In central transsection of spinal cord, last affected is proprioception. *(DNB PATTERN JUNE 2009)*
- Ankle reflex – S_1. *(DNB PATTERN JUNE 2009)*
- Ruffini end organ is associated with sensation of cold. *(DNB PATTERN 2000)*
- Inverse stretch reflex involves lengthening of Muscle. *(DNB PATTERN JUNE 2008)*
- Myoglobin is present in–Slow fibers. *(DNB PATTERN JUNE 2008)*
- Preganglionic sympathetic and parasympathetic secrete – Acetylcholine. *(DNB PATTERN JUNE 2008)*
- Circadian rhythm controlled by–Suprachiasmatic nucleus. *(DNB PATTERN JUNE 2008)*
- Superficial reflex is Corneal. *(DNB PATTERN 2000)*
- Serotonin is secreted by Argentaffin cells. *(DNB PATTERN 2006)*
- Hunger centre is located in the lateral hypothalamus. *(DNB PATTERN 2005)*

> Orexins are NOT implicated in Sexual Behaviour. *(DNB PATTERN DEC 2011)*
> Orexins are implicated in Arousal/Wakefulness and Appetite.
> Narcolepsy is caused by lack of Orexins.

- Melatonin is secreted by Pineal Gland. *(DNB PATTERN 2001)*
- Fever causes thermoregulatory centre to shift to new level. *(DNB PATTERN 2001)*
- Auditary pathway is mediated by Medial Geniculate Body. *(DNB PATTERN 2001)*
- The inverse stretch reflex is due to Golgi tendon. *(DNB PATTERN 2002)*
- Protein common to smooth and skeletal muscle: Actin and Tropomyosin. *(DNB PATTERN AUG 2013)*
- What is generator potential? – Depolarisation occurs in graded response to strength of stimulus. *(DNB PATTERN AUG 2013)*
- Nernst potential of Potassium: –90. *(NEET PATTERN 2012, DNB PATTERN AUG 2013)*
- Resting membrane potential of Neuron: –90. *(NEET PATTERN 2012)*
- Pressure receptors are: Mechanoreceptors. *(DNB PATTERN AUG 2013)*

- Which type of corpuscle are Ruffini endings? – Bulbous corpuscle, responsible for pressure sensation. *(DNB PATTERN AUG 2013)*
- Ventral spinothalamic tract carries: Pain and Temperature. *(DNB PATTERN AUG 2013)*
- Nerve fibres carrying pain: A delta/C fibres. *(DNB PATTERN AUG 2013)*
- Nucleus for Accommodation Reflex: Edinger Westphal nucleus. *(DNB PATTERN AUG 2013)*
- Phosphodiesterase hydrolyses what in the retina? – cGMP. *(DNB PATTERN AUG 2013)*
- Myelin sheath is produced by: Oligodendrocytes. *(DNB PATTERN AUG 2013)*
- Stimulation for sympathetic neuron growth: Nerve growth factor. *(DNB PATTERN AUG 2013)*
- Multiplying neurons are seen in: Hippocampus. *(DNB PATTERN AUG 2013)*
- Striatal tract mediator: Dopamine. *(DNB PATTERN AUG 2013)*
- Striatum damage affects priming of Explicit Memory. *(NEET PATTERN 2012)*
- Retinal cells which secrete Acetyl Choline: Amacrine cells. *(NEET PATTERN 2012)*
- Presynaptic facilitation is caused by: Prolonged opening of calcium channels. *(NEET PATTERN 2012)*
- Broca's area is present in: Inferior frontal gyrus. *(NEET PATTERN 2012)*
- Number of golgi tendon organs per 100 muscle fibres: 1–20. *(NEET PATTERN 2012)*
- Ion which helps in Resting Membrane Potential in Neurons: Potassium. *(FMGE PATTERN MAR 2013)*
- Synaptic potential can be recorded by: Microelectrode. *(FMGE PATTERN MAR 2012)*
- Shivering is controlled by: Posterior hypothalamus. *(FMGE PATTERN SEP 2012, MAR 2013)*
- Posterior part of Hypothalamus is concerned with: Regulation of response to smell. *(FMGE PATTERN MARCH 2013)*
- Preganglionic neurotransmitter in sympathetic division of Autonomic Nervous System is: Acetylcholine. *(FMGE PATTERN MAR 2013)*
- Blind spot of Mariotte: Optic disc. *(FMGE PATTERN MAR 2007)*
- Stretch reflex of urinary bladder is integrated at: Sacral portion of Spinal Cord. *(FMGE PATTERN MAR 2007)*

- Intention tremors are seen in lesions of: Cerebellum. *(FMGE PATTERN MAR 2013)*
- Bipolar cells are seen in: Retina. *(FMGE PATTERN MAR 2005)*
- Sweating is mediated by: Cholinergic mediated sympathetic activity. *(FMGE PATTERN MAR 2013)*
- Unmyelinated Nerve fibre: C fibre. *(DNB PATTERN NOV 2013)*
- Pronator drift test is done for lesion of: Pyramidal tract. *(DNB PATTERN NOV 2013)*
- Salt and sour taste is perceived by: Ionotrophic receptors. *(DNB PATTERN NOV 2013)*
- Structurally the type of neurons that act as sensory neurons are: Pseudounipolar neurons. *(DNB PATTERN NOV 2013)*
- Membrane potential of hair cell is: -60 Mv. *(DNB PATTERN NOV 2013)*
- Typical feature of olfactory sensation is: Stimulus required is very small. *(DNB PATTERN NOV 2013)*
- True about Type 2 muscle fibre: White, glycolytic, fast contracting. *(DNB PATTERN NOV 2013)*
- Maximum concentration of Sodium channel is at: Node of Ranvier. *(DNB PATTERN NOV 2013)*
- In action potential of nerve, the overshoot is: Above Isopotential. *(DNB PATTERN NOV 2013)*
- In a myelinated nerve fibre, the refractive period is 1/2500 seconds. What is the impulse rate? 2500 per sec. *(DNB PATTERN NOV 2013)*
- Type 1 Glomus cell secrete neurotransmitter because of oxygen sensitive: Potassium channels. *(DNB PATTERN NOV 2013)*
- Neurotrophins: include Nerve Growth Factor (NGF), Brain Derived Neurotrophic Factor (BDNF), and Neurotrophin 3 and Neurotrophin 4. *(DNB PATTERN JUNE 2014)*
- Motilin receptor: G protein coupled receptor binding Motilin, which is an intestinal peptide which causes contraction of gut smooth muscle. *(DNB PATTERN JUNE 2014)*
- Erythromycin is a Motilin receptor agonist.
- Unit of Stretch Reflex is: Reflex Arc *(DNB PATTERN NOV 2015)*
- Doll's Eye Reflex is used in Unconscious patient. *(NEET PATTERN 2015)*
- Which receptor is stimulated by sustained pressure? Ruffini's end organ. *(NEET PATTERN 2015)*
- Wallerian degeneration is for: Nerve degeneration. *(NEET PATTERN 2015)*

- Resting membrane potential in smooth muscles: –40 mv.
  (NEET PATTERN 2015)
- CSF sugar is 2/3 blood sugar. *(DNB PATTERN NOV 2015)*
- Rubrospinal tract influences: Voluntary activity.
  (DNB PATTERN NOV 2015)
- Cerebral blood flow is increased by: Increase in pCO_2
  (NEET PATTERN 2015)
- Unspecified pain pathway is for: Psychogenic pain.
  (NEET PATTERN 2015)
- Action potential in cardiac muscles has how many phases ? 5
  (NEET PATTERN 2015)
- Excitatory cells in cerebellum: Granule cells.
  (NEET PATTERN 2015)
- Somatomedin C deficiency causes: Growth retardation.
  (NEET PATTERN 2015)
- Destruction of this hypothalamic centre leads to Anorexia and Starvation: Lateral Hypothalamic Nuclei.
  (NEET 2016 PATTERN)
- Rapidly adapting capsulated receptors for Low Frequency Vibration in non-hairy skin are: Meissner's Corpuscles.
  (NEET PATTERN 2016)
- Most important stimulus for central chemoreceptors is: Increased pCO_2 in blood. *(NEET 2016 PATTERN)*
- Inability to see near objects may result from inability to contract: Ciliary Body. *(NEET 2016 PATTERN)*
- Receptors blocked in Myasthenia Gravis: Acetyl Choline Receptors. *(NEET PATTERN 2018)*
- Characteristic pattern seen in Brown Sequard Syndrome: Contralateral absence of pain sensation.
  (NEET PATTERN 2018)
- Alpha waves are seen in: Relaxed State.
  (NEET PATTERN 2018)
- Prosapagnosia is an inability to: Recognize faces.
  (NEET PATTERN 2018)

CARDIOVASCULAR SYSTEM

- Max filling of ventricles is seen in ventricular phase of diastole.
  (DNB PATTERN DEC 2011)
- Stroke volume decreases by increase in heart rate.
  (DNB PATTERN JUNE 2011)
- What happens when carotid sinus is pressed? Heart rate and peripheral resistance decreases.
  (DNB PATTERN DEC 2011)

Physiology

- Potassium in which compartment is responsible for cardiac and neural function? Intracellular compartment.
  (DNB PATTERN DEC 2011)
- MARIE'S LAW: states the relationship of Heart Rate with Arterial BP. *(DNB PATTERN JUNE 2011)*
- Decreased extracellular calcium leads to decreased membrane stability. *(DNB PATTERN JUNE 2011)*
- Coronary blood flow is maximum during isovolumetric relaxation. *(DNB PATTERN JUNE 2012)*
- Intercalated discs are present in cardiac myocytes.
  (DNB PATTERN JUNE 2012)
- In JVP, A wave is due to atrial contraction.
  (DNB PATTERN DEC 2010)
- Cardiac muscle cell does not undergo cell division.
  (DNB PATTERN DEC 2010)
- Preload measures End Diastolic Volume.
  (DNB PATTERN DEC 2009)
- Max velocity of conduction is seen in Purkinje fibres. (4 m/sec) *(DNB PATTERN DEC 2009)*
- Pulse pressure is affected by stroke volume and compliance of aorta. *(DNB PATTERN DEC 2009)*
- The result of increased preload on cardiac muscle is lengthening of muscle fibre. *(DNB PATTERN JUNE 2009)*
- Isovolumetric relaxation precedes ventricular relaxation.
  (DNB PATTERN 2000)
- Pulse pressure is systolic-diastolic BP.
  (DNB PATTERN 2000)
- Bainbridge reflex causes increased heart rate.
  (DNB PATTERN 2001)
- Cardiac output is increased by both chronotropic and ionotropic receptors. *(DNB PATTERN 2001)*
- Coronary blood flow in mL/min is 250.
  (DNB PATTERN 2003)
- Slowest conduction is in AV node. *(DNB PATTERN 2001)*
- Law relating distending pressure and tension in a blood vessel wall is called Laplace's law. *(DNB PATTERN 2003)*
- Plateau phase of action potential is due to: Influx of calcium.
  (DNB PATTERN 2002)
- All or none law refers to action potential.
  (DNB PATTERN 2001)
- Gatekeeper of the heart: AV node. *(NEET PATTERN 2012)*
- Contractility of cardiac muscle depends on: T tubules and extracellular calcium. *(DNB PATTERN NOV 2013)*

- Oxygen consumption of myocardium is: 20 mL/kg/min. *(DNB PATTERN NOV 2013)*
- Elasticity of the heart is due to: TITIN. *(NEET 2016 PATTERN)*
- C-wave is seen in: Isovolumetric Contraction phase. *(NEET 2018 PATTERN)*

BLOOD AND BLOOD VESSELS

- Predominant site of erythropoiesis during 6th month of gestation is Liver. *(DNB PATTERN DEC 2011)*
- True about thymus is consists of Hassall's corpuscles. *(DNB PATTERN DEC 2011)*
- Bicarbonate is mainly present in extracellular fluid. *(DNB PATTERN DEC 2010)*
- Hematopoiesis first starts in Yolk sac. *(DNB PATTERN DEC 2010)*
- Gamma globulins are formed by plasma cells. *(DNB PATTERN DEC 2011)*
- Milieu interior means extracellular fluid. *(DNB PATTERN DEC 2011)*
- Free fatty acid is transported in blood by albumin. *(DNB PATTERN DEC 2011)*
- NOT present in dense granules of platelets: Von Willebrand factor. *(DNB PATTERN JUNE 2011)*
- Major basic protein is secreted by Eosinophil. *(DNB PATTERN JUNE 2011)*
- Most abundant extracellular buffer is: Hemoglobin. *(DNB PATTERN JUNE 2011)*
- Plasma membrane of cell is bound to cytoskeleton by Ankyrin. *(DNB PATTERN JUNE 2012)*
- Vitamin K dependent clotting factors – 2, 7, 9, 10, Protein C, Protein S. *(DNB PATTERN DEC 2010)*
- RBC in females is less than males due to blood loss during menstruation. *(DNB PATTERN DEC 2010)*
- Ion which is needed for conversion of prothrombin to thrombin is calcium. *(DNB PATTERN DEC 2009)*
- NO is produced from endothelium. *(DNB PATTERN DEC 2009)*
- Hypoxia without cyanosis—Anemic hypoxia. *(DNB PATTERN DEC 2009)*
- Largest storage of blood is in veins. *(DNB PATTERN JUNE 2009)*

Physiology

- Clotting factor that is not affected in liver disease – Factor 8. (It is produced by vascular endothelium).
  (DNB PATTERN JUNE 2009)
- pH of blood is – 7.35 to 7.45.
  (DNB PATTERN JUNE 2008)
- Splanchnic vessels and venules contain 25–30% blood volume. *(DNB PATTERN JUNE 2008)*
- Arnith index is counting of lobes in Neutrophils.
  (DNB PATTERN 2000)
- Most important buffer in blood–Hemoglobin.
  (DNB PATTERN JUNE 2008)
- Greatest resistance in peripheral blood circulation is due to Arterioles. *(DNB PATTERN 2001)*
- The need for Vit B12 and folic acid in the formation of RBCs is primarily due to the effects on DNA synthesis in the bone marrow. *(DNB PATTERN 2004)*
- Cyanosis with normal arterial O_2 concentration causes anemic hypoxia. *(DNB PATTERN 2001)*
- Most abundant buffer in blood: Bicarbonate.
  (DNB PATTERN 2002)
- Arteriole is resistance vessel. *(NEET PATTERN 2012)*
- Windkessel effect is seen in: Large elastic vessels.
  (NEET PATTERN 2012)
- Most permissible capillaries are seen in: Liver.
  (DNB PATTERN NOV 2013)
- Lifespan of neutrophils is: 6 hrs.
  (DNB PATTERN NOV 2013)
- Life span of RBC: 120 days. *(FMGE PATTERN JUNE 2014)*
- TIBC (Total Iron Binding Capacity) is increased in: Iron deficiency anemia. *(FMGE PATTERN JUNE 2014)*
- Normal TIBC: 300–360 microgm/day
- TIBC > 400 in Iron deficiency anemia.
- TIBC is an indirect measure of circulating transferrin.
- Least in extracellular compartment: Potassium.
  (DNB PATTERN JUNE 2014)
- NOT an acute phase reactant: Trypsin.
  (DNB PATTERN JUNE 2014)
- Alpha 1 *Antitrypsin is an acute phase reactant.*
- Half life of prothrombin: 60 hours.
  (DNB PATTERN NOV 2015)
- Windkessel effect in large arteries perform: Prevention of fluctuation in BP. *(DNB PATTERN NOV 2015)*

- Poiseulle's equation states that: Blood flow is directly proportional to the 4th power of radius. *(NEET PATTERN 2015)*
- Factor which activates Prekallikrein: Factor 12. *(NEET PATTERN 2015)*
- An increase in Serum Hepcidin is caused by: Inflammation. *(NEET 2016 PATTERN)*

RENAL SYSTEM

- Effect of efferent arteriole constriction and afferent arteriole dilatation on GFR is it increases. *(DNB PATTERN JUNE 2011)*
- 100% filtration coefficient is seen in Inulin. *(DNB PATTERN DEC 2010)*
- 15% nephrons in humans have long loops. *(DNB PATTERN 2000)*
- Max absorption of glucose in a nephron is 375 mg. *(DNB PATTERN 2001)*
- Inulin clearance closely resembles GFR. *(DNB PATTERN 2003)*
- Afferent arteriolar dilator: Prostacyclin. *(DNB PATTERN 2002)*
- Organ with maximum blood flow in mL/kg/min: Kidney. *(DNB PATTERN 2002)*
- Macula Densa is part of: DCT. *(NEET PATTERN 2012)*
- Lacis cells are located at juxtaglomerular Apparatus. *(NEET PATTERN 2012)*
- Relaxation of mesangial cells is caused by: Dopamine. *(NEET PATTERN 2012)*
- At rest, blood flow is maximum in: Kidney. *(FMGE PATTERN MAR 2012)*
- Action of ADH: Regulation of reabsorption of water from collecting duct. *(NEET PATTERN 2013)*
- ADH synthesis site: Hypothalamus. *(NEET PATTERN 2013)*
- Mineralocorticoids act on: collecting duct. *(DNB PATTERN NOV 2015)*
- Renal plasma flow is measured by: PAH. *(DNB PATTERN NOV 2015)*

RESPIRATORY SYSTEM

- During underwater diving the main danger is due to oxygen and nitrogen. *(DNB PATTERN DEC 2011)*
- CO_2 causes respiratory stimulation by Central Chemoreceptors. *(DNB PATTERN JUNE 2011)*

- In a person acclimatized for high altitude, oxygen saturation is maintained because of more oxygen delivery to tissues. *(DNB PATTERN JUNE 2012)*
- In Caisson's disease, pain in the joints is due to nitrogen bubbles. *(DNB PATTERN DEC 2010)*
- Lacis cells are situated in: Macula Densa *(DNB PATTERN JUNE 2014)*
- *They are also called Polkissen cells and form the Juxtaglomerular apparatus.*
- Oliguria is defined as: < 0.5 mL/kg/hour in 24 hrs. *(DNB PATTERN JUNE 2014)*

  < 1 mL/kg/hr in 24 hrs in infants.
- Percentage of total body water in body weight at birth: 80% *(NEET PATTERN 2015)*
- Epithelial Sodium channels have 2 alpha, 1 beta and 2 gamma subunits. *(NEET PATTERN 2015)*
- Normal urinary pH: 6.5–7 *(NEET PATTERN 2015)*
- Pulmonary alveoli are kept dry due to negative interstitial pressure. *(DNB PATTERN DEC 2010)*
- Physiological dead space -150 mL. *(DNB PATTERN DEC 2010)*
- Lungs have NO role in regulating Vitamin D metabolism. *(DNB PATTERN DEC 2010)*
- Transpulmonary pressure is difference between pressure in alveoli and intra pleural pressure. *(DNB PATTERN JUNE 2009)*
- Anatomical dead space is 1/3 of tidal volume. *(DNB PATTERN JUNE 2009)*
- Parasympathetic stimulation–Increases airway resistance. *(DNB PATTERN JUNE 2008)*
- Statement NOT true about Type 2 pneumocytes: They form Air Blood Barrier. *(DNB PATTERN 2001)*
- High altitude acclimatization is facilitated by increased RBC production. *(DNB PATTERN 2000)*
- Statement NOT true about Herring Bruer inflation reflex: Protects against under inflation of the lungs. *(DNB PATTERN 2006)*
- In a normal adult, the ratio of physiological to anatomical dead space is 1:1. *(DNB PATTERN 2003)*
- Inspiratory depth is halted by: Pneumotaxic centre. *(NEET PATTERN 2012)*
- Surfactant acts on: Alveoli. *(FMGE PATTERN MAR 2013)*

- True statement regarding difference between apex and base of lung, in erect posture is: V/Q is high at the apex of lung. *(FMGE PATTERN MAR 2013)*
- Increase blood flow to lungs cause: Increased pulmonary vascular resistance. *(DNB PATTERN OCT 2013)*
- Peptide which relaxes the Bronchial Smooth Muscle: Vasoactive Intestinal Peptide. *(DNB PATTERN OCT 2013)*
- Surfactant contains: Dipalmitoyl Phosphatidyl Choline. *(DNB PATTERN OCT 2013)*
- Surfactant is secreted by: Type 2 Pneumocytes. *(DNB PATTERN OCT 2013)*
- Pulmonary alveoli is kept dry due to: Negative interstitial pressure. *(DNB PATTERN OCT 2013)*
- Best vehicle for oxygen is: Hemoglobin solution. *(DNB PATTERN OCT 2013)*
- Carbon monoxide is present maximally in: Bicarbonate form. *(DNB PATTERN OCT 2013)*
- CO_2 content in arterial blood is: 49 mL/dL. *(DNB PATTERN OCT 2013)*
- Pulmonary Lymph flow rate is: 20 mL/hour. *(DNB PATTERN OCT 2013)*
- Physiological dead space is: Equal to anatomical dead space in normal healthy adult. *(NEET PATTERN 2013)*
- Haldane effect is: CO_2 delivery by increased O_2. *(NEET PATTERN 2015)*
- Most important factor in transport across a membrane: Concentration gradient.
- Normal transpulmonary pressure during quiet breathing: +8 to +5 cm H_2O *(NEET PATTERN 2015)*
- Isocapneic buffering is normal pCO_2 with increased CO_2. *(NEET PATTERN 2015)*
- Vital capacity is measured by: Spirometer. *(NEET PATTERN 2015)*
- In zero gravity, V/Q ratio is: 1 *(NEET PATTERN 2015)*
- Compliance of lung thoracic system: 200 mL/cm H_2O *(NEET PATTERN 2015)*
- Minute Volume is: Tidal volume Respiratory Rate. *(NEET PATTERN 2015)*
- Most useful therapy in Carbon Monoxide Poisoning: Hyperbaric Oxygen. *(NEET PATTERN 2015)*
- In high altitude acclimatization, tissue oxygenation is maintained due to: More oxygen delivery to tissue. *(DNB PATTERN NOV 2015)*

- Va/Q is infinity when: There is no exchange of O_2 and CO_2.
  (NEET 2018 PATTERN)

GASTROINTESTINAL SYSTEM

- Trypsinogen is converted into Trypsin by: Enterokinase.
  (NEET PATTERN 2012)
- D cells of pancreas secrete: Somatostatin.
  (FMGE PATTERN SEP 2012)
- Folic acid is absorbed in proximal jejunum by both active and passive transport. *(DNB PATTERN JUNE 2012)*
- Statement NOT true about Stomach: Pylorus has more acid secreting cells. *(DNB PATTERN DEC 2011)*
- Enzyme with highest pH: Pancreatic Juice.
  (DNB PATTERN DEC 2011)
- Enzyme which reduces gastric secretions: Secretin.
  (DNB PATTERN JUNE 2011)
- Gastric juice secretion is 20% in cephalic phase.
  (DNB PATTERN JUNE 2012)
- Nourishment to gut is not a normal function of peritoneum.
  (DNB PATTERN DEC 2010)
- Vitamin B12 is mainly absorbed from Ileum.
  (DNB PATTERN DEC 2010)
- Ion which is more in gastric secretions compared to blood – Cl^- *(DNB PATTERN JUNE 2009)*
- Glucose is transported through Sodium cotransport.
  (DNB PATTERN 2000)
- Gastrocolic reflex is related to mass peristalsis.
  (DNB PATTERN 2006)
- Physiological gastrectomy: Ligate all major arteries.
  (DNB PATTERN 2007)
- Normal portal venous pressure is: 5–10 mm Hg.
  (DNB PATTERN 2000)
- Iron absorption is increased by Vitamin C.
  (DNB PATTERN 2000)
- HCO_3 is highest in pancreatic secretions.
  (DNB PATTERN 2001)
- Best stimulus for secretin secretion is protein and HCl.
  (DNB PATTERN 2001)
- Substance which causes increased Cyclic AMP in interstitial cells causes diarrhea via: Increased chloride secretion.
  (DNB PATTERN JUNE 2014)
- Curdling of milk is caused by: Rennin.
  (DNB PATTERN NOV 2015)

- Last discovered Taste sensation: Umami. *(NEET PATTERN 2015)*
- Umami taste sensation is due to: Glutamic acid. *(NEET PATTERN 2015)*
- Colipase is associated with Pancreatic Lipase. *(NEET PATTERN 2015)*
- Acid secretion in cephalic phase contributes to what percentage of total acid secretion? 20% *(NEET PATTERN 2015)*
- Receptive area of stomach: Fundus. *(NEET PATTERN 2015)*
- Hormone which satisfies the criteria for INCRETIN: Gastric Inhibitory Peptide. *(NEET 2016 PATTERN)*
- Other Hormone which is an Incretin : Glucagon Like Peptide 1(GLP-1)
- Glucose is absorbed in Intestine by: Facilitated Diffusion. *(NEET 2018 PATTERN)*
- Insulin Like Growth Factor is secreted by: Liver. *(NEET 2018 PATTERN)*
- Primary function of Auerbach's plexus is: Control of motility of the digestive tract. *(NEET 2016 PATTERN)*
- Iron is transported from the cytoplasm of the enterocyte to the microvillus membrane by: Divalent Metal Transporter 1(DMT 1) *(NEET 2018 PATTERN)*

GENITAL SYSTEM

- Sperm acquires motility in epidydimis. *(NEET PATTERN 2012)*
- 15 million sperm/mL of semen with total 15 % motile sperm signifies: Oligoasthenozoospermia. *(DNB PATTERN OCT 2013)*
- Androgen Binding Protein (ABP) is secreted by Sertoli cells. *(DNB PATTERN DEC 2011, DEC 2010)*
- Mullerian Inhibiting Substance (MIS) is secreted by Sertoli cell. *(DNB PATTERN DEC 2011)*
- NOT a function of estrogen: Secretory function on endometrium. *(DNB PATTERN JUNE 2011)*
- A fertilized ovum reaches uterine cavity in 3-4 days. *(DNB PATTERN JUNE 2011)*
- Most common site of fertilization is ampulla. *(DNB PATTERN JUNE 2011)*
- Post menopausal hormone that causes an increase is FSH. *(DNB PATTERN JUNE 2011)*

- Corpus Luteum secretes Progesterone. *(DNB PATTERN JUNE 2012)*
- Endometrium regeneration starts on 5th day of menstrual cycle. *(DNB PATTERN JUNE 2012)*
- Progesterone peaks on 21st day of menstrual cycle. *(DNB PATTERN JUNE 2012)*
- Sperms are released during ejaculation from epididimis. *(DNB PATTERN DEC 2010)*
- Estrogen secretion is maximum before ovulation. *(DNB PATTERN JUNE 2009)*
- HCG is secreted by syncytiotrophoblast. *(DNB PATTERN JUNE 2009)*
- Velocity of sperms in female genital tract is 1-3 mm/minute. *(DNB PATTERN JUNE 2009)*
- Daily sperm production is 120 million/day. *(DNB PATTERN JUNE 2009)*
- Sperm gets capacitated in Uterus. *(DNB PATTERN JUNE 2009)*
- Neocerebellum is concerned with motor planning. *(DNB PATTERN JUNE 2009)*
- Axillary hair growth is caused by Testosterone. *(DNB PATTERN JUNE 2009)*
- In 29 day menstrual cycle, ovulation takes place at 15th day. *(DNB PATTERN JUNE 2009)*
- Inhibin inhibits FSH. *(DNB PATTERN 2002)*
- Organelle which is NOT present in Sperm: Endoplasmic Reticulum. *(NEET PATTERN 2015)*
- Progesterone peaks on what day of the menstrual cycle ? 21st day. *(DNB PATTERN NOV 2015)*
- Ambiguous genitalia is seen in: Androgen insensitivity syndrome. *(DNB PATTERN JUNE 2014)*

MISCELLANEOUS

- Vitamin required for Hydroxylation of Proline: Vitamin C. *(NEET PATTERN 2012)*
- Most potent antioxidant: Vitamin C. *(NEET PATTERN 2012)*
- Most abundant ion in intracellular fluid: Potassium. *(FMGE PATTERN SEP 2012, MAR 2013)*
- With glucose, which ion is transported? – Sodium. *(FMGE PATTERN MAR 2013)*
- Osmolality of plasma in a normal adult: 280 -290 mOsm/kg. *(FMGE PATTERN SEP 2012)*

- BMR is dependent on: Surface area.
  (FMGE PATTERN MAR 2013)
- Milk ejection is facilitated by Oxytocin.
  (FMGE PATTERN MAR 2013)
- Level of which hormone is increased in post menopausal women: FSH. *(FMGE PATTERN MAR 2013)*
- Hyaluronic acid is present in: Synovial fluid.
  (DNB PATTERN OCT 2013)
- Method NOT used for the measurement of body fluid volumes: I-125 Albumin for blood volume.
  (FMGE PATTERN MAR 2013)
- Concentration of Sodium in ECF is: 138 -146 millimoles/lit.
  (DNB PATTERN OCT 2013)
- Hormone increased in aging: Norepinephrine.
  (NEET PATTERN 2013)
- Hormone involved in JAK/STAT pathway: Prolactin.
  (NEET PATTERN 2013)
- Immunosympathectomy in animals is due to: Nerve growth factor. *(NEET PATTERN 2013)*
- Hormone NOT derived from Pro Opio Melano Cortin: TSH. *(NEET PATTERN 2013)*
- Iodine uptake in thyroid gland is an example of secondary active transport. *(DNB PATTERN DEC 2011)*
- Wolff Chaikoff effect–Inhibition of organic binding of iodides. *(DNB PATTERN DEC 2010)*
- Calcitonin is secreted by Thyroid gland.
  (DNB PATTERN 2001)
- Role of calcitonin is decreased calcium level.
  (DNB PATTERN 2001)
- Transport of two substances in the same direction is called as Symport. *(DNB PATTERN DEC 2009)*
- TRH stimulates the release of TSH and Prolactin.
  (DNB PATTERN DEC 2009)
- Daily requirement of Potassium is 2-3 g/day.
  (DNB PATTERN JUNE 2012)
- Receptor potential is a graded change.
  (DNB PATTERN JUNE 2012)
- Umbilical vein carries oxygenated blood away from placenta.
  (DNB PATTERN JUNE 2012)
- Supra adrenal chromaffin cells secrete catecholamines.
  (DNB PATTERN JUNE 2012)
- Transducin is a protein found in retina.
  (DNB PATTERN DEC 2010)

- Acetyl Choline is secreted in eye by Amacrine cells. *(DNB PATTERN DEC 2010)*
- Adrenal Medulla secretes Epinephrine, Norepinephrine and Dopamine. *(DNB PATTERN DEC 2010)*
- Growth hormone is increased by hypoglycemia. *(DNB PATTERN JUNE 2010)*
- Most abundant extracellular ion: Sodium. *(DNB PATTERN DEC 2009)*
- Highest level of Zinc is found in prostate. *(DNB PATTERN JUNE 2009)*
- Daily requirement of Zinc in humans: 9.4 mg/day. *(DNB PATTERN JUNE 2009)*
- pH sensing receptors NOT present in Jugular bulb. *(DNB PATTERN JUNE 2008)*
- Genetic information in DNA is carried by bases. *(DNB PATTERN 2000)*
- Intracellular cation most osmotically active–Potassium. *(DNB PATTERN JUNE 2008)*
- Hyperparathyroidism associated with–Increased Alkaline phosphatase. *(DNB PATTERN JUNE 2008)*
- Non shivering thermogenesis in adults is due to thyroid hormone. *(DNB PATTERN 2006)*
- The molecule for cell signaling: Nitric Oxide. *(DNB PATTERN 2007)*
- Nernst equation deals with Chloride shift. *(DNB PATTERN 2000)*
- DNA fragment separation is done by Agarose Gel. *(DNB PATTERN 2000)*
- Major portion of body water lies in Intracellular compartment. *(DNB PATTERN 2001)*
- Hormone for breast milk feeding is: Oxytocin. *(DNB PATTERN 2001)*
- Orthodox sleep is NREM sleep. *(DNB PATTERN NOV 2015)*
- BMI considered 'LETHAL' in Men: 13 *(NEET PATTERN 2018)*

LEVEL II: HIGH YIELD FACTORS

Table 2.1: Important muscle proteins

Calmodulin	Intracellular calcium binding protein in smooth muscle
Phospholamban	Regulates the activity of Calcium pump on sarcoplasmic reticulum
Dynein and kinesin	Molecular motors

Contd...

Contd...

Table 2.1: Important muscle proteins

Titin	Provides scaffolding to the sarcomere
Troponin	Present in skeletal and cardiac muscle, NOT in smooth muscle
Tropomyosin	Covers myosin and blocks interaction of actin and myosin

Table 2.2: Important membrane potentials

Resting Membrane Potential of Smooth Muscle	– 50 mv
RMP of Nerve	– 70 mv
RMP of Skeletal and cardiac muscle	– 90 mv
End Plate Potential	Forerunner of action potential, recorded by cathode ray Oscilloscope
Action Potential	Propagatory potential
IPSP (Inhibitory Post Synaptic Potential)	Influx of calcium
EPSP (Excitatory Post Synaptic Potential)	Influx of sodium
Synaptic Potential	Recorded by microelectrodes

Table 2.3: Important brain areas and functions

Lateral nucleus of Hypothalamus	Feeding centre
Ventromedial Nucleus of Hypothalamus	Satiety centre
Suprachiasmatic Nucleus of Hypothalamus	Circadian rhythm
Supra optic Nucleus	Vasopressin secretion
Arcuate and paraventricular Nucleus	Dopamine secretion
Posterior Hypothalamus	Wakefulness/Arousal
Paraventricular Nucleus	Oxytocin secretion
Subthalamic Nucleus of Basal ganglia	Lesion causes Hemiballismus
Substantia Nigra	Lesion – Parkinsonism
Caudate Nucleus	Lesion-Chorea
Putamen	Lesion-Athetosis
Precentral Gyrus (Brodmann Area 4)	Motor Cortex/Motor Homunculus
Postcentral Gyrus and Sylvian Fissure	Sensory Cortex/Sensory Homunculus
Pretectal Area	Light Reflex

Table 2.4: Sleep stages and EEG changes

Sleep spindles	Stage II NREM
PGO spikes	REM
K complexes	Stage II NREM
Active dreams	REM
Nightmares	REM
Deep sleep	Stage IV NREM
Alpha waves	Parieto occipital lobe
Beta waves	Frontal lobe, highest frequency
Theta waves	Hippocampus, more in children
Delta waves	Deep sleep, least frequency (BAT DANCE)

Table 2.5: Hormones

Major circulating thyroid hormone	T4
Most potent/more active thyroid hormone	T3
Hormone involved in testicular descent in Males	Mullerian Inhibiting Substance
Hormone inhibiting FSH secretion produced by Sertoli cells in Males	Inhibin
Interstitial cells of Leydig secrete	Testosterone
Kidney is the major source of	Erythropoeitin

Table 2.6: Genital physiology

Hyaluronidase secreted by sperm acrosome	Penetration of corona radiata
Motility of sperms occurs in	Distal epidydimis
Sperm capacitation occurs in	Fallopian tube
Essential for Sperm Motility	Fructose
Rate of sperm movement in Female Genital tract	3 mm/min
Normal sperm count	60-100 million/ml
Fructose in sperms comes from	Seminal vesicle
Rate of sperm motility in Female Genital Tract	3 mm/min
Single spermatogonia gives rise to	512 spermatids
First Meiotic division of Graafian follicle	Completed at puberty just before ovulation
Second Meiotic division of Graafian follicle	Completed only when sperm penetrates oocyte

Table 2.7: Important points on kidney

Juxtamedullary nephrons constitute	15% of nephrons
Juxtaglomerular cells secrete	Renin
Normal urinary pH	5.85
Normal specific gravity of urine	1.015–1.025
Transport maximum of glucose	360 mg/mL
Maximum reabsorption of water and sodium occurs in	Proximal convoluted tubules
Acidification of urine	Distal convoluted tubules

Table 2.8: Gastrointestinal tract

Goblet cells	Mucus secreting cells in intestine
Enterochromaffin cells	Secretes serotonin from mucosa of small intestine
Paneth cells	In crypts of Lieberkuhn of small intestine
Chief cells	In body and fundus of stomach, secretes Pepsinogen.
G cells	Pylorus/Antrum, secretes gastrin
Neck cells	In body and fundus of stomach, secretes bicarbonate
Parietal cells	In body and fundus of stomach, secretes HCl
Brunner's gland	Duodenum, secretes mucus

UMAMI

5th basic taste

Umami represents the taste of amino acid L GLUTAMATE and 5' ribonucleotides GMP and IMP.

Other common names for Umami: SAVOURY TASTE/BROTHY TASTE/MEATY TASTE

Man tastes Umami through TASTE receptors specific to GLUTAMATE.

MONOSODIUM GLUTAMATE (MSG-Ajinomotto) exerts its action through GLUTAMATE receptors.

Existence of Umami first identified by KIKUNAE IKEDA, Japanese Scientist in 1908.

Umami rich foods: TOMATOES/SOY SAUCE/FISH SAUCE/MEAT BROTH.

USFDA considers MSG in the GRAS (Generally Recognised As Safe) category.

Taste buds in multiple areas of tongue recognize Umami, no specific geographic distribution.

3 Biochemistry

"In the real world, the smartest people are those who make mistakes and learn. In school, the smartest people don't make mistakes."
—**Robert T Kiyosaki**

REFERENCES

- *Vasudevan and Sreekumari, Textbook of Biochemistry, 8th ed.*
- *Harper's Biochemistry, 28th ed.*

LEVEL I: BASIC REPEATS

GENETICS AND PROTEOMICS

- Method used for reading 50–100 base pairs in large chromosomes: Restriction Fragment Length Polymorphism. *(DNB PATTERN 2007)*
- Primary role of chaperones is to help in Protein folding. *(DNB PATTERN 2007)*
- Base stalking of DNA is done by Hyperchromicity. *(DNB PATTERN 2006)*
- Banding of chromosome is seen in Interphase. *(DNB PATTERN 2004)*
- Chromosomal studies are done in Metaphase stage. *(DNB PATTERN 2002)*
- Folding and unfolding of DNA is done by Topoisomerases. *(DNB PATTERN JUNE 2008)*
- Telomerase: RNA dependent DNA polymerase. *(DNB PATTERN JUNE 2008)*
- Single base pair substitution is related to Restriction Fragment Length Polymorphism. *(DNB PATTERN JUNE 2010)*
- A Hormone responsive element is a: DNA sequence where hormone-binding protein complex binds. *(DNB PATTERN JUNE 2008)*
- Shine Dalgarno sequence in prokaryotes is associated with Translation. *(DNB PATTERN JUNE 2009)*
- Degeneracy of Genetic Code: for 1 amino acid, there may be more than 1 codon. *(DNB PATTERN JUNE 2008)*

- Peptidyl transferase is an example of: Ribozyme.
  (DNB PATTERN DEC 2010)
- If content of Adenine is 15%, then content of Guanine according to Chargaff's rule? 35%.
  (DNB PATTERN JUNE 2010)
- DNA microarrays allow detection of gene mutations using: Hybridisation. *(DNB PATTERN DEC 2010)*
- Enzyme responsible for unwinding of DNA is: Helicase.
  (DNB PATTERN DEC 2011)
- DNA replication occurs in which phase of cell cycle? S phase
  (DNB PATTERN DEC 2011)
- RNA polymerase recognises Promoter site.
  (DNB PATTERN JUNE 2009)
- NOT a circular DNA: Nuclear.
  (DNB PATTERN JUNE 2010)
- Tertiary structure is present in Beta keratin.
  (DNB PATTERN 2002)
- Which is obtained from Thermophilus aquaticus bacterium which is heat stable and used in PCR at high temperature? Taq polymerase. *(DNB PATTERN DEC 2011)*
- NOT a consequence of Protein denaturation: Loss of primary structure. *(DNB PATTERN DEC 2010)*
- Final product of purine metabolism is: Uric Acid.
  (FMGE PATTERN PATTERN MARCH 2010, SEP 2010)
- H_2S inhibits cytochromes in ETC complex: IV.
  (DNB PATTERN AUG 2013)
- Which protein does NOT form core of Histone? H1 and H5.
  (DNB PATTERN JUNE 2014)
- LDL reuptake in Liver associated with: Apo B100 and Apo E.
  (DNB PATTERN JUNE 2014)
- Cholesterol present in Arterial Smooth muscle mainly is: LDL. *(DNB PATTERN JUNE 2014)*
- Micro RNA is gene silencing RNA.
  (DNB PATTERN JULY 2016)
- Role of Ubiquitin in cell: Energy Dependent Protein Degradation. *(DNB PATTERN JULY 2016)*
- Function of Helicase: Unwinding of DNA.
  (NEET PATTERN 2015)
- Function of DNA Ligase: To seal and nick Okazaki fragments.
  (NEET PATTERN 2015)

- DNA Labelling is done by using: P-32.
  (DNB PATTERN NOV 2015)
- Function of Micro RNA: Gene expression Inhibition.
  (DNB PATTERN NOV 2015)
- The principle of X inactivation is explained by: Lyon's Hypothesis. *(NEET PATTERN 2016)*
- Ideal investigation for analysis of very small mutations in a chromosome is: PCR Based Assay. *(NEET PATTERN 2016)*
- TATA Box is located in: Promoter region.
  (NEET PATTERN 2016)
- CHAPERONES assist in: Protein Folding.
  (NEET PATTERN 2018)

VITAMINS AND NUTRIENTS

- Vitamin A is NOT present in: Sunflower seeds.
  (DNB PATTERN DEC 2011)
- Vitamin B12 is absorbed in: Ileum.
  (DNB PATTERN JUNE 2008)
- Hypervitaminosis A induces damage to Lysosomes.
  (DNB PATTERN 2007)
- Insulin secretion is associated with Zinc.
  (DNB PATTERN 2003)
- Activated Pantothenic Acid is found in Coenzyme A.
  (DNB PATTERN 2001)
- Allosteric activator of Acetyl CoA carboxylase: Biotin.
  (DNB PATTERN 2005)
- Activator of enzyme sulphite oxidase is: Molybdenum.
  (DNB PATTERN DEC 2011)
- Glutathione peroxidase contains Selenium.
  (DNB PATTERN 2000)
- Cytochrome oxidase contains Iron and Copper.
  (DNB PATTERN 2006)
- Absorption of iron is increased by: Vitamin C.
  (DNB PATTERN DEC 2010)
- Vitamin essential for metabolism of sulphur containing amino acids: Folic Acid. *(DNB PATTERN JUNE 2012)*
- Vitamin which prevents auto oxidation: Tocopherol.
  (DNB PATTERN 2000)
- Iron NOT present in: Ceruloplasmin.
  (DNB PATTERN JUNE 2008)
- Co factor involved in sulphur containing amino acid metabolism is: Vitamin B12. *(DNB PATTERN DEC 2011)*

- Rate limiting step in Vitamin D synthesis is 1,25 dihydroxy cholecalciferol. *(DNB PATTERN JUNE 2010)*
- Site at which 1,25 hydroxylation of Vitamin D takes place in the kidneys is Proximal convoluted tubules. *(DNB PATTERN 2003)*
- Betaquinones are involved with: Vitamin K. *(DNB PATTERN AUG 2013)*
- Mixed micelles contain which Vitamin?: Vitamin K. *(DNB PATTERN AUG 2013)*
- Most important enzyme which prevents autooxidation of PUFA in membrane: Tocopherol. *(DNB PATTERN JULY 2016)*
- Water soluble Vitamin synthesised in our body: Niacin *(DNB PATTERN JULY 2016)*
- Test to diagnose Thiamine Deficiency: RBC Transketolase. *(DNB PATTERN JULY 2016)*
- In Beri Beri higher than normal blood levels occur for: Pyruvate and Alpha Ketoglutarate. *(NEET PATTERN 2016)*

HEME/HEMOGLOBIN/MYOGLOBIN

- Quantity of Hemoglobin catabolised every day in normal adult: 8 gm. *(DNB PATTERN 2006)*
- Embryonic Hemoglobin is Alpha 2, epsilon 2. *(DNB PATTERN 2005)*
- Hemoglobin is present in Hydrophobic pocket. *(DNB PATTERN 2004)*
- Normal pH of blood is 7.4. *(DNB PATTERN 2004)*
- Hemoglobin synthesis starts with: Glycine. *(DNB PATTERN JUNE 2011)*
- The major role of 2,3 BPG in RBC is: Release of oxygen. *(DNB PATTERN DEC 2010)*
- Which is a functional enzyme? Prothrombin. *(DNB PATTERN JUNE 2011)*
- In which condition, hemolysis occurs on oxidation? G6PD deficiency. *(DNB PATTERN JUNE 2010)*
- Iron in Hemoglobin binds with: Histidine. *(DNB PATTERN NOV 2013)*
- T structure of Hemoglobin is stabilized by: 2,3 DPG. *(DNB PATTERN NOV 2013)*
- Hemoglobin M is formed by which amino acid substitution? Histidine *(DNB PATTERN NOV 2013)*

CHOLESTEROL SYNTHESIS

- Chylomicrons core is formed by: triglyceride and cholesterol. *(DNB PATTERN DEC 2011)*

- Inheritance of Familial Hypercholesterolemia is: Autosomal dominant. *(DNB PATTERN DEC 2011)*
- Squalene is the intermediate product during the synthesis of Cholesterol. *(DNB PATTERN 2006)*
- Principal apoprotein in Chylomicrons is Apo B 48. *(DNB PATTERN 2003)*
- Plasminogen domain resembles: Apolipoprotein A. *(DNB PATTERN DEC 2010)*
- Rate limiting enzyme in cholesterol synthesis is: HMG CoA reductase NOT synthetase. *(FMGE PATTERN MARCH 2010/2011/MARCH 2013)*
- Cholesterol is a form of: Steroid. *(FMGE PATTERN 2005)*
- Apo protein of cholesterol is: Apo E. *(FMGE PATTERN 2005)*
- Carrier of cholesterol is: LDL *(FMGE PATTERN MARCH 2013)*
- L CAT Activator Lipoprotein is: Apo A1. *(FMGE PATTERN 2005)*
- Wolman disease results from accumulation of: Cholesterol esters. *(DNB PATTERN AUG 2013)*
- Apoprotein associated with LCAT activation: Apo A1. *(DNB PATTERN AUG 2013)*
- Apo E is associated with: Arginine. *(DNB PATTERN NOV 2013)*
- Maximum electrophoretic mobility and least LIPID content: HDL. *(DNB PATTERN JULY 2016)*

CARBOHYDRATES

- Glycogen phosphorylase coenzyme is associated with: Pyridoxal Phosphate. *(DNB PATTERN DEC 2011)*
- PFK is allosterically activated by: fructose 2,6 biphosphate. *(DNB PATTERN DEC 2011)*.
- Insulin stimulated glucose uptake is by: GLUT4. *(DNB PATTERN JUNE 2011)*
- Normal renal threshold for glucose excretion is: 180 gm% *(DNB PATTERN 2004)*
- Dietary fibre is Non-starch Polysaccharide. *(DNB PATTERN 2002)*
- Most sensitive method for glucose estimation is Glucose Oxidase Method. *(DNB PATTERN 2003)*
- Substrate level phosphorylation in TCA cycle is in step Succinate thiokinase. *(DNB PATTERN JUNE 2009)*
- Lactose produced by glycolysis is used by: Cori cycle and TCA cycle. *(DNB PATTERN JUNE 2012)*

- Number of ATP produced per turn of TCA cycle: 10.
  (DNB PATTERN JUNE 2014)
- Major carbohydrate in the body: Hepatic Glycogen.
  (NEET PATTERN 2015)
- Insulin Dependent glucose transport is through: GLUT 4.
  (NEET PATTERN 2015)
- Anderson Disease is due to lack of: Branching enzyme.
  (FMGE PATTERN MARCH 2007)
- Alternative oxidative pathway for Glucose: Glucuronic Acid Pathway. *(FMGE PATTERN SEP 2012)*
- Muscle glycogen stores cannot be used to provide glucose into the circulation because of lack of: Glucose 6 Phosphatase.
  (FMGE PATTERN SEP 2012)
- Physiological uncoupler of oxidation and phosphorylation: Thermogenin. *(DNB PATTERN NOV 2013)*
- Preferred specimen for Glucose estimation: Fluoride Oxalated Plasma. *(NEET PATTERN 2016)*

FATS

- Hormone sensitive lipase is inhibited by Insulin.
  (DNB PATTERN JUNE 2012)
- Arachidonic Acid is synthesised from: Linoleic Acid.
  (DNB PATTERN JUNE 2012)
- Fatty liver is due to accumulation of Triglycerides.
  (DNB PATTERN JUNE 2009)
- Which of the following is a primary ketone body? Acetoacetate. *(DNB PATTERN JUNE 2009)*
- Not an omega 3 fatty acid–Linoleic acid.
  (DNB PATTERN JUNE 2008)
- Niemann Pick Disease is due to deficiency of which enzyme? Sphingomyelinase. *(DNB PATTERN DEC 2009)*
- Alpha oxidation of fatty acids takes place in: Peroxisomes
  (DNB PATTERN DEC 2011)
- Bile acids consist of all except: Taurocholic acid.
  (DNB PATTERN JUNE 2011)
- Zellweger syndrome is due to: Defect in Fatty Acid Oxidation in Peroxisomes. *(DNB PATTERN JULY 2016)*
- Beta oxidation of long chain fatty acids occur in: Peroxisomes.
  (DNB PATTERN NOV 2015)
- Most abundant end product of Fatty Acid Synthesis: Palmitic Acid. *(NEET PATTERN 2018)*

PROTEINS

- Amino acid which does NOT take part in one carbon transfer reactions: Glycine. *(DNB PATTERN 2005)*
- FIGLU is an intermediate product of Histidine. *(DNB PATTERN 2002)*
- Urea cycle is linked to Kreb's cycle by Fumarate. *(DNB PATTERN JUNE 2009)*
- Brain utilises urea in the form of Glutamine. *(DNB PATTERN 2001)*
- NOT an essential amino acid: Alanine. *(DNB PATTERN DEC 2010)*
- Boiled cabbage or rancid butter smelling urine is seen in: Tyrosinemia. *(DNB PATTERN JUNE 2011)*
- Source of norepinephrine is: Tyrosine. *(DNB PATTERN DEC 2009)*
- End product of purine metabolism is: Uric Acid. *(DNB PATTERN JUNE 2012)*
- Amino acid used in Carnitine synthesis is: Lysine. *(DNB PATTERN DEC 2011)*
- Which hormone is synthesised from Tyrosine: Thyroxine. *(DNB PATTERN DEC 2011)*
- Which among the following is not an example of Steroid hormone? Thyroxine. *(DNB PATTERN DEC 2010)*
- Hormone substrate concentration affects the velocity of enzymatic action. This is Michaelis Menten Reaction. *(DNB PATTERN 2000)*
- Shortest peptide among Angiotensin I,II,III and vasopressin is Angiotensin III. *(DNB PATTERN 2001)*
- Fenton reaction leads to free radical generation when ferrous ions are converted into ferric ions. *(DNB PATTERN 2007)*
- Amino acid involved in urea synthesis: Aspartic Acid. *(FMGE PATTERN SEP 2011)*
- Ubiquitin Proteosome pathway is involved in Proteolysis. *(DNB PATTERN AUG 2013)*
- Chaperonins are involved in: Protein Folding. *(DNB PATTERN AUG 2013)*
- Proper folding of newly synthesised proteins in Endoplasmic Reticulum is carried out due to: Chaperone. *(NEET PATTERN 2016)*
- Middle level protein based on molecular weight: Albumin/Transferrin. *(DNB PATTERN AUG 2013)*
- Protein-protein interaction is best studied by: Mass Spectrometry. *(NEET PATTERN 2013)*

- True about Glutathione: Glutamate is linked to cysteine through gamma carboxyl bond. *(DNB PATTERN JUNE 2014)*
- Serine is produced in human body from: Glycine. *(DNB PATTERN JULY 2016)*
- Urea cycle is linked to TCA cycle by: Fumarate. *(DNB PATTERN JULY 2016)*
- Tyrosinemia Type 1 is due to deficiency of Fumaryl Acetoacetate Hydroxylase. *(DNB PATTERN JULY 2016)*
- Enzyme defect in Krabbe's Disease: Beta Galactosidase. *(DNB PATTERN JULY 2016)*
- Histidine is the most important amino acid for buffering in normal conditions because: pKa value is closer to pH *(DNB PATTERN NOV 2015)*
- OTC Deficiency causes: Hyperammonemia Type 2 *(DNB PATTERN NOV 2015)*
- HHH syndrome is due to defect in: Ornithine Transporter. *(DNB PATTERN JULY 2016)*
- Rancid butter smell of Urine is seen in: Tyrosinemia. *(NEET PATTERN 2015)*
- Lysyl Oxidase requires which cofactor ? Copper. *(NEET PATTERN 2015)*
- NO is synthesised by: Arginine. *(NEET PATTERN 2015)*
- GlcNAc-P-P oligosaccharide is: Glycoprotein. *(NEET PATTERN 2015)*
- Enzyme deficient in Hers Disease: Liver Phosphorylase *(NEET PATTERN 2015)*
- Hartnup Disease is due to defective transport of: Tryptophan. *(NEET PATTERN 2015)*
- Hunter Syndrome is due to deficiency of: Iduronate Sulfatase. *(DNB PATTERN NOV 2015)*
- Earliest symptom of Tay Sach's disease; Exaggerated startle response. *(DNB PATTERN NOV 2015)*
- Buffering capacity of Proteins and Hemoglobin is due to: Histidine. *(NEET PATTERN 2016)*
- TYROSINOSIS is due to the deficiency of : Fumaryl Acetoacetate Hydrolase. *(NEET PATTERN 2018)*
- NOT excreted in Cystinuria: Still searching !!. *(NEET PATTERN 2018)*
- Lysine, Ornithine, Arginine and Cystine are excreted in large quantities in Cystinuria.

MISCELLANEOUS

- NADPH oxidase deficiency causes: Chronic Granulomatous Disease. *(DNB PATTERN DEC 2010)*

- In monoclonal antibody production, monoclonal cells are differentiated from: Myeloma cell lines.
  (DNB PATTERN DEC 2010)
- Accumulation of Homogentisic acid causes Ochronosis.
  (DNB PATTERN JUNE 2010)
- Ethanol is used in the treatment of ethylene glycol poisoning because it is: Competitive inhibitor of alcohol dehydrogenase.
  (DNB PATTERN DEC 2009)
- Most common deficiency responsible for Galactosemia: Galactose 1 phosphate uridyl transferase.
  (DNB PATTERN DEC 2009)
- Hyperammonemia blocks which phase of the cell cycle? Alpha ketoglutarate dehydrogenase. *(DNB PATTERN JUNE 2009)*
- Enzyme deficiency seen in Tay Sach's disease: Hexosaminidase A. *(DNB PATTERN JUNE 2014)*
- Which does NOT cause Cataract? Phenylketonuria.
  (DNB PATTERN JUNE 2014)
- NOT seen in Von Gierke's disease: Hyperglycemia.
  (DNB PATTERN JUNE 2014)
- Hyperammonemia Type 1 is due to deficiency of CPS 1.
  (DNB PATTERN NOV 2015)
- Which of the following requires NAD as co factor? Alpha ketoglutarate dehydrogenase. *(DNB PATTERN JUNE 2009)*
- Only tissue where NAD and NADP are equally distributed– Liver. *(DNB PATTERN 2000)*
- Precursor of Adrenaline and Noradrenaline: Tyrosine.
  (FMGE PATTERN MARCH 2011)
- Norepinephrine to epinephrine conversion requires which enzyme? – Phenylethanolamine N methyl transferase.
  (FMGE PATTERN MARCH 2011)
- Cytochrome B5 is located on: CYTOPLASMIC side of smooth Endoplasmic Reticulum.
  (DNB PATTERN AUG 2013)
- Selenocysteine is part of: Thioredoxene reductase.
  (DNB PATTERN NOV 2013)
- Enzyme deficiency in Tay Sach's Disease: Hexominidase A.
  (DNB PATTERN NOV 2013)
- Hallervorden Spatz Disease is otherwise called: Pantothenate Kinase associated Neurogeneration.
  (DNB PATTERN NOV 2013)

MRI Finding in Hallervorden Spatz Disease: Eye of the tiger sign

- Protein having an axial ratio more than 200 is: Collagen.
  (DNB PATTERN NOV 2013)
- Enzyme deficiency in McArdle's disease: Muscle Phosphorylase Deficiency. *(DNB PATTERN NOV 2013)*

- Natural steroid with glucocorticoid property: Cortisol. *(DNB PATTERN AUG 2013)*
- Natural anticoagulant which is a glycosaminoglycan: Heparin. *(DNB PATTERN AUG 2013)*
- Barth Syndrome is due to defect in: Cardiolipin. *(DNB PATTERN NOV 2015)*
- Edman's Reagent is: Phenyl Isocyanate. *(DNB PATTERN NOV 2015)*
- Both lipid and protein content are equal in membrane of which organelle? Mitochondria. *(DNB PATTERN JULY 2016)*
- MELAS is due to: Defect in Complex 1 of Electron Transport Chain. *(DNB PATTERN JULY 2016)*
- Sweaty Feet Odour of Urine is for: Glutaric Acidemia. *(NEET PATTERN 2016)*
- Sweaty Feet Odour of Urine is also seen in: Isovaleric Acidemia.
- Serotonin is also known as: 5 Hydroxy Tryptamine. *(NEET PATTERN 2018)*
- Fish Odour Syndrome is caused due to the deficiency of: Monoxygenase 3. *(NEET PATTERN 2018)*
- Fish Odour Syndrome is also known as Trimethylaminuria.
- Fishy odour of body occurs due to deficiency of this vitamin: Riboflavin. *(NEET PATTERN 2018)*
- Riboflavin Deficiency causes Trimethylaminuria which causes Fishy Odour.
- Galactosemia is due to the deficiency of: Galactose 1 Phosphate Uridyltransferase. *(NEET PATTERN 2018)*
- Vanilyl Mandelic Acid is excreted in urine in: Phaeochromocytoma. *(NEET PATTERN 2018)*
- HIAA is secreted in Urine in: Carcinoid. *(NEET PATTERN 2018)*
- Fibrinopeptide A and Fibrinopeptide B are acidic due to the presence of these aminoacids in their structure: Glutamate and Aspartate. *(NEET PATTERN 2018)*

LEVEL II: HIGH YIELD FACTORS

Table 3.1: Amino acids—high yield

Imidazole group	Histidine
Protonation and deprotonation at neutral pH	Histidine
Most basic AA	Arginine
Precursor of Heme	Glycine
Optically inactive	Glycine
Only ketogenic AA	L leucine
Semi essential AA	Arginine, Histidine

Biochemistry

Table 3.1: Amino acids—high yield

Imino acid	Proline/Hydroxyproline/**Selenocysteine**

Table 3.2: Minerals

Cytochrome oxidase contains	Copper
Carbonic Anhydrase contains	Zinc
Xanthine oxidase contains	Molybdenum
Keshan's disease, KashinBeck disease-deficiency	Selenium
Glutathione peroxidase contains	Selenium
Acrodermatitis Enteropathica deficiency of	Zinc
Glucose tolerance factor	Chromium
Manganese toxicity	Parkinsonism
Aluminium toxicity	Alzheimer's disease
Ouch Ouch disease	Cadmium
Black foot disease	Thallium
Fanconi like syndrome	Copper excess

Table 3.3: Vitamins

Increased RBC transketolase activity in deficiency of	Thiamine
Konig reaction is used to assess deficiency of	Niacin
Constituent of Coenzyme A	Pantothenic acid
Burning Feet syndrome	Pantothenic acid deficiency
Leiner's disease	Biotin deficiency
Antagonist of Biotin	Avidin
RBC maturation factor	Vitamin B12
Most heat labile vitamin	Vitamin C
Chromane ring	Vitamin E
Necrotizing enterocolitis in newborn	Vitamin E excess
Halibut liver oil is richest source of	Vitamin D
Vitamin synthesised in skin	Vitamin D
Hartnup disease is associated with	Niacin deficiency

Table 3.4: Hemoglobin

Heme in haemoglobin is present in	Hydrophobic pockets
Hemoglobin resistant to Alkali denaturation	Hb F
1 gm of hemoglobin binds	1. 34 ml of O_2
1 gm of heme contains	3. 34 mg of Iron
Rectangular hyperbola dissociation curve	Myoglobin

Table 3.4: Hemoglobin

Sigmoid dissociation curve	Hemoglobin
Normal hemoglobin level in newborn	16-18 gm%
Level of HbA2 is increased in	Beta thalassemia trait

Table 3.5: Protein structure and separation techniques

Primary structure of proteins is formed by	Peptide bond
Secondary and tertiary structure of Proteins is determined by	X-ray crystallography
Separation of proteins at isoelectric pH	Iso electric Focussing
Separation of proteins on the basis of electric charge	Ion exchange Chromatography
Amino acid sequence of proteins are identified by	Edman reaction
Alpha helix and Beta pleats are examples of	Secondary structure
Peptide bonds do NOT take part in	Quaternary structure

Table 3.6: Insulin and glucagon

Insulin does NOT cause	Gluconeogenesis
Glucose utilisation without insulin takes place in	RBC, WBC, Brain, Kidney Tubules, Intestine, Liver
Insulin is	Anabolic hormone
Epinephrine has glucagon like action	On muscles during exercise
Glucagon is released	Between meals, during starvation, during fasting

Table 3.7: Rate limiting enzymes

Cholesterol synthesis	HMG CoA reductase
Ketone body synthesis	HMG CoA synthetase
Krebs cycle	Isocitrate dehydrogenase
Catecholamine synthesis	Tyrosine hydroxylase
Glycolysis	Phosphofructokinase
Gluconeogenesis	Pyruvate carboxylase
Bile acid synthesis	7 alpha hydroxylase
Fatty acid synthesis	Acetyl CoA carboxylase

Table 3.8: Plasma lipoproteins

Lipoprotein absent in serum	Chylomicron
Lipoprotein with max size	Chylomicron
Apoprotein present in chylomicron	Apo B 48
Major transporter of cholesterol in blood	LDL

Table 3.8: Plasma lipoproteins

Lipoprotein with minimum size	LDL
Lipoprotein with scavenging action	HDL
Apolipoprotein in LDL and VLDL	Apo B100
Lipoprotein which transports cholesterol from peripheral tissues to liver	HDL

GENETICS

Features of the Genetic Code: UNAMBIGUOUS	Each codon specifies only 1 amino acid.
DEGENERATE/REDUNDANT	More than 1 codon may code for the same Amino Acid.
NONOVERLAPPING	Read from a fixed point as a continuous sequence.
UNIVERSAL	Conserved throughout Evolution
Fluorescence In Situ Hybridisation (FISH)	Used for specific localisation of genes and direct detection of anomalies.at molecular level.
GENETIC PHENOMENON IN:	
Angelman and Prader Willi Syndrome	IMPRINTING
Retinoblastoma	LOSS OF HETEROZYGOSITY
KNUDSON'S DOUBLE HIT HYPOTHESIS.	
Huntington's Disease	ANTICIPATION
Phenylketonuria	PLEIOTROPY
Marfan's Syndrome /MEN2B/ HOMOCYSTINURIA(All three have Marfanoid Habitus)	LOCUS HETEROGENEITY
Most abundant RNA	rRNA
Longest RNA	mRNA
Smallest RNA	tRNA

4. Pathology

"I think it is possible for ordinary people to choose to be extraordinary"
—*Elon Musk*
CEO, Tesla/SpaceX

REFERENCES
- *Robbins Basic Pathology, 9th ed.*
- *Harrison's Internal Medicine, 19th ed.*

LEVEL I: BASIC REPEATS

CELLULAR ADAPTATION AND CELL INJURY

- Decrease in cell size refers to Atrophy.
  (NEET PATTERN 2013;2014, FMGE PATTERN 2009)
- Hypertrophy is increase in cell size.
  (NEET PATTERN 2013;2014, DNB PATTERN AUG 2015)
- Replacement of columnar epithelium of respiratory tract to squamous epithelium is Metaplasia.
  (NEET PATTERN 2014;2015, 2016, FMGE PATTERN 2013)
- In cell death myelin figures are derived from cell membrane
  (NEET PATTERN 2013;2014;2015)
- The sign of reversible injury in a case of alcoholic liver disease- cytoplasmic vacuole. *(NEET PATTERN 2013;2014;2016)*
- Organelle where H_2O_2 is produced and destroyed is peroxisome. *(DNB PATTERN NOV 2013, NOV 2015)*
- Anaplasia is: Lack of Differentiation.
  (NEET 2018 PATTERN)

APOPTOSIS

- Programmed cell death is called Apoptosis.
  (DNB PATTERN JUNE 2008, NEET PATTERN 2013;2014)
- Example of apoptosis is Councilman Bodies.
  (DNB PATTERN DEC 2009, JUNE 2009, NEET PATTERN 2013;2014)
- Apoptosis is cell self-initiated.*(DNB PATTERN JUNE 2009)*
- Characteristic feature of apoptosis-cell membrane intact.
  (NEET PATTERN 2013;2014;2016)
- Organelle which plays a pivotal role in Apoptosis: Golgi complex. *(DNB PATTERN 2008)*

Pathology

- False about Apoptosis–Inflammation is present.
  (DNB PATTERN JUNE 2010)
- Annexin V is associated with Apoptosis.
  (DNB PATTERN Dec 2011, 2015, FMGE PATTERN 2014).
- Which has a direct role in apoptosis–Cytosolic Cytochrome C.
  (DNB PATTERN DEC 2011, NEET PATTERN 2014;2015;2016)
- In apoptosis cytochrome c acts through–Apaf-1.
  (NEET PATTERN 2013;2014;2015)
- True about Caspases–they are involved in apoptosis.
  (DNB PATTERN JUNE 2011, FMGE PATTERN 2014)
- CD 95 is a marker of death receptor.
  (NEET PATTERN 2014;2015)
- CD 95 has a major role in Apoptosis.
  (DNB PATTERN JUNE 2014)
- Apoptotic bodies are–cell membrane bound with organelles.
  (NEET PATTERN 2013;2014;2016)
- All are true regarding apoptosis except–smear pattern in
  > P for P & M for N: steP ladder pattern in aPoptosis & sMear pattern in Necrosis]
- Pro-apoptotic factor is Bax. *(NEET PATTERN 2014, 2016)*
- Antiapoptotic gene is BCL 2.
  (NEET PATTERN 2013;2014;2015;2016, DNB PATTERN DEC 2012;2015;2016)
- Antiapoptotic gene is FLIP. *(NEET PATTERN 2015;2016)*
- Caspases are involved in Apoptosis.
  (NEET PATTERN 2014, 2016)
- [Apoptosis & caspases-in initiation phase-caspase 10, 9, 8; in Execution phase-caspase **3**-"**E** for **3**"]
- Defective apoptosis and increased cell survival is seen in- Autoimmune disease. *(NEET PATTERN 2014)*

NECROSIS

- Liquefactive necrosis is seen in BRAIN.
  (DNB PATTERN 2002;2006;2008, FMGE PATTERN 2014)
- Liquefactive necrosis on necrotic tissue results in GANGRENE. *(NEET PATTERN 2013;2014)*
- Type of necrosis occurring in Brain-Liquefactive.
  (NEET PATTERN 2013;2014)
- Coagulative necrosis is NOT seen in CNS.
  (DNB PATTERN 2000)
- Eosinophilia in necrosed tissue is due to–coagulation of proteins.
  (NEET PATTERN 2013;2014;2016)

- Coagulative necrosis is due to denaturation of protein.
  (NEET PATTERN 2013;2014, DNB PATTERN DEC 2015)
- Caseous necrosis is not seen in CMV.
  (DNB PATTERN AUG 2013)
- FIBRINOD necrosis is seen in all except-diabetes mellitus.
  (DNB PATTERN NOV 2014, DEC 2015, NEET PATTERN 2015;2016)
- Fat necrosis is common in omentum, breast and retroperitoneal fat. *(NEET PATTERN 2013;2014)*
- Fat necrosis occurs in omentum.
  (NEET PATTERN 2015;2016)
- Type of necrosis in pancreatitis-FAT necrosis.
  (NEET PATTERN 2013;2014)

CELLULAR PATHOLOGY AND CALCIFICATION

- Brown atrophy is due to accumulation of Lipofuscin.
  (DNB PATTERN DEC 2009, FMGE PATTERN 2015, NEET PATTERN 2014;2015)
- Steatosis means fatty change. *(NEET PATTERN 2013;2014)*
- Oncocytes are found in all except pineal gland.
  (DNB PATTERN NOV 2014)
- Dysrophic calcification is seen in Atheromatous plaque.
  (NEET PATTERN 2014;2015)
- Dysrophic calcification is seen in all except LUNGS.
  (NEET PATTERN 2013;2014)
- Psammomma bodies show which type of calcification-dysrophic. *(DNB PATTERN JUN 2008, NOV 2015)*
- True about psammoma bodies are all except–seen in teratoma.
  (NEET PATTERN 2013;2014;2016)
- Metastatic calcification is most often seen in LUNGS.
  (DNB PATTERN DEC 2007:2014)

> [Tissue is Dead in Dystrophic calcification and calcium is More in Metastatic calcification.]

- Warthin Finkledy Cells are seen in: Measles.
  (NEET 2018 PATTERN)

INFLAMMATION

- Rubor in inflammation is due to-dilation of arterioles.
  (DNB PATTERN 2008)
- All are celsus signs of inflammation except-cyanosis.
  (NEET PATTERN 2014;2015)

ACUTE INFLAMMATION

- Most characteristic feature of acute inflammation-vasodilation and increased vascular permeability.
(DNB PATTERN NOV 2014)
- Increased permeability in acute inflammation is due to– histamine. *(NEET PATTERN 2013;2014;2016)*
- Increased permeability in acute inflammation is due to all except-lytic enzymes.
(NEET PATTERN 2013, DNB PATTERN NOV 2015)
- Sequence of events in acute inflammation: Transient vasoconstriction->vasodilation->increased permeability->stasis.
(NEET PATTERN 2014:2016)
- All of the following are family of selectins except-A-selectin.
(NEET PATTERN 2013;DNB PATTERN JUNE 2015)
- Cell matrix adhesions are mediated by-integrins.
(NEET PATTERN 2014:2015;2016)
- Most important adhesion molecule for diapedesis-PECAM.
(NEET PATTERN 2014;2015;2016; DNB PATTERN NOV 2015)
- Rolling of leucocytes on endothelial cell is mediated by: P-selectin. *(NEET PATTERN 2015;2016)*
- Which among the following is not an adhesion molecule? Transferrin. *(DNB PATTERN DEC 2010)*

CHRONIC INFLAMMATION

- Macrophages are converted to epithelioid cells by–IFN gamma.
(NEET PATTERN 2013;2014;2016, FMGE PATTERN 2015)
- Principal cell in granuloma is–histiocytes.
(DNB PATTERN JUNE 2014)
- Vasoconstricting mediator is thromboxane A2.
(NEET PATTERN 2013;2014)
- Necrotizing epithelioid granuloma is seen in all except-leprosy.
(NEET PATTERN 2014;2015, FMGE PATTERN 2010:2015)
- Stellate granuloma is seen in–cat-scratch disease.
(NEET 2014, 2018 PATTERN)
- The most important source of histamine-Mast cell.
(NEET PATTERN 2013;2014)
- Lipoxins synthesized from Arachidonic acid act by: decrease leucocyte migration, adhesion, chemotaxis.
(NEET PATTERN 2013;2014;2016)

- All are chemokines except-histamine.
  (NEET PATTERN 2013;2014, DNB PATTERN JUNE 2016)

COMPLEMENT SYSTEM

- Complement responsible for activation of bacterial lysis is: c5-9. *(NEET PATTERN 2014;2015;2016)*
- C3 convertase acts on: c3. *(DNB PATTERN NOV 2014)*

INFLAMMATORY MEDIATORS

- Increased vascular permeability is caused by all except-renin.
  (NEET PATTERN 2013:2014:2015;2016)
- Which is not caused by platelet activation factor: vasoconstriction. *(NEET PATTERN 2013;2014)*

PHAGOCYTOSIS

- Phagocytosis is the function of: microglia.
  (NEET PATTERN 2013;2014;2016)
- Chediak Higashi syndrome defect is: fusion of lysosome.
  (NEET PATTERN 2013;2014)
- Oxygen dependent killing is done through: NADPH oxidase.
  (NEET PATTERN 2014;2015;2016)
- The process increasing the ability for phagocytosis of foreign body is called: opsonization. *(DNB PATTERN NOV 2014)*

EXTRACELLULAR MATRIX AND TYPES OF CELL

- Triple helix is found in: collagen.
  (NEET PATTERN 2013:2014:2016)
- Oval cells seen in stem cells of: liver.
  (NEET PATTERN 2013;2014;2016)
- Stem cells are taken from all except-liver.
  (NEET PATTERN 2013;2014)
- [Sources of adult stem cells in humans-BABU (Blood, Adipose tissue, Bone marrow, Umbilical cord blood)]
- Which of the following is a labile cell? Surface epithelium.
  (DNB PATTERN AUG 2013)
- During angiogenesis recruitment of pericytes and periendothelial cells is due to: angiopoetins, PDGF and TGF.
  (NEET PATTERN 2013;2014)
- In wound injury sequence of appearance of cells is: platelet->neutrophil->macrophages->fibroblast hint-reverse alphabet order-p, n, m, f. *(NEET PATTERN 2013:2014;2016)*
- Complete wound strength is gained by–it is never regained.
  (DNB PATTERN DEC 2011)

Pathology

- Maximum collagen in wound healing is seen at: end of 2nd week. *(NEET PATTERN 2013;2014;2015)*
- Fibrosis is due to TGF-beta. *(NEET PATTERN 2013;2014;2015)*
- Formation of granulation tissue is due to–budding of new capillaries. *(NEET PATTERN 2014;2015)*
- Which of the following is a chemokine? IL–8. *(DNB PATTERN DEC 2011)*
- Interleukin responsible for pyrexia: IL–1. Cytokine causing fever-IL1. *(DNB PATTERN JUNE 2011, NOV 2015, NEET PATTERN 2013;2014;2016)*
- Procalcitonin is considered as marker for SEPSIS. *(DNB PATTERN DEC 2010)*
- The primary function of Toll-like receptors is activation of immune system. *(DNB PATTERN DEC 2010)*
- All of the following are angiogenic factors except Interferon. *(DNB PATTERN DEC 2010)*
- First sign of wound injury is capillary dilatation. *(DNB PATTERN 2000)*
- Resolution of inflammation is caused by TNF Alpha, IL-10, IL-1 receptor antagonist. *(DNB PATTERN DEC 2010)*
- All of the following are angiogenic factors except Interferon. *(DNB PATTERN DEC 2010)*
- Granulomatous inflammation is type 4 hypersensitivity. Three variants of Type IV. *(DNB PATTERN DEC 2009)*
- Hypersensitivity–contact/tuberculin (within 72 hrs)/granulomatous (B/W 21-28th day). *(DNB PATTERN DEC 2009)*
- Delayed type of hypersensitivity is associated with–Memory CD4 cells. *(DNB PATTERN JUNE 2008)*
- Mediator that is NOT formed in Mast cells: Leukotriene C4. *(DNB PATTERN AUG 2013)*
- Labile Cells are: cells which multiply constantly through out life. *(DNB PATTERN AUG 2013)*
- L Selectin on neutrophils binds to what on endothelium? Gly Cam 1. *(NEET PATTERN 2013)*
- Cyclin D is related to: G1S phase. *(NEET PATTERN 2013)*
- Cyclin B is essential for G2M transition. *(ROBBINS 9/e p181)*

CHEMICAL MEDIATORS

- Which of the following is a chemokine? IL-8. *(DNB PATTERN DEC 2011)*

- Interleukin responsible for pyrexia: IL-1.
  (DNB PATTERN JUNE 2011)
- Which of the following is a chemotactic factor? Leukotrienes.
  (DNB PATTERN DEC 2011)
- Not a mediator in Allergic rhinitis–PG E2.
- Cytokines are released by: T cells.
  (FMGE PATTERN SEP 2012)

STAINS AND FIXATIVES

- Amyloid is stained by Congo red.
  (DNB PATTERN JUNE 2012)
- Staining characteristics used for demonstration of Amyloid: Apple Green Birefringence under polarised light.
  (DNB PATTERN 2009)
- Amyloid gives Brilliant Pink colour with Congo Red Dye.
  (DNB PATTERN 2003)
- Stain for fat cells: Sudan IV. *(DNB PATTERN DEC 2009)*
- Stain for Heart failure cells: Prussian blue.
  (DNB PATTERN DEC 2009)
- PAS stain shows black positivity in Lymphoblasts.
  (DNB PATTERN 2008)
- Color of Hemosiderin: Brown. *(DNB PATTERN DEC 2009)*
- Fixative used for bone histopathology is 10% formalin.
  (DNB PATTERN DEC 2011)
- Substance commonly used for organ/tissue preservation for histopathological examination is Formalin.
  (DNB PATTERN JUNE 2009)
- Stain used for Carcinoma Oral cavity: Toluidine Blue.
  (DNB PATTERN AUG 2013)
- Myelin sheath is stained by: Luxol Fast Blue.
  (NEET PATTERN 2013)
- Barrett's epithelium stains: Alcian Blue positive.
  (NEET PATTERN 2013)

AMYLOIDOSIS

- Most common feature of death in primary amyloidosis is Cardiac failure. *(DNB PATTERN JUNE 2011)*
- Confirmatory test for the diagnosis of Amyloidosis is Rectal Biopsy. *(DNB PATTERN DEC 2010)*
- Secondary Amyloidosis is a complication of Chronic Osteomyelitis. *(DNB PATTERN 2002)*
- Least common cause of calcification in the lung is Amyloidosis.
  (DNB PATTERN 2007)

- Lardaceous spleen is due to deposition of amyloid in sinusoids of red pulp. *(DNB PATTERN 2007)*
- Birefringence is seen in: Polarized Microscope. *(DNB PATTERN AUG 2013)*

NAMED BODIES AND STRUCTURES IN PATHOLOGY

- Zellballen pattern on histopathology is observed in Carotid body tumor. *(DNB PATTERN DEC 2010)*
- **Auer Rods** are formed from Primary granules. *(DNB PATTERN DEC 2010)*
- **Pappenheimer Bodies** are composed of Iron. *(DNB PATTERN JUNE 2010)*
- **Asteroid bodies** are seen in Sarcoidosis. *(NEET PATTERN 2016, DNB PATTERN JUNE 2010)*
- **Neurofibrillary Tangles** are seen in Alzheimer's disease. *(DNB PATTERN JUNE 2010)*
- **Cabot's ring** is seen in RBC is seen after splenectomy. *(DNB PATTERN DEC 2009)*
- **Michaelis-Gutmann** bodies are found in Malakoplakia. *(DNB PATTERN DEC 2009)*
- **Hutchinson's Secondaries** in skull are due to tumors in Adrenals. *(DNB PATTERN 2000, 2003)*
- **Hurthle cells** are seen in Hashimoto's thyroiditis. *(DNB PATTERN 2000)*
- **APUD cells** are seen in Bronchial carcinoid. *(DNB PATTERN 2000)*
- **Echinocytes** are types of RBCs. *(DNB PATTERN 2001)*
- **Kupffer cells** are found in Liver. *(DNB PATTERN 2003, 2006)*
- **Psammoma bodies** show Dystrophic calcification. *(DNB PATTERN 2003, 2006)*
- **Heart Failure cells** are found in Lungs. *(DNB PATTERN 2003)*
- **Linzenmeter** is used to measure ESR. *(DNB PATTERN 2003, 2006)*
- **Gamma Gandy bodies** contain Hemosiderin and Calcium. *(DNB PATTERN 2003, 2007)*
- **Mallory hyaline** NOT seen in Primary Biliary Cirrhosis. *(DNB PATTERN 2004)*
- **Mallory Hyaline** is a characteristic feature of Alcoholic liver disease. *(NEET PATTERN 2016, DNB PATTERN JUNE 2011)*
- **Perioral pallor and Dennie's lines** are seen in Atopic Dermatitis. *(DNB PATTERN 2008)*

- **Paneth cells** contain Zinc. *(DNB PATTERN 2008)*
- **Onion peel** appearance of splenic capsule is seen in SLE. *(DNB PATTERN 2007)*
- **Lardaceous spleen** is due to deposition of amyloid in sinusoids of red pulp. *(DNB PATTERN 2007)*
- **Oncocytes** are NOT found in Pineal body. *(DNB PATTERN 2000)*
- **Alder-Reilly bodies** are seen in: Mucopolysaccharidoses. *(NEET PATTERN 2016)*
- Dominantly inherited condition with large platelets and Dohle Bodies in Neutrophils is: MAY HEGGLIN ANOMALY. *(NEET PATTERN 2016)*
- **Zellballen pattern** is NOT seen in: Acoustic Neuroma. *(NEET PATTERN 2016)*

ONCOPATHOLOGY

- Biopsy of opposite breast is done in which histological subtype of breast cancer? Lobular. *(DNB PATTERN JUNE 2012)*
- Chromosomal translocation seen in CML is 9:22. *(DNB PATTERN DEC 2011)*
- High risk of malignancy is seen in Complex hyperplasia with atypia. *(DNB PATTERN JUNE 2011)*
- Small round cell tumors does NOT include Synovial carcinoma. *(DNB PATTERN DEC 2010)*
- CD 99 is a marker of Ewing sarcoma. *(DNB PATTERN DEC 2010)*
- Burkitt's lymphoma arises from B cell lymphoma. *(DNB PATTERN DEC 2010)*
- DIC is seen most commonly in AML which type? AML M3. *(DNB PATTERN DEC 2010)*
- Most common extranodal site of lymphoma in HIV is CNS. *(NEET PATTERN 2015;2016, DNB PATTERN DEC 2010)*
- Most commonly associated human papilloma virus with cancer cervix is HPV 16. *(DNB PATTERN DEC 2010;2015)*
- HPV associated with laryngeal papilloma are 6 and 11. *(DNB PATTERN DEC 2010)*
- Orphan Annie eye nuclei are seen in Papillary carcinoma thyroid. *(DNB PATTERN DEC 2010, NEET PATTERN 2015)*
- Zellballen pattern on histopathology is observed in Carotid body tumor. *(DNB PATTERN DEC 2010)*
- Rb gene is located on chr 13q14. *(DNB PATTERN JUNE 2009)*

Pathology

- Burkitt lymphoma shows 8:14 translocation.
  (DNB PATTERN JUNE 2009;2014;NEET PATTERN 2016)
- BCR ABL gene is seen in CML.
  (DNB PATTERN JUNE 2009)
- Chromosomal translocation seen in CML is 9:22.
  (DNB PATTERN JUNE 2009)
- Marker for Hairy cell Leukemia: CD 103.
  (DNB PATTERN JUNE 2009)
- Mycosis fungoides is T cell lymphoma.
  (DNB PATTERN JUNE 2009)
- S100 is a marker of melanoma, schwannoma and histiocytoma. *(DNB PATTERN JUNE 2009)*
- Tumor Markers of Malignant Melanoma: HMB 45 and S100. *(DNB PATTERN JUNE 2009)*
- HTLV is not a DNA oncogenic virus.
  (DNB PATTERN JUNE 2009)
- Chemotherapeutic agent which is procarcinogenic: alkylating agents, aromatic amines and azo dyes, nitrosamines and amides. *(DNB PATTERN JUNE 2009)*
- Spontaneous regression is seen in Neuroblastoma.
  (DNB PATTERN 2000)
- Bone tumor arising from epiphysis is Giant cell tumor.
  (DNB PATTERN 2001)
- Commonest Malignant bone tumor is: Multiple Myeloma.
  (DNB PATTERN 2001)
- Deletion of short arm of chromosome 11 in Wilms tumor.
  (DNB PATTERN 2001)
- Mycosis fungoides is Cutaneous lymphoma.
  (DNB PATTERN 2002)
- Low grade non-Hodgkin's lymphoma is Follicular NHL.
  (DNB PATTERN 2002)
- Commonest benign tumor of the liver is a Hemangioma.
  (DNB PATTERN 2003)
- Most common primary tumor of heart is Myxoma.
  (DNB PATTERN 2004)
- BRCA 1 gene on chromosome 17. *(DNB PATTERN 2008)*
- CD 10 is seen in Acute Lymphoblastic Leukemia.
  (DNB PATTERN 2007)
- Paraneoplastic syndrome not seen in renal cell cancer is SLE.
  (DNB PATTERN DEC 2011)
- All are markers of Mantle cell lymphoma except CD23.
  (DNB PATTERN DEC 2011)
- Gastric carcinoma is associated with all except over expression of C-erb. *(DNB PATTERN DEC 2011)*

- Essential for tumor metastasis is Angiogenesis. *(DNB PATTERN 2008)*
- Cells like Reed Sternberg are seen in–Infectious Mononucleosis. *(DNB PATTERN JUNE 2008)*
- HMB 45 is a tumor marker of Malignant Melanoma. *(DNB PATTERN JUNE 2008)*
- Ann Arbor classification is used for: Hodgkin's Lymphoma. *(DNB PATTERN NOV 2013)*
- Most common cause of pathological nipple discharge: Intraductal Papilloma. *(DNB PATTERN AUG 2013)*
- Scrotal skin cancer is associated with: Chimney Sweepers. *(DNB PATTERN AUG 2013)*
- Metastasis to liver is UNCOMMON in malignancy of: Prostate. *(FMGE PATTERN MAR 2013)*
- Ames Test in Neoplasia is for: Chemical Mutagenicity. *(NEET PATTERN 2013)*
- Erb B2 is related to: Breast Malignancy. *(NEET PATTERN 2013)*
- Paraneoplastic syndrome NOT seen in renal cell cancer is SLE. *(DNB PATTERN DEC 2011)*
- Gastric carcinoma is NOT associated with over expression of C-erb. *(DNB PATTERN DEC 2011)*
- H and L variety is seen in: Lymphocyte Predominant Hodgkins' Lymphoma. *(NEET 2018 PATTERN)*
- CYFRA 21-1 Test is positive in: Small Cell Lung Cancer. *(JIPMER 2017 PATTERN)*
- It detects Cytokeratin Fragment 19.
- Good prognosis in Neuroblastoma: TrK A expression. *(JIPMER 2017 PATTERN)*
- Van Nuys Prognostic Index (VNPI) is not based on: Estrogen Receptor Status. *(NEET PATTERN 2018)*
- Van Nuys Prognostic Index for Ductal Carcinoma In Situ (DCIS) takes into account size and grade of DCIS, margins and age of patient.

GENETICS

- Which of the following has X-linked recessive inheritance? G6PD. *(DNB PATTERN JUNE 2012)*
- Inheritance pattern of hemophilia is X-linked recessive. *(DNB PATTERN JUNE 2012)*
- DNA replication occurs in which phase of cell cycle? S phase. *(DNB PATTERN JUNE 2012)*
- No of Barr bodies in XXY males is 1. *(DNB PATTERN JUNE 2012)*

- Barr body first detected in—Buccal mucosa.
  (DNB PATTERN JUNE 2008)
- Mutation in Keratin 1 and 10 are associated with Epidermolytic hyperkeratosis.
  (DNB PATTERN JUNE 2011)
- Which of the following is NOT a tumor marker: HLA A2.
  (DNB PATTERN DEC 2010)
- Bloom syndrome is a DNA repair defect.
  (DNB PATTERN DEC 2010)
- In xeroderma pigmentosum, the defect is in Nucleoside excision repair. *(DNB PATTERN DEC 2010)*
- Which among the pair of oncogenes is activated by translocation? ABL and C-MYC. *(DNB PATTERN DEC 2010)*
- All of the following are characteristic of Turner syndrome except Umbilical hernia. *(DNB PATTERN DEC 2010)*
- Gaucher's disease is inherited as Autosomal recessive.
  (DNB PATTERN JUNE 2010)
- Which of the following is inherited as autosomal recessive form? Sickle cell anemia. *(DNB PATTERN JUNE 2010)*
- Rb gene is located on chr 13q14.
  (DNB PATTERN JUNE 2009)
- AFP is not elevated in Down's syndrome.
  (DNB PATTERN JUNE 2009)
- HTLV is not a DNA oncogenic virus.
  (DNB PATTERN JUNE 2009)
- HLA complex in man is located on Chromosome 6.
  (DNB PATTERN 2000)
- Mutation in Marfan syndrome is fibrillin.
  (DNB PATTERN JUNE 2011)
- An enzyme which recognizes a palindromic sequence and cuts within a DNA molecule is Restriction endonuclease.
  (DNB PATTERN JUNE 2012)
- Deletion in Thymic Hypoplasia: 22q11.2
  (JIPMER 2017 PATTERN)
- Chromosome responsible for the production of Mullerian Inhibiting Substance: Y Chromosome.
  (NEET 2018 PATTERN)
- Protein involved in Cowden's Syndrome: PTEN.
  (NEET 2018 PATTERN)
- Chromosome involved in Myotonic Dystrophy: Chromosome 19. *(NEET 2018 PATTERN)*
- Wiskott Aldrich Syndrome gene is located on the: Short arm of X chromosome. *(JIPMER 2017 PATTERN)*

SLE AND OTHER CONNECTIVE TISSUE DISORDERS

- Onion peel appearance of splenic capsule is seen in SLE. *(DNB PATTERN 2007)*
- Libman Sacks endocarditis is associated with SLE. *(DNB PATTERN JUNE 2010)*
- Best marker of SLE is Anti-DS DNA antibodies. *(DNB PATTERN JUNE 2010)*
- Paraneoplastic syndrome not seen in renal cell cancer is SLE. *(DNB PATTERN DEC 2011)*
- Anti-U1RNP antibody is seen in Mixed Connective tissue disorder. *(DNB PATTERN DEC 2009)*

RENAL SYSTEM

- Increased levels of C3NeF are associated with Type 2 MPGN. *(DNB PATTERN DEC 2010)*
- Periglomerular fibrosis is considered typical of chronic pyelonephritis. *(DNB PATTERN 2000, 2006)*
- Crescent forming glomerulonephritis is RPGN. *(DNB PATTERN 2002)*
- Diabetes is NOT a cause of Granular contracted kidneys. *(DNB PATTERN 2000)*
- One side kidney normal, other side contracted with scar, what is the probable diagnosis? Chronic pyelonephritis. *(DNB PATTERN JUNE 2010)*
- Paraneoplastic syndrome not seen in renal cell cancer is SLE. *(DNB PATTERN DEC 2011)*
- An emerging organism responsible for causing Pyelonephritis in Renal allografts is Polyoma virus. *(DNB PATTERN DEC 2010)*
- Takayasu disease most commonly affects renal artery. Subclavian > common carotis > Abdominal Aorta > renal > aortic arch > vertebral > celiac axis. *(DNB PATTERN DEC 2009)*
- Thrombosis is seen in which stage of lupus nephritis? Class iii. *(DNB PATTERN NOV 2013)*
- Michaelis Guttmann Bodies are seen in: Malakoplakia. *(DNB PATTERN AUG 2013)*
- Von Hippel-Lindau Syndrome is associated with: Renal Cell Carcinoma. *(DNB PATTERN AUG 2013)*
- Predisposing factor for Wilms' tumor: WAGR syndrome. *(DNB PATTERN AUG 2013)*
- False about Alports' syndrome: Autosomal Recessive. *(NEET PATTERN 2013)*
- Laxative abuse iproduces this kind of stones: Ammonium Urate Stones. *(NEET 2018 PATTERN)*

HEMATOLOGY

- If blood is left to stand for one day, which clotting factor is reduced? Factor VIII. *(DNB PATTERN JUNE 2012)*
- Adding glucose to stored blood causes prevention of hemolysis. *(DNB PATTERN DEC 2011)*
- Increased PT and normal PTT are found in Factor 7 deficiency. *(DNB PATTERN DEC 2011)*
- All are seen in Sickle cell Anemia except High hematocrit. *(DNB PATTERN JUNE 2011)*
- Autosplenectomy is seen in Sickle cell Anemia. *(DNB PATTERN JUNE 2010)*
- Autonephrectomy is seen in TB Kidney.
- Prothrombin time is NOT used to assess platelet function. *(DNB PATTERN JUNE 2010)*
- Cabot's ring in RBC is seen after splenectomy. *(DNB PATTERN DEC 2009)*
- Shape of RBC is biconcave due to spectrin. *(DNB PATTERN DEC 2009)*
- Leukoerythroblastic reaction is NOT seen in Hemolytic Anemia. *(DNB PATTERN 2000)*
- Sideroblastic Anemia is seen in chronic poisoning of Lead. *(DNB PATTERN 2001)*
- Echinocytes are types of RBCs. *(DNB PATTERN 2001)*
- Increased Erythropoeitin level is NOT a feature of Polycythemia vera. *(DNB PATTERN 2001)*
- Increase in Alkaline Phosphatase is seen in a Leukemoid Reaction. *(DNB PATTERN 2001)*
- To test hepatic function in evaluation of bleeding disorder, test done is aPTT. *(DNB PATTERN 2001)*
- In sickle cell anemia, defect can be seen in alpha chain or beta chain. *(DNB PATTERN 2001)*
- Tissue thromboplastin activates Factor 7. *(DNB PATTERN 2001)*
- Beta macroglobulin is derived from B cells. *(DNB PATTERN 2001)*
- ESR is NOT elevated in Polycythemia Rubra Vera. *(DNB PATTERN 2002, 2005)*
- Increased Haptoglobulin is NOT a feature of Hemolytic Anemia. *(DNB PATTERN 2002)*
- Decreased Fibrinogen products is NOT a feature of DIC. *(DNB PATTERN 2002)*
- Earliest feature of correction in Iron Deficiency Anemia is Reticulocyte count. *(DNB PATTERN 2002)*

- Blood stored at 4 degrees can be stored for 21 days.
  (DNB PATTERN 2003)
- Bone infarcts are seen in Sickle cell Anemia.
  (DNB PATTERN 2008)
- Common complement component for both pathways: C3.
  (DNB PATTERN 2008)
- Abnormal complement levels are NOT seen in TTP.
  (DNB PATTERN 2008)
- Sickling protects blood cells against Malaria.
  (DNB PATTERN 2008)
- Histamine causes all except Platelet aggregation.
  (DNB PATTERN JUNE 2010)
- Which among the following is not an adhesion molecule? Transferrin. *(DNB PATTERN DEC 2010)*
- Anemia in humans is caused by Hook Worm.
  (DNB PATTERN 2001, 2006)
- Patient having VWF deficiency. Abnormalities he is having– Normal PT/PTT. *(DNB PATTERN DEC 2009)*
- CO poisoning leads to Anemic hypoxia.
  (DNB PATTERN JUNE 2010)
- In hereditary spherocytosis, mutation not seen in Na^+K^+ channel protein. *(DNB PATTERN DEC 2010)*
- Most common cause of Hereditary Spherocytosis: Ankyrin.
  (DNB PATTERN DEC 2011)
- Most potent stimulator of Naïve T cells is: Mature Dendritic cells. *(DNB PATTERN 2008)*
- Which among the following is true about iron deficiency anemia? Marrow is normoblastic.
  (DNB PATTERN DEC 2010)
- Cryoprecipitate contains–Factor VIII and fibrinogen.
  (DNB PATTERN JUNE 2008)
- Thrombosthenin is–A contractile protein of platelets.
  (DNB PATTERN JUNE 2008)
- Donath Landsteiner Test is used in the diagnosis of: Paroxysmal Cold Hemoglobinuria. *(DNB PATTERN NOV 2013)*
- Lacunar variant of Reed Stenberg cells are seen with: Nodular Sclerosis. *(DNB PATTERN AUG 2013)*
- CD marker of Angiosarcoma: CD 31.
  (DNB PATTERN AUG 2013)
- BCL positivity is seen in Follicular Lymphoma.
  (NEET PATTERN 2013)
- Pseudo Pelger-Huet Syndrome is seen in: AML/CML/ Multiple Myeloma/Myelodysplastic Syndrome.
  (DNB PATTERN AUG 2013)

- Von Willebrand's Disease is associated with this tumor: Lung Cancer. *(JIPMER 2017 PATTERN)*
- Dactylitis occurs in: Sickle Cell Anaemia. *(NEET 2018 PATTERN)*
- Sialylated Lewis Antigen is: Ca19-9. *(JIPMER 2017 PATTERN)*
- Bernard Soullier Syndrome is due to the deficiency of: Glycoprotein IB. *(NEET 2018 PATTERN)*
- CD59 is a marker of: Paroxysmal Nocturnal Hemoglobinuria. *(NEET 2018 PATTERN)*
- Opsonin is: C3b. *(NEET 2018 PATTERN)*

HEPATOLOGY

- Kupffer cells are found in Liver. *(DNB PATTERN 2003, 2006)*
- Mallory hyaline NOT seen in Primary Biliary Cirrhosis. *(DNB PATTERN 2004)*
- Micronodular cirrhosis is NOT a feature of Wilson's disease. *(DNB PATTERN 2004)*
- White infarcts are NOT seen in Liver. *(DNB PATTERN 2004)*
- Focal diffuse gall bladder thickening with comet tail reverberation artifacts on USG is in: Adenomyomatosis of Gallbladder. *(DNB PATTERN 2008)*
- Councilman bodies are seen in Viral Hepatitis. *(DNB PATTERN DEC 2009)*
- Nutmeg liver is seen in Chronic venous congestion. *(DNB PATTERN DEC 2009)*
- On stopping alcohol, the stage of disease which is irreversible is cirrhotic stage. *(DNB PATTERN DEC 2010)*
- Mallory Hyaline is a characteristic feature of Alcoholic liver disease. *(DNB PATTERN JUNE 2011)*
- Mallory Hyaline consists of intermediate filaments.
- First antibody to appear in plasma/blood in acute hepatitis B is IgM Anti-HBc. *(DNB PATTERN JUNE 2010)*
- Recumbent stage of Hepatitis B is characterized by Anti-HBc. *(DNB PATTERN JUNE 2010)*
- Hepatocytes are stable cells. *(DNB PATTERN JUNE 2008)*
- Most common subtype of Hepatitis B in North India: ayw. *(DNB PATTERN NOV 2013)*

- Most common subtype of Hep B in Southern India: ayw3.
- Most common subtype of Hep B in Eastern India: adr. *(Ref: International Journal of Infectious Diseases, March 2014)*
- Number of genotypes of Hep B: 8 (A-H Genotypes).
- Most common genotype of Hep B in India: Genotype D.
- Most common type of gallbladder carcinoma: Adenocarcinoma with Infiltrating pattern. *(DNB PATTERN AUG 2013)*
- Cholemic cardiomyopathy occurs in association with: Cirrhosis/Hepatic Dysfunction. *(DNB PATTERN AUG 2013)*
- Incubation period of Hepatitis A is: 2–4 weeks. *(FMGE PATTERN MAR 2013)*
- Area of the Liver most sensitive to ischaemic injury: Centrilobular. *(NEET PATTERN 2016)*
- Periportal Fibrosis is NOT a feature of SNOVER'S TRIAD of Acute Cellular Rejection. *(NEET PATTERN 2016)*
- Periportal Fibrosis is a feature of Chronic cellular Rejection.

LUNGS

- APUD cells are seen in Bronchial carcinoid. *(DNB PATTERN 2000)*
- Pneumonia alba is caused by Treponema Pallidum. *(DNB PATTERN 2000)*
- SHOCK LUNG is characterised by: Diffuse Alveolar Damage. *(NEET PATTERN 2016)*
- Characteristic finding in Chronic Radiation Pneumonitis: Foam cells in vessel wall. *(NEET PATTERN 2016)*
- MOC 31 in Immunohistochemistry is used to differentiate between: Adenocarcinoma and Malignant Mesothelioma. *(JIPMER 2017 PATTERN)*
- TRALI (Transfusion Associated Acute Lung Injury) occurs during/within how many hours of transfusion? 6 hrs. *(NEET 2018 PATTERN)*

OBSTRUCTIVE LUNG DISORDER

- Commonest type of emphysema-centriacinar. *(NEET PATTERN 2014;2015;2016)*
- Emphysema pathologically involve beyond the-terminal bronchiole. *(NEET PATTERN 2014;2015)*
- Reid's index is increased in chronic bronchitis. *(DNB PATTERN DEC 2010)*
- Curschmanns spirals are seen in–Bronchial asthma. *(NEET PATTERN 2016, DNB PATTERN NOV 2013)*

Pathology

- Creola bodies are seen in–bronchial asthma.
(NEET PATTERN 2013;2014)
- [3C IN BRONCHIAL ASTHMA-curschmanns spirals, charcoat leyden crystals and creola bodies) Bronchiectasis means Dilation] *(NEET PATTERN 2013;2014)*
- Sweat chloride in cystic fibrosis-increased.
(NEET PATTERN 2013;2014;2016)

PNEUMOCONIOSIS

- Cut surface of lung in silicosis shows-pleural thickening, nodules and hard collagenous scars.
(DNB PATTERN JUNE 2009)
- Asbestosis is a premalignant condition.
(DNB PATTERN 2001)
- The dangerous particle size causing pneumoconiosis varies from 1 to 5 micrometer. *(NEET PATTERN 2014;2015)*
- Anthracosis is due to inhalation of coal dust.
(NEET PATTERN 2014;2015;2016, FMGE PATTERN 2015)
- Ferruginous bodies are seen in asbestosis.
(FMGE PATTERN 2009;2012)

SARCOIDOSIS

- Asteroid bodies are seen in Sarcoidosis.
(DNB PATTERN JUNE 2010)
- Schaumann bodies are seen in–sarcoidosis.
(NEET PATTERN 2013;2014:2015)
- Good Pasteurs syndroime is characterised by–necrotising hemporrhagic interstitial pneumonitis.
(NEET PATTERN 2013;2014;2016)

SARCOIDOSIS
↓
Schaumann bodies   Aster**oid** bodies

- Alpha one antitrypsin deficiency causes Emphysema.
(DNB PATTERN 2000, DNB PATTERN 2008)
- Alpha 1 antitrypsin deficiency is associated with PANACINAR emphysema.
- Grey Hepatization of lungs is seen on day 3–5.
(DNB PATTERN 2000)
- Metastatic calcification most often seen in Lungs.
(DNB PATTERN 2000, 2006)
- Scar in lung tissue develops into squamous cell carcinoma.
(DNB PATTERN 2001)

- Earliest feature of Tuberculosis is lymphocytic proliferation.
  (DNB PATTERN 2002, 2007)
- Heart failure cells are found in Lungs.
  (DNB PATTERN 2003)
- Reactivated TB commonly occurs near Apex.
  (DNB PATTERN 2004)
- Cut surface of lung in silicosis shows palpable nodules in early stage, hard collagenous scars (later), pleural thickening.
  (DNB PATTERN JUNE 2009)

HEART AND BLOOD VESSELS

- Factor responsible for Cardiac Hypertrophy is c-Myc.
  (DNB PATTERN DEC 2010).
- In Polyarteritis nodosa, there is no raised ANCA.
  (DNB PATTERN JUNE 2009)
- Atrial Myxoma most commonly arises from Left Atrium.
  (DNB PATTERN 2000)
- Onion skin thickening of arteriolar walls is seen in Hyperplastic Arteriolosclerosis. *(DNB PATTERN 2008)*
- Hypersensitivity vasculitis is seen in Post-capillary venules.
  (DNB PATTERN 2008)
- In Myocardial infarction, microscopic picture of coagulation necrosis with neutrophilic infiltration is seen in 1–3 days.
  (DNB PATTERN 2008)
- Least common cause of calcification in the lung is Amyloidosis.
  (DNB PATTERN 2007)
- Ascending aorta involvement is a feature of Syphilitic Aneurysm. *(DNB PATTERN 2001)*
- Most common cause of aortic aneurysm is Atherosclerosis.
  (DNB PATTERN 2000)
- Color of Hemosiderin: Brown.
  (DNB PATTERN DEC 2009)
- Edema is caused by a fall in plasma proteins below 50%.
  (DNB PATTERN 2003)
- Fibrinoid Necrosis is seen in: Malignant Hypertension.
  (DNB PATTERN AUG 2013)
- Dallas Myocarditis Criteria is based on: Lymphocytes and Necrosis. *(JIPMER 2017 PATTERN)*

GIT

- Most significant site for Amoebiasis: Sigmoid colon.
  (DNB PATTERN 2000)

- Inflammatory bowel disease with transmural involvement and skip lesions is Crohn's disease.
(DNB PATTERN JUNE 2011)
- True about Barrett's esophagus is Columnar metaplasia.
(DNB PATTERN JUNE 2011)
- Anti-Saccharomyces cerevisiae antibodies are seen in Crohn's disease. *(DNB PATTERN JUNE 2011)*
- Paneth cells contain Zinc. *(DNB PATTERN 2008)*
- Pseudopolyposis is seen in Ulcerative colitis.
(DNB PATTERN 2000)
- Commonest site of diverticulosis is Sigmoid colon.
(DNB PATTERN 2000)
- In Werner syndrome, most common site of Gastrinoma is small intestine. *(DNB PATTERN DEC 2010)*
- Anti-transglutaminase antibody is seen in Celiac disease.
(DNB PATTERN DEC 2009)
- Epithelial tumor of Stomach: Gastric Adenocarcinoma.
(NEET 2018 PATTERN)

CNS

- The macrophage in the brain is microglia.
(NEET PATTERN 2014;2015;2016)
- Phagocytosis in brain is caused by microglia.
(NEET PATTERN 2013;2014)
- The cell type which do not take part in repair after brain infarction-fibroblasts. *(NEET PATTERN 2013;2014)*
- Perivascular lymphocytes and microglial nodules are seen in– HIV encephalitis. *(NEET PATTERN 2013;2014)*
- Commonest cause of intracranial bleed-hypertension.
(NEET PATTERN 2013;2014, FMGE PATTERN 2012;2014)
- Which is the most common tumor associated with type 1 neurofibromatosis? Optic nerve glioma.
(NEET PATTERN 2013;2014;2015)
- Ash leaf macules are seen in Bourneville's Disease.
(NEET PATTERN 2013;2014)
- Koenen tumor is seen in: Tuberous Sclerosis.
(DNB PATTERN JUNE 2014)
- Most common site of glioblastoma multiforme is–Frontal Lobe. *(NEET PATTERN 2013;2014)*
- Rosenthal fibres are seen in–pilocytic astrocytoma.
(NEET PATTERN 2013;2014;2016)
- Rosenthal fibres are intracytoplasmic inclusions.
(NEET PATTERN 2013;2014)

Contd...

- Which of the following is a pathological calcification? Suprasellar calcification. *(DNB PATTERN JUNE 2010)*
- Hutchinson's secondaries in skull are due to tumors in Adrenals. *(DNB PATTERN 2000, 2003)*
- Rosette shaped arrangement of cells are seen in Ependymoma. *(DNB PATTERN 2000, 2006, 2007)*
- Commonest type of intracranial tumor is: Secondaries. *(DNB PATTERN 2000)*
- Brain changes in Creutzfeldt Jakob Disease–Spongiform encephalopathy. *(DNB PATTERN JUNE 2008)*
- Herring bodies are seen in: Neurohypophysis. *(DNB PATTERN AUG 2013)*
- Inclusion Bodies seen in Alzheimer's Disease: HIRANO BODIES. *(NEET PATTERN 2016)*
- Level of Prolactin which definitely suggests a Prolactinoma: 200 ng/ml. *(NEET 2018 PATTERN)*

MISCELLANEOUS

- Mechanism of oxygen toxicity is free radicals. *(DNB PATTERN DEC 2009)*
- True about gp120 is it is important in HIV Virus attachment. *(DNB PATTERN JUNE 2011)*
- Mosaic appearance is seen in Paget's disease. *(DNB PATTERN JUNE 2012)*
- Xenograft means transplanting organs from one species to another. *(DNB PATTERN JUNE 2012)*
- Plasmodium falciparum binds to which receptor molecule in brain vascular endothelium–ICAM 1. *(DNB PATTERN JUNE 2008)*
- Row of Tombstones appearance is seen in: Pemphigus vulgaris. *(DNB PATTERN AUG 2013)*
- Dent Disease is due to the defect of: Chloride channel. *(DNB PATTERN NOV 2013)*
- Guardian Angel against Obesity is a name given to: Adiponectin. *(DNB PATTERN NOV 2013)*
- Guardian Angel Adipocytokine: Adiponectin.
- Guardian Angel against Breast Cancer: Adiponectin.
- Thiazolidinediones increase Adiponectin activity.
- Rosiglitazone increases Adiponectin activity and decreases Leptin induced tumorigenesis in breast cancer.
- Most common gene responsible for Hereditary Hemochromatosis is: HFE gene. *(DNB PATTERN NOV 2013)*

- Intraepidermal deposits are seen in: Neutrophilic IgA dermatosis. *(DNB PATTERN AUG 2013)*
- Row of Tombstones appearance is seen in: Pemphigus vulgaris. *(DNB PATTERN AUG 2013)*
- Obesity is a risk factor for: Ca Endometrium and Adenocarcinoma Esophagus. *(DNB PATTERN AUG 2013)*
- Owl's eye inclusions are seen in: CMV. *(DNB PATTERN AUG 2013)*
- Rod Bodies are seen in: Congenital Nemaline Myopathy. *(DNB PATTERN NOV 2013)*
- Biphasic cellular pattern is seen in: Synovial Sarcoma. *(DNB PATTERN NOV 2013)*
- Biphasic Pattern also in: Schwannoma (Antoni A and Antoni B areas).
- Triphasic pattern classically in: Wilms Tumor (Nephroblastoma).
- Triphasic waves in EEG: Non-specific, can indicate Hepatic Encephalopathy.
- Ach receptor antibodies are seen in: Myasthenia Gravis. *(FMGE PATTERN SEP 2012)*
- Nude Mice is NOT resistant to Xenograft due to absence of: T-cells. *(NEET 2018 PATTERN)*
- Nude Mice have greatly reduced number of T cells and they lack body hair. Hence called Nude Mice.
- ABCD 1 mutations occur in: Adrenoleukodystrophy. *(JIPMER 2017 PATTERN)*
- CADASIL is associated with: NOTCH 3 mutations. *(JIPMER 2017 PATTERN)*

LEVEL II: HIGH YIELD FACTORS

Table 4.1: Apoptosis

Apoptotic bodies	Consist of membrane bound vesicles Containing cytoplasm and organelles
Anti-apoptotic genes	Bcl-2, Bcl-XL, MCL-1 [a/w drug resistance] FLIP, IAPs
Apoptotic genes	Bcl-Xs, BAX, BAK, BH3 only proteins
Death receptors	Type 1 TNF receptor/CD 95 (Fas)
Pathways of apoptosis	Mitochondrial (Intrinsic pathway)/Death receptor(Extrinsic pathway)

Table 4.2: Cell injury

Enlargement of uterus during Pregnancy	Combination of both hyperplasia and hypertrophy
Atrophy	Involves ubiquitin protease pathway
Squamous metaplasia of respiratory epithelium	Vit A deficiency, Cigarette smoking
Myelin figures are seen in	Necrosis
Coagulative necrosis occurs in infarcts of all solid organs except the	Brain
Liquefactive necrosis occurs primarily in the	Brain
Fibrinoid Necrosis occurs	Immune mediated diseases (PAN, SLE) and Malignant hypertension
Fat necrosis occurs in	Acute pancreatitis
Triggered effect of heart is seen in	Fatty change
Hemosiderin is	A golden yellow to brown colored pigment and contains ferritin micelles

Table 4.3: Cell death

Telomere shortening	Is associated with cell death
Telomerase enzyme	Prevents shortening and maintains chromosome length
Telomerase	Is absent in somatic cells, present in germ cells and in low levels in stem cells
Only effective intervention to date which increases life span	Calorie restriction
Lipofuscin	Is a marker of past free radical injury
Wear and Tear pigment	Lipofuscin

Table 4.4: Stains and fixatives

Amyloid produces apple green birefringence due to	Cross beta pleated configuration of Amyloid fibrils
Amyloid tissue produces Mahogany Brown staining	With iodine and sulfuric acid
Histopathological confirmation of Amyloid	Is by Electron Microscopy which reveals amorphous non-oriented thin fibrils
Stain used for identifying viable myocardium in myocardial injury	Triphenyltetrazolium Chloride
Fat is stained orange red by	Sudan black or Oil Red O
Glycogen is stained by	PAS

Table 4.5: Amyloidosis

Carpel Tunnel Syndrome in a patient undergoing long term dialysis is commonly due to	Amyloid deposition in carpel ligaments
Sago spleen is	Amyloid limited to splenic Follicles
In liver, amyloid deposits initially occur in the	Space of Disse
In kidney, amyloid deposits are found principally in the	Glomeruli
There is NO inflammatory response in amyloidosis and on cells and tissues	Mainly causes pressure effects
Amyloid fibrils are produced by	Extracellular aggregation of misfolded proteins including proteoglycans, glycosaminoglycans, and plasma proteins including Serum Amyloid P component (SAP)

Table 4.6: Wound healing

Most important growth factors involved in Angiogenesis	VEGF/FGF 2
Carefully sutured wounds have	70% strength of normal unbroken skin
When sutures are removed	Wounds have 10% strength of normal skin
After 3 months	Wounds regain up to 70–80% of normal skin strength
Wound strength	Never regained 100%; never improves more than 80%
Healing by second intention	Has more inflammation/more granulation tissue/more scarring and wound contraction

Table 4.7: Named structures

Status spongiosus	Creutzfeldt Jakob Disease
Perivascular Pseudorosettes	Ependymoma
Verocay Bodies	Schwannoma
Lisch Nodules	Type 1 Neurofibromatosis
Subungual Fibromas	Tuberous Sclerosis
Kogoj pustules/Munro Microabscesses	Psoriasis
Civatte Bodies	Lichen Planus
Cherry Red nuclei	Malignant Melanoma

Table 4.8: CVS

Weibel-Palade bodies	Storage organelles for Von Willebrand Factor found in Endothelial cells
Framingham study or Massachusetts study has identified	Risk factors for ischaemic heart disease
The most extensively involved vessels in Atherosclerosis	Are the lower abdominal aorta, the coronary arteries, the popliteal arteries, the internal carotid arteries, and the vessels of the circle of Willis
Fibrous cap of Atheroma is	Smooth Muscle cells and Collagen
Necrotic core contains	Lipid, Debris, foam cells, fibrin and other plasma proteins
Fibrous plaques are composed	smooth muscle cells, fibrous tissue, No lipid
Most common site of left atrial myxoma	Fossa ovalis
Ball valve obstruction is caused by	Left atrial myxoma, mobile enough to swing into mitral and tricuspid valves
Spider cells are characteristic of Cardiac rhabdomyomas	Rhabdomyoma of heart occur in high incidence with Tuberous Sclerosis
Constitutional symptoms in Myxoma	is due to elaboration of IL-6
Critical coronary stenosis is defined	as 70–75% obstruction of vessel lumen

Table 4.9: CNS

Tuberous Sclerosis	Cysts in *lungs, liver, kidney and pancreas*
Von Hippel-Lindau disease	Cysts in *liver, kidney and pancreas*
Von Hippel-Lindau	Predisposed to develop Renal cell carcinoma of kidney
Rosenthal fibres	Typically seen in Pilocytic Astrocytoma
Exquisitively radiosensitive brain tumor which occurs exclusively in the cerebellum	Medulloblastoma

TUMOR MARKERS

Bombesin	Neuroblastoma, Lung and Gastric Cancer
Tartrate Resistant Acid Phosphatase (TRAP)	Hairy Cell Leukemia
CA 19-9	Pancreatic Adenocarcinoma
Calcitonin	Medullary Carcinoma Thyroid
Alpha Fetoprotein	Hepatocellular Carcinoma
Beta HCG	Hydatidiform Mole, Choriocarcinoma, Gestational Trophoblastic Disease
Alkaline Phosphatase	Paget's disease
CA 125	Ovarian Malignant Epithelial Tumors

5. Microbiology

"Let me tell you the secret that has led me to my goal. My strength lies solely in my tenacity."
—Louis Pasteur

REFERENCES
- *Harrison's Textbook of Internal Medicine, 19th ed.*
- *Textbook of Microbiology by Ananthanarayan and Jayaram Panikker, 10th ed.*

LEVEL I: BASIC REPEATS

GENERAL MICROBIOLOGY

- Ig in Peyer's patch – Ig A. *(2011)*
- Macrophages are sources of IL – 1. *(2010)*
- Major component of Complement system – C3. *(2011)*
- Complement which acts as an opsonin – C3B. *(2011)*
- Rheumatoid factor is 19S globulin. *(2000, 2001)*
- Surgical blade is sterilized by Hot air oven. (Dry Heat) *(2009)*
- Human anatomical waste is disposed by incineration. *(2009)*
- Heat labile instruments are best sterilized by Ethylene oxide gas. *(2007)*
- Proctoscope is sterilized by Glutaraldehyde. *(2002)*
- Mantoux Test is an example of: Type 4 Hypersensitivity. *(2001)*
- Interferon gamma is secreted by CD4 T cells. *(2009)*
- Snake venom acts by classical and alternate pathways. *(2010)*
- Exotoxins are highly antigenic. *(2000)*
- Okazaki fragment is DNA. *(2000)*
- Examples of continuous cell line – He la, Hep 2, Vero, KB. *(2011)*
- Commonest Immunoglobulin deficiency is IgA deficiency. *(2000)*
- Cell mediated immunity is by virtue of helper T cells, cytotoxic T cells and suppressor T cells. *(2011)*
- IgA is the main immunoglobulin in secretions such as saliva, milk, tears and in secretions of respiratory, intestinal and genital tracts. *(2011)*

Microbiology

- Epsilon Aminocaproic Acid given prophylactically is useful if used in: C1 inhibitor deficiency. *(2007)*
- Serum concentration of IgG Subclass which is maximum is IgG1. *(2007)*
- Type 1 hypersensitivity is mediated by IgE. *(2007)*
- IgM activates classical complement pathway. *(2001)*
- Widal test is an example of Agglutination test. *(2001)*
- Bilirubin metabolism is NOT a function of the reticuloendothelial system. *(2002, 2008)*
- Immunoglobulin which acts as a receptor on B cell – IgM. *(2010)*
- Wheal and flare reaction is Type 1 hypersensitivity reaction. *(2010)*
- Conditions required for autoclaving–121 degree celsius for fifteen minutes. *(2012)*
- Secretions are rich in IgA. *(2009)*
- Innate immunity is stimulated by which part of bacteria– carbohydrate sequence in cell wall. (Bacterial lipopolysaccharide) *(2011)*
- LPS is connected to outer membrane by Lipid A. It stimulates innate immunity. *(2011)*
- Father of Microbiology: Antoni Van Leuwenhoek. *(NEET 2018 PATTERN)*
- Father of Modern Microbiology: Louis Pasteur. *(2003)*
- Disinfectant which works by plasma membrane damage = quaternary ammonium compounds. *(2011)*
- Action of papain on an IgG molecule produces one Fc fragment and two Fab fragments. *(2010)*
- Nitroblue Tetrazolium test is for Phagocytes. *(2008)*
- Pentameric antibody with J chain – IgM. *(2010)*
- Dimeric Antibody with J chain: Secretory Ig A
- Multiple drug resistance spreads by Conjugation. *(2007)*
- Blood agar is an example of enriched media. *(2012)*
- Bacillus used to test efficacy of sterilization by autoclave – Bacillus stearothermophilus. *(2010)*
- In transduction, DNA transmitted by the vector to the bacteria belongs to another bacterium. *(2010)*
- Immunoglobilin Pentamer is: IgM. *(2009)*
- Germ Theory was given by: Louis Pasteur. *(2013)*
- Settle culture plate method: simple and inexpensive method for qualitative assessment of microbial contamination of Air. *(2013)*
- Thickness of Bacterial cell wall is: 20 -80 nm. *(2013)*

- Concentration of Glutaraldehyde used for sterilization: 2%. *(2013)*
- Glassware sterilization is done by: Hot Air Oven. *(2013)*
- Alcohol destroys bacteria by which mechanism? Cell membrane defect. *(2013)*
- Sterilization of heat labile media is done by: Tyndallization. *(2013)*
- Th1 forms: IL2. *(2013)*
- MHC 1 is recognized by: CD8 T cells. *(2013)*
- Processes of dendritic cells contain which MHC? MHC 11. *(2013)*
- Double diffusion in two dimesions is known as: Ouchterlonyprocedure. *(2013)*
- Intravenous IgG to Rh negative mother confers which type of immunity? Passive immunity. *(2013)*
- Membranous unfolding in bacteria that initiates DNA replication are: Mesosomes. *(2013)*
- Oakley Fulthorpe procedure is: Double Diffusion in one dimension. *(2016)*
- Most commonly used method for using Antibiotic susceptibility of Bacteria: Kirby Bauer Disc Diffusion Method. *(2016)*
- Shadow Casting is used in: Electron Microscopy. *(2016)*
- Rose-Waaler Test is: Passive Hemagglutination Test. *(2016)*
- Glutaraldehyde is used to sterilize: Endoscopes, Corrugated rubber anesthetic tubes, plastic endotracheal tubes. *(2015)*
- Prausnitz-Kustner Reaction is used to demonstrate: IgE. *(2015)*
- Prausnitz-Kustner Reaction is used to demonstrate: Type 1 hypersensitivity. *(2015)*
- Function of Gp120: Attachment of CD4 receptor *(2015)*
- Indicator for sterilization by autoclave: Bacillus stearothermophilus. *(2016)*
- > 100 colony forming unit per mL of urine is significant in: Suprapubic aspiration. *(2016)*
- Inspissation is used for: Protein containing culture medium. *(2016)*
- Nosocomial infection occurs in hospital in more than 48 hrs. *(2016)*
- Real Time PCR is used for: quantitative detection of PCR material. *(2016)*
- In Rideal-Walker method, plates are incubated for 2–3 days. *(2016)*
- Phenol Coefficient test for testing the efficiency of disinfectants in the presence of organic matter: Chick Martin Test. *(NEET 2016 PATTERN)*

- Whole Blood is used for: Interferon Gamma Release Assay. *(NEET 2018 PATTERN)*

VIROLOGY

- True about Polio – Man is only reservoir. *(2008)*
- Yellow fever virus is – Flavi virus. *(2008)*
- Torres bodies are seen in Yellow fever. *(2003)*
- SARS is – Corona virus. *(2008, 2009)*
- Dengue virus belongs to family of Flaviviridae. *(2008)*
- Most sensitive diagnostic test for Dengue: IgM ELISA. *(2008)*
- Acute HIV infection is diagnosed by – p24 Ag capture assay. *(2008)*
- HIV can be detected and confirmed by Reverse Transcriptase PCR. *(2007)*
- HIV virus has a predilection for infecting CD4+ T cells. *(2002)*
- HIV primarily replicates in CD4 HELPER T cells. *(2012)*
- Enzyme NOT present in HIV: Endonuclease. *(2007)*
- Highly specific test for HIV antibodies is: Western Blot. *(2000)*
- Epstein-Barr virus is NOT causative in Slow Virus Disease. *(2000)*
- Epstein-Barr virus CAUSES Burkitt lymphoma, Hodgkins lumphoma, Nasopharyngeal Ca, NOT Verrucous lymphoma. *(2009)*
- Epstein-Barr virus causes Nasopharyngeal carcinoma. *(2001, 2007)*
- Epstein-Barr virus is NOT implicated in Leukaemia. *(2002)*
- Epstein-Barr virus is NOT transmitted transplacentally. *(2001)*
- Paul-Bunnell test – EBV. *(2010)*
- Oral hairy leukoplakia is associated with EBV. *(2010)*
- Hepatitis A can be restrained by boiling over 120-degree Celsius over 1 minute. *(2009)*
- Marker of Hepatitis B infectivity is: Anti HBc +, HBsAg + *(2000)*
- Chronic Hepatitis is seen in infection with Hepatitis C. *(2001)*

- Hepatitis B surface antigen may be present in Saliva. *(2002)*
- Not a RNA virus – Hepatitis B. *(2008)*
- NOT true about Hepatitis A virus: Carrier rate 2%. *(2008)*
- Route of transmission of Hepatitis E virus is Faeco-oral. *(2001)*
- Carrier state in liver disease is due to infection with Hepatitis B. *(2001)*
- RSV does NOT cause ARDS. *(2009)*
- Treatment of Varicella in immunocompetent host is prevention of complications. *(2010)*
- Antigenic variation is not seen in Influenza Type C. C is antigenically stable. *(2011)*
- Age group most prone to Rubella–women of childbearing age. *(2009)*
- Continuous cell line for virus not present for WT38. *(2011)*
- Antigenic drift is commonly seen in Influenza virus. *(2000)*
- Cause of acute laryngotracheal bronchitis–Parainfluenza virus. *(2009)*
- Kaposi sarcoma is related to HHV 8. *(2010)*
- Viral inclusion bodies–Negri, molluscum, Bollinger NOT PSAMMOMA BODY. *(2010)*
- Suckling mice is used in the isolation of Arbovirus. *(2010)*
- Hemorrhagic fever caused by viruses–yellow fever, dengue, Kyasanur forest. *(2010)*
- Pharyngoconjunctival fever is caused by Adenovirus subgroup (type 3,7). *(2009)*
- Northern blotting is used for separation of RNA. (South–dosa, North–roti, West–pizza.) *(2012)*
- Not an RNA virus: Simian virus 40. *(2008)*
- HIV Type E is most prevalent in: Thailand. *(2013)*
- HIV most prevalent in India: Type C.
- Average incubation period of HIV: 10 yrs. *(FMGE PATTERN MAR 2011)*
- Most common HIV strain in North India: ayw strain. *(2013)*
- Chance that a health worker gets HIV from an accidental needle prick is: 0.3%. *(FMGE PATTERN MAR 2013)*

- Most common cause of Cervical cancer: HPV 16. *(2013)*
- Oncoproteins produced by HPV: E6/E7. *(2013)*
- HPV was found to be the causative organism for Carcinoma cervix by: Harald Van Hausur. *(2013)*
- Speed of travel of Rabies Virus: 3 mm/hr. *(2013)*
- Incubation period of Mumps: 16-18 days. *(2013)*
- Intestinal Pathogen in HIV: Cryptosporidium. *(2013)*
- Herpes simplex has: Linear DS DNA. *(2013)*
- A negative strand virus: Bunya virus. *(2013)*
- Hemagglutination showing viruses are: Influenza virus. *(2013)*
- Most common cause of common cold is: Virus. *(2013)*
- Most important cause of severe diarrhea is: Rota virus A. *(2013)*
- Intranuclear basophilic inclusion body with halo is seen in: CMV. *(2013)*
- Most common viral infection after Kidney Transplantation: Cytomegalovirus. *(NEET PATTERN 2018)*
- H PV does not cause: Condyloma Lata. *(2013)*
- Common warts are caused by: HPV 2,7. *(2013)*
- Oral Hairy Leukoplakia is associated with: Epstein-Barr Virus *(2013)*
- Vector for Chandipura virus is: Sandfly. *(2013)*
- Dane particles are seen in: Hepatitis B. *(2013)*
- Australian Antigen is: HBsAg. *(NEET 2018 PATTAERN)*
- Hallmark for diagnosis of Hepatitis B is: HBsAg. *(2013)*
- Feco-Oral transmission occurs in: Polio. *(FMGE PATTERN MAR 2013)*
- Infection common after organ transplantation: Cytomegalovirus. *(FMGE PATTERN MAR 2010)*
- Acute Hemorrhagic Conjunctivitis seen with: Adenovirus. *(2015)*
- Acute Hemorrhagic Conjunctivits is associated with: Enterovirus 70. *(NEET 2018 PATTERN)*
- Included in Biohazard Risk Group 4: Herpes Simiae. *(2016)*
- HPV 6 is implicated in the causation of: Condyloma Acuminata. *(2016)*
- Shingles is caused by: Varicella Zoster. *(NEET PATTERN 2018)*

MYCOLOGY

- Lipophilic fungus Cryptococcus. *(2008)*
- Cryptococcus diagnostic test–India ink. *(2008)*
- Cryptococcus Neoformans is visualized by India ink preparation. *(2009)*
- NOT a yeast form in Tissue: Aspergillus. *(2008)*
- Aflatoxin is secreted by Aspergillus. *(2009)*
- Malt worker's lung is caused by Aspergillus clavatus. *(2008)*
- Histoplasma capsulatum is Dimorphic fungus. *(2002)*
- Not a dimorphic fungi: Cryptococcus. *(2010, 2011)*
- Candida is NOT an example of Dimorphic fungi. *(2000)*
- Dimorphic fungi–Histoplasma, Blastomycosis, Paracoccoidosis, Coccydiodes, Sporothrix, Pencillium.
- Asteroid bodies and Cigar shaped globi are characteristic of Sporotrichosis. *(2000)*
- MC deep mycosis in India–Histoplasmosis. *(2011)*
- Mucormycosis–caused by Rhizopus, Rhizomucor, Cunninghamella, common in India, nose is the common site. *(2011)*
- Sclerotic bodies are found in Chromoblastomycosis. *(2010)*
- Fungus which cannot be grown on artificial media is rhinosporidium seeberi.
- Most common fungal infection–Deuteromycetes. *(2009)*
- Negative staining technique–India Ink. *(2010)*
- Which is coenocytic fungus? Zygomycetes. *(2013)*
- Which is dimorphic fungus? Histoplasma. *(2013)*
- Fungus with Aseptate hyphae with branching at 90 degree: Mucor. *(2015)*
- Tuberculous spores are characteristic of: Histoplasma. *(2016)*
- Fungus which infects Reticuloendothelial cells: Histoplasma *(2016)*
- 1,3 Beta D Glucan Assay (FUNGITELL Assay) is NOT useful to detect: Cryptococcosis. *(AIIMS 2017 PATTERN)*
- Bodies in Chromoblastomycosis: Sclerotic Bodies *(2015)*
- Most common cause of Orbital Cellulitis in patients associated with Diabetic KetoAcidosis: Mucor.

(NEET 2018 PATTERN)

PARASITOLOGY

- Intermediate host of Malarial parasite: Human. *(2011)*
- Schizonts are not seen in peripheral smear in Plasmodium falciparum malaria. *(2011)*

- Parasite causing myocarditis: Trichinella spiralis *(2011)*
- Parasite which can enter through intact skin: Strongyloides. *(2011)*
- Chagas disease is caused by Trypanosoma cruzi. *(2011)*
- Skin test useful in Hydatid disease: Casoni's test. *(2011)*
- Trichuris does not affect EYES. *(2010)*
- Sabin Feldman test is used for Toxoplasmosis. *(DNB PATTERN 2001, NEET PATTERN 2018)*
- Route of transmission of Toxoplasma is: Blood. *(2001)*
- Casoni's test is positive in Echinococcus. *(2000)*
- Hydatid cyst occurs most commonly in the Liver. *(2004)*
- Congenital toxoplasmosis occurs if – infection acquired in later half of pregnancy in non-immune mother. *(2008)*
- Leishman-Donovan bodies are seen in Spleen. *(2002)*
- Trichinella spiralis does not cause pulmonary eosinophilia. *(2002)*
- Intermediate host for Taenia Saginata is: Cattle *(2002)*
- Toxoplasma teratogenicity is maximum during first trimester of pregnancy. *(2002)*
- Non-sheathed Microfilaria are: Mansonella ozzardi. *(2000)*
- Plasmodium falciparum the number of life cycles in the liver is 1. *(2000)*
- Giardiasis is best diagnosed by Presence of both cysts and trophozoites in stools. *(2000)*
- Visceral larva migrans is due to Toxocara canis. *(2000, 2001)*
- Man is an intermediate host of Malaria. *(2009)*
- Duffy blood group antigen confers protection form infections by Plasmodium vivax. *(2008)*
- Cryptosporidial cyst is identified by acid fast stain in stool sample. *(2012)*
- R2 type of drug resistance in Malaria is decline by 75% in 72 hrs followed by persistence. *(2000, 2007)*
- Primary amoebic Meningoencephalitis (brain eating Amoeba). *(2011)*
- Treatment given to Entamoeba cyst carriers – Paromomycin *(2009)*
- Meningoencephalitis caused by amoeba: Naegleria fowleri. *(2001)*
- Cat acts as reservoir in Toxoplasma gondii. *(2009)*
- Largest protozoan ia Balantidium coli. *(2009)*
- Aldehyde test is used for Leishmania. *(2008)*

- Ova in stool are NOT of diagnostic significance in Strongyloides. *(2009)*
- Cerebral Malaria is caused bt Plasmodium falciparum. *(2010)*
- Parasite causing myocarditis–Trichinella spiralis RPT. *(2010)*
- Nematode which resides in Caecum and appendix is Enterobius vermicularis. (Pin worm) Trichuris trichura (Whip worm). *(2010)*
- Largest protozoal infection is: Balantidium coli. *(2002, 2008)*
- Ascaris lumbricoides causes deficiency of Vit A. *(2010)*
- Trichinella does not enter human body via skin. (It infects by ingestion of undercooked pork which contains encysted larva in the striated muscle.) *(2010)*
- Loeffler's syndrome is caused by: Ascaris. *(2013)*
- Maculae cerulae is seen in: Pubic Lice. *(2013)*
- Cutaneous Larva Migrans is caused by: Ancylostoma braziliense. *(NEET PATTERN 2018)*

FOOD POISONING

- Food poisoning in canned food is caused by Clostridium Botulinum. *(2011)*
- Food poisoning that does not present within 6 hrs is due to Salmonella.(presents after 12 hrs). *(2011)*
- E. coli causes food poisoning which occurs late ie after 6 hrs. *(2011)*
- Shortest incubation period food poisoning: Staphylococcus aureus. *(2008)*
- Pea soup stool is characteristically seen in typhoid. *(2004)*
- Enterobacterium faecalis does not produce acute infectious diarrhea. *(2010)*
- Preformed toxin produces diarrhea in Staphylococcus. *(2010)*
- Fecal leucocytes are absent in Campylobactor infections. *(2008)*
- Nagler reaction is positive for: Clostridium perfringens. *(2013)*
- Clostridium perfringens toxemia is caused by which toxin? Alpha toxin. *(2013)*
- Bacteria causing vomiting and diarrhea within 6 hours of food intake: Staphylococcus aureus. *(FMGE PATTERN MAR 2005)*

- Best test for diagnosis of typhoid in the first week–Blood culture. *(FMGE PATTERN MAR 2007)*

VIBRIO

- Vibrio cholerae characteristic feature–growth in alkaline medium. *(2008)*
- Cholera is caused by Vibrio cholerae 01, vibrio cholerae 0139. *(2009)*
- Transport Medium for Vibrio Cholerae: Venkataraman Medium. *(2013)*
- MONSUR'S MEDIUM is used for isolation of Vibrio cholerae.
- Seventh pandemic of Cholerae was due to which strain of Vibrio Cholerae? Vibrio cholerae El Tor. *(2013)*
- EL TOR was earlier called PARACHOLERA.

DIPHTHERIA AND DIPHTHEROIDS

- Lysogenic conversion occurs in Diphtheria. *(2008)*
- Diphtheria TOXIN–toxin production depends on optimum concentration of iron. *(2010)*
- Diphtheria will NOT produce maculopapular rash. *(2011)*
- Types of Diphtheria–Respiratory, cutaneous and invasive. *(2011)*
- Elek test is used in Diphtheria. *(2007)*
- Pleomorphism is most commonly seen in Corynebacterium Diphtheriae. *(2006, 2007)*
- Metachromatic granules are seen in Corynebacterium. *(2011)*

LEGIONELLA

- In Legionnaire's disease, culture medium used is: BCYE medium. *(2007)*
- Legionella pneumonia can be isolated from lung biopsy. *(2002)*
- Legionella pathogenicity is due to failure of oxidative burst. *(2010)*
- Pontiac fever is caused by: Legionella. *(2013)*

RABIES

- Anti-rabies vaccine is prepared by fixed virus. *(2012)*
- Pasteur developed the vaccine for Anthrax and Rabies. *(2008)*

- Intracytoplasmic inclusion bodies are diagnostic of Rabies. *(2002)*
- Negri bodies are commonly found in Hippocampus. *(2006)*

PROTOZOA

- MCC dysentery in Adults: Entamoeba. *(2011)*
- Most common extra intestinal manifestation of Amoebiasis is: Liver. *(2001)*
- Acute meningoencephalitis is caused by Naegleria. *(2011)*
- A patient with history of travel to Burma came with fever and was admitted with a GCS of 7. The most probable diagnosis is: Cerebral malaria. *(2013)*

RICKETTSIAE

- Most common cause of Bacillary Angiomatosis: Bartonella henselae. *(2011)*
- Diagnostic test for rickettsial infection is Weil-Felix reaction. *(2002)*
- Causative agent of Lyme's disease is: Borrelia burgdorferi. *(2002)*
- Rocky Mountain spotted fever is a rickettsial disease NOT VIRAL. *(2010)*
- Endemic typhus is transmitted by Rat flea. *(2001)*
- Neil Mooser reaction or Tunica reaction is used to differ-entiate between R. prowazekii and R. typhi. *(2010)*
- Q fever is caused by Coxiella burnetii. *(2010)*
- Rickettsiae is resistant to which antibiotics Penicillin. *(2013)*

SPIROCHETES

- Causative agent of YAWS–Treponema pertenue. *(2011)*
- Pneumonia alba is due to Treponema pallidum. *(2008)*
- Treponema is most difficult to isolate from gumma. *(2010)*
- Weil's disease–caused by Leptospira. *(2011)*
- Dark Ground illumination helps to detect–Leptospira, Treponema and Borrelia. *(2000)*
- Lyme disease–Borrelia burgdorferi. *(2009)*
- Dark Field Microscopy is used for: Syphilis. *(2013)*
- Spirochetes are: Flexible spirals. *(2013)*
- Spirochetes can be identified by: Dark Field Microscopy. *(FMGE PATTERN MAR 2005)*
- Culture medium for Leptospira for laboratory diagnosis: EMJH Medium. *(JULY 2016)*

- Fletcher's medium containing rabbit serum is used for: Leptospira. *(JULY 2016)*
- VDRL is which type of reaction? Slide Flocculation Test. *(2013)*
- NOT a feature of Anicteric Leptospirosis: High mortality. *(FMGE PATTERN MAR 2013)*

STAPHYLOCOCCUS

- Localized myogenic infection is caused by: Staphylococcus. *(2011)*
- Most common cause of pyomyositis: Staph. aureus. *(2011)*
- Commonest pathogen isolated from abscess of the jaw is: Staphylococcus aureus. *(2002)*
- TSS caused by–Staphylococcus aureus. *(2008)*
- Ritter's disease is caused by: Staph. aureus. *(2013)*
- Oil Paint appearance on Nutrient agar is seen in: Staphylococcus aureus. *(2016)*

STREPTOCOCCUS

- Pike's medium is used for the transport of Streptococci. *(2003)*
- Subacute Bacterial Endocarditis is caused by Streptococcus viridians. *(2000)*
- Strain of streptococci implicated in Neonatal Meningitis is: Group B. *(2002)*
- Draughtsman concentric rings on culture are produced by Pneumococci. *(2008)*
- Group A hemolytic pharyngitis is due to local infection. *(2010)*
- MC streptococcus in neonatal meningitis–Lancefield Group B. *(2008)*

MYCOBACTERIA

- Number of Mycobacteria required to be seen by AFB staining: 10000–20000. *(2004)*
- John's Bacillus is Mycobacterium paratuberculosis. *(2003)*
- NOT a mycobacterium tuberculosis complex organism–M. kansasii. *(Photochromogen)* *(2010)*
- Buruli ulcer is caused by Mycobacterium ulcerans. *(2008)*
- NOT a method of testing resistance to drugs in TB–Disc diffusion method. *(2010)*

LISTERIA

- DOC for Listeria – Ampicillin. *(2009)*
- Tumbling motility is shown by Listeria. *(2007)*

CHLAMYDIA

- Chlamydia escapes killing by–molecular mimicry. *(2011)*

CLOSTRIDIUM

- Clostridium tetani is Gram positive spore forming. *(2002)*
- A dead end infection-TETANUS. *(2010)*
- Clostridia is Gram positive, obligate, anaerobe. *(2010)*
- Botulinum toxin acts by inhibiting acetyl choline release. *(2003)*
- NOT true about Infant Botulism–preformed toxin. *(2008)*
- Endotoxin does NOT cause Tetanus. *(2001)*
- Most common cause of Antibiotic associated Colitis is: Clostridium difficile. *(2000)*
- Pseudomembanous colitis is caused by Clostridium difficile *(2002, 2008, 2012)*

PSEUDOMONAS

- Strict aerobic bacterium: Pseudomonas. *(2011)*
- Burkholderia cepacea is resisitant to: Cefotetan. *(NEET PATTERN 2018)*

E. COLI AND PROTEUS

- E. coli is not a capsulated pathogen. *(2011)*
- E157 strain of E. coli can be grown in: Sorbitol Mc Conkey Agar. Agar. *(2008)*
- L form phenomenon occurs in Proteus. *(2006)*
- Most common organism detected in Ischiorectal fossa: E. coli. *(2001)*

GONOCOCCI

- Gonorrhea can be identified by fermentation of glucose. *(2011)*
- Differentiating feature of Neisseria Meningitidis from Neisseria gonorrhea–it ferments maltose. *(2010)*

MYCOPLASMA

- Atypical pneumonia is caused by Mycoplasma, Chlamydia, Adenovirus. *(2011)*
- Eaton agent is Mycoplasma. *(2008)*
- Fried egg colony is seen in culture of Mycoplasma. *(2000)*
- Colour of granules produced by Actinomycetes: Yellow. *(DNB 2010 PATTERN)*
- Sulfur Granules are diagnostic of: Actinomycosis. *(DNB 2002 PATTERN)*
- BREAD CRUMB COLONY appearance is seen in: Actinomyces israelii. *(DNB 2007 PATTERN)*
- Nocardia and Actinomycetes can be differentiated by: Acid Fast Staining. *(DNB 2013 PATTERN)*
- Nocardia is weakly Acid Fast.
- DOC Nocardia: Cotrimoxazole. *(DNB 2009 PATTERN)*
- Anaerobic organism producing multiple discharging abscesses with sulfur granules: Actinomycosis. *(NEET 2018 PATTERN)*

MISCELLANEOUS

- Characteristic of Anaerobic bacteria is–fail to grow in aerobic media, gas in tissue in aerobic infections, foul smelling discharge. *(2011)*
- Meningococci does not have plasmid. *(2009)*
- Test for diagnosis of Pyogenic Meningitis–CSF examination. *(2009)*
- Best rapid test for etiology of Acute pyogenic meningitis – Latex agglutination. *(2009)*
- Nocardia DOC is NOT penicillin but Septran. *(2009)*
- Community acquired Pneumonia – Strep Pneumonia, H. influenza, Moraxella catarrhalis, NOT KLEBSIELLA. *(2010)*
- Satellitism is seen in culture of Hemophilus. *(2000, 2001)*
- H. pylori is found in mucus layer. *(2010)*
- Not a COCCYDEAN–Enterocytozoon. *(2010)*
- Vibrio parahaemolyticus is seen in undercooked shell fish. *(2009)*
- Prion is a protein. *(2009)*
- In carrier state of Typhoid, O titre < 1:40, H titre <1:40, Vi titre >1:40. *(2000)*

- Prions basic defect is in folding of proteins. *(2008)*
- Stalactite growth is a feature of Pasteurella. *(2006)*
- Ito's test is used for the diagnosis of Chancroid. *(2006)*
- Fermentation of glycerol is the basis of the classification of Yersinia. *(2003)*
- Mad Cow disease – protein-prion. *(2008)*
- Diagnostic in 1st week of typhoid – blood culture. *(2008)*
- Typhoid incubation period – 3–21 days. *(2008)*
- Petroff's method for sputum microscopy. *(2008)*
- Earliest diagnostic test for H. pylori infection – C14 Breath test. *(2008)*
- Ecthyma Gangrenosum was caused by: Pseudomonas aeruginosa. *(2013)*
- Organism which shows motility at 25 degrees but NOT at 37 degrees: Listeria monocytogenes. *(2013)*
- Urea Breath Test is positive for: Helicobactor pylori. *(2013)*
- Carcinoma caused by Epstein-Barr virus: Nasopharyngeal Carcinoma. *(2013)*
- Meliodosis is caused by: Burckholderia pseudomallei. *(2013)*
- Rat bite fever is caused by: Spirillum Minus. *(2013)*
- C3b deficiency causes: Recurrent pyogenic infections. *(2013)*
- Hereditary angioneurotic edema is caused by deficiency of: C1 inhibitor. *(2013)*
- NOT an opsonin: C5a. *(2013)*
- Chancroid is caused by: Hemophilus ducreyi. *(2013)*
- Mec A gene confers resistance to which gene? Nafcillin. *(2013)*
- Minimum concentration of Tetanus Antiserum in blood to protect against Tetanus is: 0.1 IU/mL. *(2013)*
- Differentiating feature of Neisseria gonococcus from Neisseria meningitidis is: Maltose Fermentation. *(2013)*
- Peliosis Hepatis is caused by: Bartonella. *(2013)*
- Most common cause of complicated UTI: Escherischia coli. *(2013)*
- Campylobactor jejuni can be isolated in culture at what temperature? 42-degree celsius. *(2013)*
- Cold agglutinins hemolysins are seen in pneumonia caused by: Mycoplasma. *(2013)*
- Hebra Nose is caused by: Frisch bacillus. *(2016)*
- Izumi Fever is caused by: Yersinia pseudotuberculosis. *(2016)*
- Satellitism is seen in cultures of: Hemophilus. *(2016)*

- Urease Breath Test is used for: Helicobactor Pylori.

(NEET PATTERN 2018)

LEVEL II: HIGH YIELD FACTORS

Table 5.1: Immunoglobulins

Each immunoglobulin molecule is digested by Papain into	One Fc and two Fab fragments
Each immunoglobulin molecule is digested by Pepsin into	F(ab)2 and smaller fragments of Fc.
L chain is attached to H chain by most abundant IgG subclass	Disulphide bond IgG1
Only maternal immunoglobulin transported across the placenta	IgG
IgA found in mucosal surfaces and secretions is	A dimer with a J chain
Phylogenetically oldest immunoglobulin class	IgM
Earliest immunoglobulin to be synthesized by the fetus	IgM
IgM secretion starts at Millionaire molecule	20 weeks of age in the fetus IgM
Major antibody receptor on the surface of B lymphocytes for antigen recognition	Monomeric IgM
Homocytotropism is exhibited by	IgE
Prausnitz-Kustner reaction is mediated by	IgE
Mast cell affinity is exhibited by	IgE
IgM producing cells are selectively involved in	Waldenstrom's Macroglobulinemia
Cryoglobulins consist of	IgG/IgM or their mixed precipitates
Bence Jones proteins are	Light chains of immunoglobulins and may occur as kappa or lambda forms
Least concentration among total antibodies is for	IgE
In Wiskott-Aldrich syndrome	Serum IgM is low, IgG and IgA are normal or elevated

Table 5.2: Microbiological tests frequently asked

Ascoli's thermoprecipitin test is	a Ring test which is a type of Precipitation test
VDRL test for syphilis is	a type of slide flocculation test which is a precipitation test

Contd...

Contd...

Kahn test for syphilis is	a type of tube flocculation test which is a precipitation test
Elek's test for Diphtheria is	a type of immunodiffusion test which is a precipitation test
Blood grouping and cross matching	are examples of slide agglutination tests
Widal test, Weil-Felix test, Paul-Bunnell test	are examples of tube agglutination tests
Rose-Waaler test for Rheumatoid Arthritis	is a passive agglutination test
Coombs test or antiglobulin test	is also example of agglutination test
Wassermann reaction for serological diagnosis of syphilis is	an example of Complement Fixation test
Schick's test for Diphtheria	is an example of Neutralization test

Table 5.3: Grafts

Grafts from self	Autograft
Grafts from different genetically identical individual	Isograft
Grafts from different non-identical person of the same species	Allograft or Homograft
Grafts from different species	Xenograft or Heterograft
Non-living grafts	Structural or Static grafts
Living grafts or live organs	Vital grafts
Unilateral sex linked incompatibility	Eichwald-Silmser effect

Table 5.4: Mycology

Only pathogenic yeast	Cryptococcus neoformans
Pseudomycelium	Candida
Tinea Pedis	Epidermophyton Floccosum and Trichophyton rubrum
Tinea cruris	Trichophyton Rubrum and Epidermophyton Floccosum
Commonest predisposing factor for Candida	Diabetes
Chlamydospores on Corn Meal Agar	Candida
Germ tube test (Reynolds Braude phenomenon)	Candida albicans
Botryomycosis	Staphylococcus aureus
Sclerotic bodies	Chromoblastomycosis
Asteroid bodies	Sporotrichosis
Only deep mycosis common in India	Cryptococcosis

Contd...

Contd...

Fungal infection transmitted through bird faeces	Histoplasmosis
Tuberculate spores	Histoplasmosis
Commonest human disease caused by Aspergillus	Otomycosis
Aflatoxin	Aspergillus Flavus
Fungus which has not been cultivated in any media	Rhinosporidium seeberi
India Ink Negative staining	Cryptococcus
Fungi without any known sexual reproduction	Fungi imperfecti or Deuteromycetes
Vascular invasion	Mucormycosis

Table 5.5: FAQ – Immune system

Schultz-Dale reaction	In vitro anaphylaxis
Prausnitz-Kutzner reaction	Type 1 hypersensitivity
Arthus reaction	Local manifestation of Type 3 Hypersensitivity
Serum sickness	Systemic manifestation of Type 3 Hypersensitivity
Giant peroxidase positive inclusions	Chediak-Higashi syndrome
Nitroblue Tetrazolium test	screening test-Chronic Granulomatous Disease
Multiple large cold Staphylococcal abscesses	Job's syndrome
Primary lymphoid organs	Thymus and bone marrow
Secondary Lymphoid organs	Lymph nodes, Spleen and Mucosa associated Lymphoid tissue (MALT)

IMMUNODIFFUSION PROCEDURES (ANANTHANARAYAN, 8TH ED.)

Immunodiffusion is	Precipitation in gel
Single Diffusion in 1 DIMENSION	Oudin procedure (Mnemonic single 'O')
Single Diffusion in 2 DIMENSIONS	Radial Immunodiffusion
Double Diffusion in 1 DIMENSION	Oakley Fulthorpe Procedure *(Two 'O's in two words)*
Double Diffusion in 2 DIMENSIONS	Ouchterlony Procedure *(Two 'O's in single word)*
Special variety of Double Diffusion in 2 DIMENSIONS	Elek's test
Elek's test is used for	toxigenicity in Diphtheria Bacilli

Contd...

Contd...

Resolving power of Immunodiffusion is greatly enhanced by:	Immunoelectrophoresis (Grabar and Williams)
Electrophoresis combined with Immunodiffusion	Immunoelectrophoresis
1 DIMENSIONAL double electroimmunodiffusion	Counter Immunoelectrophoresis (CIE)
1 DIMENSIONAL Single Electroimmunodiffusion	Rocket Electrophoresis
Laurell's two-dimensional Electrophoresis is a variant of	Rocket Electrophoresis

CHLAMYDIAE

Most common sexually transmitted infection worldwide	Chlamydia
Chlamydia implicated to have a causative role in Vascular Atheromatous disease	Chlamydia pneumoniae
Chlamydial strain isolated from Taiwan and named TWAR (Taiwan Acute Respiratory)	Chlamydia pneumoniae
Ornithosis is caused by	Chlamydia psittaci
Levinthal Cole Lillie (LCL) Bodies are seen in	Chlamydia psittaci
Chlamydial Infection presenting as a Typhoid-like syndrome	Chlamydia psittaci
Miyagawa's granulocorpuscles are seen in	Lymphogranuloma venereum (Chlamydia trachomatis)
Most common strain of Chalmydia trachomatis causing LGV	L2
Perihepatitis as a part of Genital Chlamydiasis is called	Fitz-Hugh-Curtis syndrome.
Most commonly used cell culture methods for isolation of CHLAMYDIAE	McCoy and HeLa cells
Frei's test for diagnosis of LGV by skin testing is no longer used because of	High false positive

HISTORY OF MICROBIOLOGY

Antiseptic Techniques	Joseph Lister
Proposition of contagion vivum as a cause of Infectious Disease	Fracastorius
First observation and reporting of Bacteria	Leeuwenhock

Contd...

Term Vaccine was coined by	Louis Pasteur
Rabies Vaccine	Louis Pasteur
Discovery of Tubercle Bacillus and Cholera Vibrio	Robert Koch
Leprosy Bacillus	Hansen
Syphilis spirochete was identified by	Schaudinn and Hoffman
Gonococcus	Neisser
Staphylococcus	Ogston
Steam Steriliser/Autoclave/Hot Air Oven	Louis Pasteur
Biological Standardisation	Paul Ehlrich
First identified Viral disease	Yellow Fever
Electron Microscope	Ruska
Antibody	Von Behring and Kitasato
Term Virus was coined by:	Beijerinck
Phagocytosis was discovered by	Metchnikoff

ACTINOMYCOSIS

Most prevalent form of Actinomyces	Actinomyces israelii
Actinomycetes	Traditionally considered to be transitional forms between bacteria and fungi. Currently, they are recognized as **True Bacteria** with a superficial resemblance to fungi.
Name is derived from	Ray fungus or **Sun Ray Appearance** of the organism in the granules that characterise the lesions.
Actinomyces spp. are	*Gram Positive bacilli* Nonmotile, Nonsporing, Non-capsulated filaments. *Facultative Anaerobes*
Actinomyces	Normally colonise the human mouth, digestive and genital tracts.
Molar tooth colony on Agar	Actinomyces israelii
Bread Crumb Colonies	Actinomyces israelii
On Solid media, Actinomyces israelii produces	Spidery Colonies
Colour of Sulfur granules	Yellow
Size of Sulfur granule	0.1–1 mm in diameter

Contd...

Contd...

Sulfur granules are composed of	Internal tangle of mycelial fragments and a rosette of peripheral clubs.
DOC Actinomycosis	Penicillin G or Amoxicillin for prolonged periods (6-12 months in some cases)
Most common clinical form of Actinomycosis	Cervicofacial Actinomycosis or Lumpy Jaw Syndrome.
Pelvic Actinomycosis associated with	IUD (Intrauterine Device) Use
Actinomyces are also involved in pathogenesis of	Bisphosphonate Osteonecrosis of Jaw (BONJ)
Typical presentation of Actinomycosis	Multiple Abscesses with draining sinus tracts on the skin surface or mucosa, with thick yellow exudate with characteristic Sulfur granules.
How to Differentiate Actinomycotic Mycetoma from Eumycetoma.	**Actinomycotic Mycetoma** • Granules white to yellow. • Examination of crushed smears of granules – Thin filaments (1 micron size) **Eumycetoma** • Black granules • Examination of crushed smears of granules – Stout filaments (4–5 micron size)

6 Pharmacology

" When I woke up just after dawn on September 28,1928 I certainly didn't plan to revolutionize all medicine by discovering the world's first antibiotic, or bacteria killer, but I guess that was exactly what I did...."
—*Alexander Fleming*

REFERENCE

❏ *Essentials of Medical Pharmacology by KD Tripathi 7th ed.*

LEVEL I: BASIC REPEATS

GENERAL

❏ Drug binding to the receptor and causing opposite action of the agonist is called as an Inverse agonist.
(DNB PATTERN DEC 2009)

❏ Zero Order Kinetics is independent of total drug concentationj in plasma. *(DNB PATTERN DEC 2009)*

❏ cAMP is NOT the second messenger for Insulin.
(DNB PATTERN 2004)

❏ First pass metabolism is seen in Propranalol.
(DNB PATTERN 2004)

❏ Clearance of a drug is the unit volume of the plasma which is cleared off the drug in unit time. *(DNB PATTERN 2002)*

❏ Elimination of alcohol follows Zero order kinetics.
(DNB PATTERN 2000)

❏ As per drugs and cosmetic act, prescription drugs are included in SCHEDULE H. *(DNB PATTERN JUNE 2011)*

❏ Therapeutic index is a measure of safety.
(DNB PATTERN JUNE 2011)

❏ Systemic Antacid is: Sodium Hydroxide.
(DNB PATTERN JUNE 2014)

❏ Therapeutic use in Human subjects comes under which phase of clinical trial? Phase IV. *(DNB PATTERN JUNE 2014)*

❏ Zero order kinetics is seen with: Alcohol.
(DNB PATTERN 2003)

❏ Zero order kinetics at higher doses is followed by: Propranalol, Phenytoin. *(DNB PATTERN 2000)*

❏ ORPHAN DRUGS: includes drugs for some common diseases in developing countries. *(NEET PATTERN 2016)*

- ORPHAN RECEPTORS: are receptors for which there is NO endogenous ligand. *(NEET PATTERN 2016)*
- BIOAVAILABILITY is defined as: AUC (oral)/AUC (intravenous)* 100. *(NEET PATTERN 2016)*
- Logarithmic graded dose response curve is: Sigmoid. *(NEET PATTERN 2016)*
- At pKA = pH: Concentration of Drug is 50% Ionic AND 50% Non Ionic. *(NEET PATTERN 2018)*

ANESTHETICS

- Emergence delirium is characteristic of Ketamine. *(DNB PATTERN JUNE 2009)*

ANTIEPILEPTICS

- Nephrotoxicity is NOT a side effect of Valproic Acid. *(DNB PATTERN 2008)*
- DOC Absence seizure–Valproate. *(DNB PATTERN JUNE 2012)*
- Phenobarbitone does NOT cause thrombocytopenia *(DNB PATTERN 2000)*
- NOT a side effect of Valproic acid: Hirsutism. *(DNB PATTERN JUNE 2011)*
- Dilantin causes folic acid deficiency. *(DNB PATTERN JUNE 2011)*
- Drug which is highly albumin bound–Barbiturate. *(DNB PATTERN JUNE 2012)*
- Drug recommended for Absence Seizures: Lamotrigine. *(NEET PATTERN 2014)*
- Drug preferred for Resistant Rheumatic Chorea: Valproate *(NEET PATTERN 2018)*

ANTIBIOTICS

- Drugs whose dose need NOT be reduced in renal failure: Penicillins. *(DNB PATTERN 2000)*
- Long post antibiotic effect is seen in Quinolones. *(DNB PATTERN JUNE 2012)*
- Prophylaxis of Meningococcal Meningitis: Rifampicin. *(DNB PATTERN JUNE 2009)*
- Drug used in prophylaxis of meningococcal meningitis: Rifampicin. *(DNB PATTERN DEC 2011)*
- False about Rifampicin: used in treatment of meningococcal meningitis. *(DNB PATTERN DEC 2011)*
- Treatment of non-specific urethritis is: Erythromycin. *(DNB PATTERN 2000)*

Pharmacology

- Drug used in the treatment of resistant Gonorrhea: Spectinomycin. *(DNB PATTERN 2000)*
- Penicillin does NOT precipitate G6PD deficiency. *(DNB PATTERN 2000)*
- Which tetracycline can be used in renal failure without dose adjustment? Doxycycline. *(DNB PATTERN DEC 2011)*
- Mechanism of Action of Quinolones is DNA gyrase inhibitors. *(DNB PATTERN JUNE 2011)*
- In treatment of Pseudomonas infection, Carbenicillin toxicity is frequently combined with Gentamycin. *(DNB PATTERN 2001)*
- Antibiotic causing Pseudomembranous colitis: Clindamycin. *(DNB PATTERN 2000)*
- NOT used in treatment of Helicobactor Pylori: Cisapride. *(DNB PATTERN JUNE 2009)*
- DOC of malaria in pregnancy: Chloroquine. *(DNB PATTERN JUNE 2011)*
- Niclosamide is NOT a treatment of Neurocysticercosis. *(DNB PATTERN 2000)*
- Probenecid does NOT decrease the renal excretion of Cephaloridine. *(DNB PATTERN 2003)*
- Pseudolymphoma is caused by Penicillin. *(DNB PATTERN DEC 2011)*
- Drug that inhibits cell wall synthesis is: Penicillin. *(DNB PATTERN DEC 2011)*
- Penicillinase resistant Penicillin is Methicillin. *(DNB PATTERN 2001)*
- Treatment of choice for Legionnaires' disease: Azithromycin/Ciprofloxacin. *(DNB PATTERN 2003)*
- Cholestatic jaundice is a side effect of Erythromycin. *(DNB PATTERN 2004)*
- Drug which can cause hypertrophic pyloric stenosis is: Erythromycin. *(DNB PATTERN DEC 2011)*
- Metrifonate is effective against Schistosomiasis. *(DNB PATTERN 2008)*
- Extended activity of beta lactamases inactivate cephalosporins 3rd generation. *(DNB PATTERN 2002)*
- The ratio of concentration of drug in cotrimoxazole of trimethoprim and sulfamethoxazole is 1:5. *(DNB PATTERN 2002)*
- Drug of choice of rickettsial infections in pregnancy: chloramphenicol *(NEET PATTERN 2014)*

- Antibiotic with Antiplatelet action: Cephalosporins. *(NEET PATTERN 2014)*
- Most sensitive marker for CARBAPENEMASE production is: Resistance to ERTAPENEM. *(NEET PATTERN 2014)*
- ERTAPENEM is NOT effective against Pseudomonas. *(NEET PATTERN 2015)*
- ERTAPENEM is not recommended for the treatment of Nosocomial infections. *(NEET PATTERN 2015)*
- Aminoglycoside with more cochlear toxicity than Vestibular toxicity: Kanamycin. *(NEET PATTERN 2016)*
- Pill Induced Esophagitis is most commonly associated with: DOXYCYCLINE. *(NEET PATTERN 2016)*
- Mycoplasma is resistant to: Ceftriaxone. *(NEET PATTERN 2018)*
- NOT a bacteriostatic Antibiotic: Vancomycin. *(NEET PATTERN 2018)*
- Anaerobes are intrinsically resistant against: Aminoglycosides. *(NEET PATTERN 2018)*

ANTIVIRAL DRUGS

- Cidofovir can be used for: Respiratory papillomatosis, Herpes zoster, Herpes simplex. *(DNB PATTERN DEC 2011)*
- NOT a prodrug: Valacyclovir. *(DNB PATTERN JUNE 2009)*
- Podophyllin is used to treat which type of wart? Genital wart. *(DNB PATTERN 2007)*
- Neuraminidase inhibitor: Oseltamivir. *(NEET PATTERN 2013)*
- Antiretroviral drug with antihepatitis activity: EMTRICITABINE. *(NEET PATTERN 2018)*
- Antihepatitis Drug with anti HIV action: ENTECAVIR.

ANTIPSYCHOTICS

- Drug with both antidepressant and antipsychotic properties: Amoxapine. *(DNB PATTERN JUNE 2009)*
- Lithium produces Hypothyroidism. *(DNB PATTERN 2003)*
- Appetite is NOT decreased by Olanzapine. *(DNB PATTERN 2001)*
- Antipsychotic with partial agonist action on D2/5HT1A – Aripiprazole. *(DNB PATTERN JUNE 2012)*

ANTITUBERCULAR DRUGS

- Rifampicin acts by: DNA dependent RNA polymerase. *(DNB PATTERN DEC 2011)*

- Which of the following causes OCP failure? Rifampicin. *(DNB PATTERN JUNE 2011)*
- A bacteriostatic antitubercular drug? Ethambutol. *(DNB PATTERN DEC 2011)*
- NOT a cause of Gynecomastia: Pyrazinamide. *(DNB PATTERN 2005)*
- Most effective antitubercular drug against slow multiplying intracellular mycobacteria: Rifampicin. *(DNB PATTERN 2002)*
- NOT a hepatotoxic antitubercular drug: Ethambutol. *(DNB PATTERN 2002)*
- DNA dependent RNA synthesis is inhibited by Rifampicin. *(DNB PATTERN 2001)*
- Resistance to drugs in Tuberculosis develops by Mutation. *(DNB PATTERN 2003)*
- NOT a cause of gynecomastia: Pyrazinamide. *(DNB PATTERN 2001)*
- A person on ATT complained of deafness and tinnitus in one ear. Drug implicated is Streptomycin. *(DNB PATTERN JUNE 2011)*
- NOT a side effect of Isoniazid: Thrombocytopenia. *(DNB PATTERN DEC 2011)*
- ATT entering caseous tissue: Rifampicin. *(DNB PATTERN AUG 2013)*
- Gene for Rifampicin resistance: rpoB. *(FMGE PATTERN JUNE 2014)*
- Antitubercular Drug contraindicated in Pregnancy: Streptomycin. *(FMGE PATTERN JUNE 2014)*
- Streptomycin is contraindicated in pregnancy because it is known to cause 8th cranial nerve damage to the fetus. *(HARRISON 17/e p864)*
- Antitubercular Drug which causes side effect of suicidal tendency? Isoniazid. *(FMGE PATTERN JUNE 2014)*
- Antitubercular agents which DOES not induce a LAG phase: Thioacetazone. *(NEET PATTERN 2014)*
- Most common type of gene resistance to Isoniazid in patients with Tuberculosis: katG. *(NEET PATTERN 2014)*
- XDR TB implies resistance to: INH/Rifampicin, any Quinolone and one injectable second line drug. *(NEET PATTERN 2014)*
- Treatment of choice of Tuberculosis in Pregnancy: HRE 2 months + HR 7 months. *(NEET PATTERN 2015)*
- Antitubercular Drug with highest sterilizing action: Rifampicin. *(NEET PATTERN 2016)*

- Antitubercular Drug with highest ability to prevent resistance to Isoniazid: Rifampicin. *(NEET PATTERN 2016)*

ANTIDIABETICS

- In diabetes mellitus with increased HbA1c, drug that is NOT used in treatment is Biguanides. *(DNB PATTERN DEC 2011)*
- Drug used in Postprandial sugar control is Repaglinide. *(DNB PATTERN DEC 2011)*
- Long acting insulin is: Insulin glargine. *(DNB PATTERN DEC 2011)*
- Peakless Insulin is: Insulin Glargine. *(NEET PATTERN 2015)*
- True about cause of lactic acidosis: Biguanides. *(DNB PATTERN 2000)*
- NOT true about Acarbose: useful for both pre- and postprandial hyperglycemia. *(DNB PATTERN 2008)*
- Drug used in Diabetes: Acetohexamide. *(DNB PATTERN 2001)*
- Drug used in Diabetic Neuropathy: Pregabalin. *(DNB PATTERN AUG 2013)*

ANTIHYPERTENSIVES

- Antihypertensive agent which decreases libido: Methyldopa. *(DNB PATTERN 2002)*
- Antihypertensive drug contraindicated in pregnancy is: Enalapril. *(DNB PATTERN JUNE 2011)*
- Beta-blockers are indicated in Hypertension. *(DNB PATTERN 2000)*
- Alpha 1 adrenergic blocker without any effect on blood pressure: Tamsulosin. *(DNB PATTERN JUNE 2011)*
- SLE like reaction is caused by: Hydralazine. *(DNB PATTERN JUNE 2011)*
- Antihypertensive which causes decreased libido and impotence: Atenolol. *(DNB PATTERN 2001)*
- Antihypertensive which can be used in Gout and diabetes mellitus is: Enalapril. *(DNB PATTERN 2001)*
- NOT an adverse effect of Losartan: Cough. *(DNB PATTERN JUNE 2011)*
- ACE inhibitors may aggravate renovascular hypertension. *(DNB PATTERN JUNE 2009)*
- Spironolactone should NOT be given with ACE inhibitors. *(DNB PATTERN 2007)*

- Diuretic which is a sulfonamide: Acetazolamide.
  (DNB PATTERN AUG 2013)
- Loop Diuretics have what action with Thiazides? Synergistic Action. *(DNB PATTERN AUG 2013)*
- Potassium sparing Drug: Spironolactone.
  (FMGE PATTERN MAR 2013)
- Spironolactone is least commonly used in: Hypertension.
  (FMGE PATTERN SEP 2011)
- Diuretic causing maximum loss of Potassium in urine: Acetazolamide. *(FMGE PATTERN MAR 2010)*
- Drug of Choice for hypertension in Systemic Sclerosis: ACE inhibitor. *(NEET PATTERN 2013)*
- Acetazolamide decreases intraocular pressure by: Decreased aqueous humor production. *(FMGE PATTERN SEP 2010)*
- Antihypertensive contraindicated in pregnancy: ACE inhibitors. *(NEET PATTERN 2013)*
- DRUG OF CHOICE for Hypertension in patients with Metabolic Syndrome and no Diabetes Mellitus: ACE Inhibitor. *(NEET PATTERN 2014)*

ANTICANCER DRUGS

- Anticancer drug causing lung fibrosis: Bleomycin.
  (DNB PATTERN JUNE 2009)
- Treatment for chronic phase of CML: Imatinib.
  (DNB PATTERN JUNE 2009)
- Microtubule formation is inhibited by Vincristine.
  (DNB PATTERN DEC 2011)
- Imatinib primarily acts on: Tyrosine kinase.
  (DNB PATTERN DEC 2011)
- Bevacizumab is Monoclonal antibody against Vascular Endothelial Growth Factor. *(DNB PATTERN JUNE 2011)*
- Cladarabine belongs to the class of Alkylating agents.
  (DNB PATTERN JUNE 2009)
- True about Azathioprine: It selectively affects differentiation of T cells. *(DNB PATTERN JUNE 2009)*
- Ifosfamide is an Alkylating agent. *(DNB PATTERN 2008)*
- Abciximab is NOT a tumor necrosis factor blocking agent.
  (DNB PATTERN 2008)
- Antineoplastic agent which is also an antifolate drug: Methotrexate. *(DNB PATTERN 2002)*
- Drug of choice in choriocarcinoma is: Methotrexate.
  (DNB PATTERN 2001)

- Drug used to counteract Methotrexate toxicity: Folinic Acid. *(DNB PATTERN 2001)*
- Drug which acts by binding to P site in Prokaryotes: Actinomycin D. *(DNB PATTERN 2001)*
- Cyclosporin A acts on CD 4 cells and lymphocytes. *(DNB PATTERN 2003)*
- Monoclonal antibody used in Renal Cell Carcinoma: Sunitinib. *(DNB PATTERN AUG 2013)*
- Anti cancer drug causing Noncardiogenic Pulmonary Edema: GEMCITABINE. *(JIPMER PATTERN 2017)*
- Mechanism of action of BORTEZOMIB: Proteasome Inhibitor. *(JIPMER PATTERN 2017)*
- Bortezomib: Inhibits the mammalian 26S Proteasome. Used in Multiple Myeloma.

CARDIAC DRUGS

- NOT a contributing factor to Digoxin toxicity: Hyperkalemia. *(DNB PATTERN 2008)*
- Digoxin can accumulate to toxic levels in patient with Renal insufficiency. *(DNB PATTERN 2008)*
- NOT a cardioselective beta-blocker – Pindolol. *(DNB PATTERN 2002)*
- Drug NOT used in Prinzmetal's Angina: Propranalol. *(DNB PATTERN 2000, 2001)*
- Isovolumic diuretic: Indacrinone. *(DNB PATTERN 2001)*
- Dialysis is NOT indicated in Digitalis toxicity. *(DNB PATTERN 2000)*
- Hemodialysis is NOT effective in Nifedipine poisoning. *(DNB PATTERN 2000)*
- HIT syndrome–occurs commonly in about a week, less common with fractionated heparin, causes both arterial and venous thrombosis, LMWH should not be used for treatment. *(DNB PATTERN JUNE 2011)*
- Drugs used in atrial arrhythmias: Digoxin, Verapamil, Quinidine NOT Lignocaine. *(DNB PATTERN JUNE 2011)*
- Beta-blocker with Beta 2 receptor agonism–Celiprolol *(DNB PATTERN JUNE 2012)*
- Pulsus Bigeminy is seen in: Digitalis Toxicity. *(DNB PATTERN AUG 2013)*
- CLOPIDOGREL is NOT to be used in oral anticoagulation in high risk patients with Atrial Fibrillaton. *(NEET PATTERN 2014)*

MISCELLANEOUS

- NOT a GABA A agonist: Buspirone.
  (DNB PATTERN JUNE 2009)
- NOT a cause of Gynecomastia: Levodopa.
  (DNB PATTERN JUNE 2009)
- Carbidopa is used in the treatment of Parkinsonism because it decreases peripheral utilization of L dopa.
  (DNB PATTERN 2002)
- Drug of choice in Theophylline poisoning: Charcoal Hemoperfusion. *(DNB PATTERN 2007)*
- NOT a bronchodilator: Steroids.
  (DNB PATTERN JUNE 2009)
- Neostigmine increases gastrointestinal motility.
  (DNB PATTERN 2007)
- Drug useful in the prophylaxis of Migraine: Propranalol.
  (DNB PATTERN 2007)
- Formula for parenteral iron therapy: 4.4 * body weight * Hemoglobin deficit. *(DNB PATTERN 2008)*
- Thallidomide is NOT useful in HIV-related Neuropathy.
  (DNB PATTERN 2008)
- Rate limiting enzyme for the biosynthesis of dopamine is Tyrosine Hydroxylase. *(DNB PATTERN 2004)*
- Treatment of choice of cyanide poisoning is: Sodium Nitrite followed by thiosulfate. *(DNB PATTERN 2004)*
- Aspirin is contraindicated for patient on Warfarin.
  (DNB PATTERN 2005)
- Hyperprolactinemia is a side effect of Metoclopramide.
  (DNB PATTERN 2005)
- Antidote of Heparin: Protamine sulfate.
  (DNB PATTERN 2000)
- Drug causing Parkinsonism: Metoclopramide.
  (DNB PATTERN 2001)
- Antihelminthic also acting as immunomodulator: Levamisole.
  (DNB PATTERN 2001)
- Mechanism of action of Colchicine: Suppresses immunity.
  (DNB PATTERN 2001)
- Glucocorticoids does NOT cause reduced appetite.
  (DNB PATTERN 2001)
- Octreotide is NOT an absorbent. *(DNB PATTERN 2001)*
- Corticosteroid given by inhalation route: Beclomethasone.
  (DNB PATTERN 2001)

- Drug in Bronchial asthma which needs monitoring: Theophylline. *(DNB PATTERN 2001)*
- Corticosteroid which needs least systemic monitoring: Budesonide. *(DNB PATTERN 2001)*
- Antiemetic frequently used in cancer chemotherapy induced vomiting: Ondansetron. *(DNB PATTERN 2001)*
- Chronic steroid therapy does NOT cause Optic Neuritis. *(DNB PATTERN 2000)*
- Botulinum acts by inhibiting acetylcholine release. *(DNB PATTERN 2000)*
- Flumazenil is opiate agonist. *(DNB PATTERN 2000)*
- Theophyllin levels in blood are increased by Phenylbutazone. *(DNB PATTERN 2000)*
- Aspirin is contraindicated in a case who is on treatment with Warfarin. *(DNB PATTERN 2000)*
- Hyperprolactinemia is a side effect of Metoclopramide. *(DNB PATTERN 2000)*
- Uricosuric drug used for Gout: Sulfinpyrazone. *(DNB PATTERN 2003)*
- Drug of choice for Addison's Disease: Hydrocortisone. *(DNB PATTERN 2003)*
- Most potent cardiac stimulant is Adrenaline. *(DNB PATTERN 2003)*
- Action of Dapsone is antagonized by Para-aminobenzoic Acid. *(DNB PATTERN 2003)*
- Clomiphene is Anti-estrogen. *(DNB PATTERN 2003)*
- Epinephrine does NOT cross plasma membrane. *(DNB PATTERN 2003)*
- Which is not an alkaloid? Neostigmine. *(DNB PATTERN DEC 2011)*
- Effect of morphine which has least tolerance is: Constipation. *(DNB PATTERN DEC 2011)*
- Bisphosphonates are NOT used in Vitamin D intoxication. *(DNB PATTERN JUNE 2011)*
- Alpha 1 adrenergic blocker given for symptomatic relief in BPH: Tamsulosin. *(DNB PATTERN JUNE 2011)*
- Peripheral neuropathy not caused by antiretroviral drug: Lamivudine. *(DNB PATTERN JUNE 2011)*
- True about Bicalutamide is: Binds to Androgen receptor, causes gynecomastia, can be given as monotherapy in prostatic carcinoma. *(DNB PATTERN JUNE 2011)*
- Most common side effect of Salbutamol is: Tremors. *(DNB PATTERN JUNE 2011)*

- Nicotine replacement therapy is available in the following forms: gum, patches, lozenges NOT tablets. *(DNB PATTERN JUNE 2011)*
- Not a side effect of Prostaglandin–Convulsions. *(DNB PATTERN JUNE 2012)*
- An opioid with antitussive action–Codeine. *(DNB PATTERN JUNE 2012)*
- Loop diuretics act on Ascending limb of loop of Henle. *(DNB PATTERN JUNE 2012)*
- Sibutramine belongs to which group of drugs? Anti-obesity. *(DNB PATTERN JUNE 2012)*
- Allopurinol inhibits which enzyme? Xanthine oxidase. (Allopurinol and gout are another of examiners tasteless obsessions–suffer). *(DNB PATTERN JUNE 2012)*
- Which is an ADP receptor inhibitor? Clopidogrel. *(DNB PATTERN JUNE 2012)*
- Dose of mebendazole for the treatment of Ascariasis: 100 mg bd * 3 days. *(DNB PATTERN JUNE 2012)*
- Atropine is most sensitive to mucous and pharyngeal secretions. *(DNB PATTERN DEC 2011)*
- Which is not an effect of atropine? Bradycardia. *(DNB PATTERN DEC 2011)*
- HbA1c is decreased most by Sulfonylureas. *(DNB PATTERN DEC 2011)*
- Drug which should not be given with Apomorphine is Ondansetron. *(DNB PATTERN DEC 2011)*
- In anaphylactic shock, epinephrine is given by which route? Intramuscular. *(DNB PATTERN DEC 2011)*
- Which of the following is an example of endogenous/physiological antagonism? Prostacyclin thromboxane. *(DNB PATTERN DEC 2011)*
- In the treatment of shock, Dibutamine is preferred over Dopamine because it is beta 1 specific, does not cause vasoconstriction and is less arrythmogenic, and does not affect renal vasculature. *(DNB PATTERN DEC 2011)*
- Drug used in treatment of obesity are: Sibutramine, Orlistat, Rimonabant. *(DNB PATTERN DEC 2011)*
- All are true about estrogen except: used in treatment of gynecomastia. *(DNB PATTERN DEC 2011)*
- Most hepatotoxic anabolic steroid is: Stanozolol. *(DNB PATTERN DEC 2011)*
- Fastest acting antithyroid drug is: Potassium iodide. *(DNB PATTERN DEC 2011)*

- NOT a topical steroid: Prednisolone.
  (DNB PATTERN DEC 2011)
- Treatment of choice in Maduramycosis: Ketoconazole.
  (DNB PATTERN AUG 2013)
- Intranasal Calcitonin is used for: Postmenopausal Osteoporosis.
  (DNB PATTERN AUG 2013)
- Bosentan mechanism of action: Endothelin 1 antagonist at ET1 and ET2 receptor, Primarily used as a treatment for Pulmonary Arterial Hypertension.
  (DNB PATTERN AUG 2013)
- Mechanism of action of Montelukast: Leukotriene antagonist.
  (DNB PATTERN AUG 2013)
- Sulfasalazine is used in: Ulcerative Colitis.
  (FMGE PATTERN MAR 2011)
- Laboratory monitoring of which is desirable with Low Molecular Heparin Therapy? Anti Factor Xa activity.
  (FMGE PATTERN MAR 2012)
- Statin having longest half life: Rosuvastatin.
  (FMGE PATTERN SEP 2012)
- Thrombolytics are least useful in: Hemorrhagic Stroke.
  (FMGE PATTERN MAR 2013)
- Mechanism of action of Statins: HMG-CoA Reductase inhibitor.
  (FMGE PATTERN MAR 2013)
- Drug of choice of NSAID induced gastric ulcer: Misoprostol.
  (FMGE PATTERN SEP 2008, MAR 2012)
- Montelukast acts via: Cys Leukotriene receptor.
  (DNB PATTERN JUNE 2014)
- TERIPARATIDE is used in: Osteoporosis.
  (DNB PATTERN JUNE 2014)
- CAPECITABINE acts via: converts to 5 Fluorouracil.
  (DNB PATTERN JUNE 2014)
- Aspirin acts via: Irreversible COX inhibition.
  (DNB PATTERN JUNE 2014)
- HAND-FOOT-MOUTH SYNDROME a variant of Hand-Foot-Mouth Disease is a potential side effect of: SORAFENIB.
  (NEET PATTERN 2014)
- SILDENAFIL is contraindicated in patients taking NITRATES.
  (NEET PATTERN 2014)
- ALISKIREN (Direct Renin Inhibitor) IS CURRENTLY NOT A FIRST LINE Antihypertyensive Drug.
  (NEET PATTERN 2014)
- VARENICLINE is: a partial agonist on Acetylcholine Receptors.
  (NEET PATTERN 2014)

Pharmacology

- Recommended dose of TAMIFLU for the treatment of Swine Flu in Adults is: 75 mg B.I.D * 5 days.
  (NEET PATTERN 2014)
- GRAMICIDIN S is a cyclic decapeptide.
  (NEET PATTERN 2015)
- TORCETRAPIB is: Cholesteryl Ester Transfer Protein Inhibitor (CETP) for the treatment of Dyslipidemia.
  (NEET PATTERN 2015)
- Effect of Adrenaline after alpha receptor blockade: Fall in BP.
  (NEET PATTERN 2016)
- Mechanism of Action of LEVOSIMENDAN: Calcium Sensitizer. *(NEET PATTERN 2016)*
- This treatment is a type of Placebo: Sham Surgery.
  (AIIMS PATTERN 2017)
- General advice to Lactating mothers with regard to drug intake: Give breast feed just before next dosage as drug levels would be minimum. *(AIIMS PATTERN 2017)*
- Patient on Haloperidol, very restless and moving about for the last few days. Condition to be suspected is: Akathisia.
  (AIIMS PATTERN 2017)
- OLCEGEPANT is an example of: Calcitonin Gene Related Peptide (CGRP) Antagonist. *(JIPMER PATTERN 2017)*
- Example of Bi specific T cell Engagers (BiTEs): BLINATUMOMAB. *(JIPMER PATTERN 2017)*
- Site of action of Amphotericin B: Cell Wall.
  (NEET PATTERN 2018)
- Site of action of Amphotericin B: Plasma membrane.
  (NEET PATTERN 2018)
- Amphotericin B acts through pore formation at the cell membrane after binding to Ergosterol.
- Tadalafil cannot be combined with: Vasodilators.
  (NEET PATTERN 2018)
- Tadalafil when combined with Nitrates may produce serious hypotension.
- Tadalafil and Sildenafil can cause a rare side effect called Non Arteritic Ischemic Optic Neuropathy. (NAION)
- Tadalafil is also useful in Pulmonary Arterial Hypertension.
- Melanosis Coli is caused by long term use of: Senna.
  (NEET PATTERN 2018)
- APIXABAN is: Direct Factor Xa inhibitor.
  (NEET PATTERN 2018)
- Centrally acting alpha 2 agonist muscle relaxant: Tizanidine.
  (NEET PATTERN 2018)

- ❏ Endothelin acts through: Cyclic GMP.
  (NEET PATTERN 2018)
- ❏ BASILIXIMAB is an IL-2 receptor antagonist.
  (NEET PATTERN 2018)
- ❏ Metyrapone is: Glucocortcoid Synthesis Inhibitor.
  (NEET PATTERN 2018)
- ❏ SACUBITRIL is a: Neutral Endopeptidase Inhibitor.
  (NEET PATTERN 2018)
- ❏ Sacubitrilat, the active form of Sacubitril inhibits the enzyme NEPRILYSIN or Neutral Endopeptidase.
- ❏ Niacin therapy is contraindicated in Diabetics because: It increases blood sugar levels. *(NEET PATTERN 2018)*
- ❏ INCORRECT regarding PRASUGREL: NOT a prodrug.
  (NEET PATTERN 2018)
- ❏ PRASUGREL is a prodrug, similar to Clopidogrel.
- ❏ PIRENZIPINE is used for: Gastric Ulcer.
  (NEET PATTERN 2018)
- ❏ Physiological dose of Hydrocortisone is: 10 mg/m^2/day.
  (NEET PATTERN 2018)

LEVEL II: HIGH YIELD FACTORS

Table 6.1: Antihypertensives – FAQ

Antihypertensive agent of choice in Diabetes Mellitus	ACE inhibitors
Antihypertensive of choice in post-MI patient	Beta-blockers
Antihypertensives contraindicated in Pregnancy	ACE inhibitors/beta-blocker/Diuretics
Antihypertensive agent of choice in Heart failure	ACE inhibitors
Antihypertensive of choice in Pregnancy	Methyldopa
Antihypertensive of choice in Isolated Systolic Hypertension	Diuretics

Table 6.2: Antitubercular drugs

Primary antitibercular drug resistance in India is maximum due to	Isoniazid
Most common Antitubercular drug causing Sideroblastic Anemia	Isoniazid
Antitubercular Drug frequently causing Lupus like symptoms	Isoniazid

Contd...

Contd...

Drug most active on Spurters	Rifampicin
Drug obtained from Streptomyces Mediterraneaas	Rifampicin
Drug causing Orange urine/sweat	Rifampicin
Drug which acts within caseous material	Rifampicin
Most hepatotoxic Antitubercular drug	Pyrazinamide
Optic Neuritis is a side effect of	Ethambutol
Antitubercular drug absolutely contraindicated in Pregnancy	Streptomycin
Antitubercular Drug which does not cross the Blood brain barrier	Streptomycin
Tuberculostatic Ist line Antitubercular drug	Ethambutol
Drug given with Isoniazid to prevent Neurotoxicity	Pyridoxine

Table 6.3: Antibiotics

Linezolid	Binds to 23S fraction of 50S ribosome and interferes with formation of N formyl Methionine-t RNA-70S initiation complex
Macrolides	Inhibits Translocation by binding to 50S ribosome
Chloramphenicol	Binds to 50S ribosome and inhibits prokaryotic peptidyl transferase
Streptomycin	Binds to 30S ribosome and brings about its structural distortion
Most nephrotoxic Cephalosporin	Cephaloridine
Fluoroquinolone with highest CSF penetration	Pefloxacin
Most nephrotoxic Aminoglycoside	Gentamycin
Most ototoxic Aminoglycoside	Streptomycin
Broadest spectrum Aminoglycoside	Amikacin
4th generation cephalosporins	Cefpirome/Cefepime
5th generation cephalosporins	Ceftobipirole/Ceftaroline

Table 6.4: Antiparasitic drugs

Schistosomiasis	Praziquantel
Strongyloidiasis	Ivermectin
Toxoplasmosis	Pyrimethamine with Clindamycin
Chagas Disease	Nifurtimox or Beznidazole
East African Trypanosomiasis	Melarsoprolol
West African Trypanosomiasis	Pentamidine
Cryptosporidiosis	Nitazoxanide
Kala Azar	Antimony
Cerebral Malaria	Intravenous Quinine

Table 6.5: Antiepileptic drugs

Phenytoin	Zero order kinetics
Lamotrigine	Inhibits voltage gated sodium channels
Vigabatrin	Irreversible inhibitor of GABA transaminase
Topiramate	Carbonic anhydrase inhibitor
Zonisamide	Blocks T type Calcium channels
Levitiracetam	Binds to synaptic vesicular protein
Vigabatrin	Drug of choice in infantile spasms associated with tuberous Sclerosis

Table 6.6: Antifungal drugs

Only oral use antifungals	Griseofulvin/Itraconazole
Mechanism of Action of Griseofulvin	Inhibits Mitosis
Voriconazole	Broad spectrum triazole effective against Invasive Aspergillosis
Cryptococcosis (Pulmonary)	Fluconazole for 3–6 months
Mucormycosis	Amphotericin B
Onychomycosis	Terbenafine/Itraconazole(Oral) * 3 months
Dermatophytosis	Terbenafine/Itraconazole * 1–2 weeks

Table 6.7: CNS drugs

Once daily transdermal patch used in Parkinson's disease	Rotigotine (Dopamine Agonist)
MAO B inhibitors used in Parkinsonism	Selegeline/Rasagiline
COMT inhibitors used in Parkinsonism	Tolcapone/Entacapone

Contd...

Contd...

NMDA Glutamate receptor Antagonist used in Alzheimer's disease	Memantine
Cholinesterase inhibitors used in Alzheimer's disease	Donepezil/Tacrine/Gallantamine
Direct thrombin inhibitors used in Stroke prevention	Dabigatran/Ximelogatran
Monoclonal Antibody used for Multiple Sclerosis	Natalizumab
Melatonergic drug used in the treatment of Insomnia	Ramelteon

7. Preventive and Social Medicine

"Every 10 seconds, we lose a child to hunger. This is more than HIV/AIDS, Malaria and Tuberculosis combined."
—**Josette Sheeran, Former Executive Director, UN World Food Programme.**

REFERENCES
- *Park's Textbook of Preventive and Social Medicine, 24th ed.*

LEVEL I: BASIC REPEATS

WASTE DISPOSAL

- Plastic covers are disposed in black bag. *(DNB PATTERN DEC 2009)*
- Plastic covers of syringes should be deposited in black bag. *(DNB PATTERN DEC 2011)*
- Discarded cytotoxic medicines should be discarded in black bag. *(DNB PATTERN DEC 2010)*
- Waste sharps should be discarded in blue bag. *(DNB PATTERN DEC 2010)*
- Red bag should not be incinerated because it contains Cadmium. *(DNB PATTERN DEC 2010)*
- Syringes and glassware are sterilised by hot air oven. *(DNB PATTERN JUNE 2011)*
- Bangalore method is anaerobic decomposting. *(DNB PATTERN NOV 2015)*
- Indore method is for aerobic decomposting.
- Coimbatore Method: Anaerobic decomposition first, followed by aerobic fermentation.

SCREENING METHODS

- Screening of disease is secondary prevention. *(DNB PATTERN DEC 2011)*
- Breast self-examination is NOT primary prevention. *(DNB PATTERN DEC 2011)*
- Increased false positives in a screening test is due to low prevalence. *(DNB PATTERN DEC 2011)*
- Most important factor in a good screening test is sensitivity. *(DNB PATTERN DEC 2011)*

Preventive and Social Medicine

- Screening of cervical cancer in PHC is done by PAP smear. *(DNB PATTERN JUNE 2011)*
- Ability of a test to correctly diagnose the percentage of people who have the disease is Positive Predictive Value (PPV). *(DNB PATTERN DEC 2009)*
- Missing cases are detected by Sentinel Surveillance. *(DNB PATTERN DEC 2011)*
- Type of surveillance included in the Integrated Disease Control Programme for non-communicable diseases is Periodic Regular Survey. *(DNB PATTERN DEC 2010)*
- 2 standard deviation—95.4%. *(FMGE PATTERN SEP 2012)*
- Frequently repeated value: mode. *(FMGE PATTERN SEP 2012)*
- The incidence of a disease is 4/1000 for a period of 2 years. The prevalence is: 8. *(NEET PATTERN 2018)*
- Prevalence = Incidence Rate x Average Duration of Disease.
- In a screening test for 1000 people for Diabetes, 90 were positive. The gold standard test was then done in which 100 were found to be positive for the disease. The sensitivity of the test is: 90/100. *(NEET PATTERN 2018)*
- Risk among exposed compared to the risk among non exposed is known as: Relative Risk. *(NEET PATTERN 2018)*
- Susceptible persons get disease in range of incubation period from the primary case. This is known as: Secondary Attack Rate. *(NEET PATTERN 2018)*

MOSQUITO

- Number of holes per square inch in a standard mosquito net is 150 (156 is the number as per WHO website). *(DNB PATTERN DEC 2009)*
- Japanese Encephalitis is transmitted by Culex. *(DNB PATTERN DEC 2010)*
- Not caused by Aedes Aegypti: Japanese Encephalitis. *(DNB PATTERN JUNE 2011)*
- Cyclopropagative life cycle is seen in malaria. *(DNB PATTERN JUNE 2011)*

BIOSTATISTICS

- Cause to effect progression is NOT seen in Case control study. *(DNB PATTERN DEC 2011, JUNE 2010)*
- NRR to be 1, Couple Protection Rate should be 60%. *(DNB PATTERN DEC 2011)*

- Strong correlation is implied by a correlation coefficient of 1.
  (DNB PATTERN JUNE 2011)
- Degree of freedom in a 2/2 contingency table is 1.
  (DNB PATTERN JUNE 2011)
- In a left skewed curve, Mean < mode.
  (DNB PATTERN JUNE 2011)
- Chi-square test is used for determination of standard error of difference between proportions.
  (DNB PATTERN DEC 2010)
- Rejecting a null hypothesis when it is true is called a TYPE 1 error.
  (DNB PATTERN DEC 2010)
- When an association between variables is explained by a third association, it is called a confounding bias.
  (DNB PATTERN DEC 2009)
- Berksonian bias is due to differing rates of hospital admissions.
  (DNB PATTERN DEC 2010)
- Simple random sampling is for homogeneous population.
  (DNB PATTERN DEC 2010)
- Hypothesis is not tested by descriptive studies.
  (DNB PATTERN JUNE 2011)
- In a standard normal curve, one standard deviation on either side will be 68%.
  (DNB PATTERN 2000)
- Interval between primary and secondary case is Serial interval.
  (DNB PATTERN JUNE 2011)
- First case that comes to the attention of the physician is the index case.
  (DNB PATTERN JUNE 2011)
- Children surveyed in cluster sampling for coverage of immunisation programme is 30 clusters of 7 children each.
  (DNB PATTERN JUNE 2011)
- Randomised Controlled Trial is not an analytical study.
  (DNB PATTERN JUNE 2011)
- Selection bias can be eliminated by Randomisation.
  (DNB PATTERN DEC 2011)
- In a standard normal curve, one standard deviation on either side will be 68%.
  (DNB PATTERN 2000)
- Village Health Guide is for a population of 5,000.
  (DNB PATTERN 2000)
- NRR = 1, CPR should be 60% *(DNB PATTERN JUNE 2014)*
- Most effective way of eliminating standard error is: Large sample size.
  (NEET PATTERN 2015)
- Ogive is: Cumulative Frequency Curve
  (DNB PATTERN JULY 2016)
- The sensitivity of a diagnostic test is very high. It means that: If the disease is prevalent in the population and the test becomes positive, the patient is likely to have the disease.
  (AIIMS PATTERN 2017)

- When comparing the relationship between two variables, a significant correlation was found between them (p value <.5) though none existed in reality. Type of error seen in the study: Alpha Error. *(AIIMS PATTERN 2017)*
- For NRR to be 1, the couple protection rate must be 60%. *(NEET PATTERN 2018)*
- Out of 100 women who were offered OCP for contraception, 10 people got pregnant when followed for 24 months. The Pearl Index is: 5. *(NEET PATTERN 2018)*
- Study Unit for Ecological Study: Population. *(NEET PATTERN 2018)*

SCALES

- Socioeconomic/Housing scale developed for rural area: Pareek scale *(DNB PATTERN DEC 2009)*
- Ideal Socioeconomic Scale developed for urban Area: Kuppuswamy Scale.
- Kuppuswamy scale DOES NOT include Living/Housing conditions. *(DNB PATTERN DEC 2011)*
- Kuppuswamy Scale includes: Education/Occupation/Income.
- Father of public health: Cholera. *(DNB PATTERN JUNE 2011)*

NFHS (NATIONAL FAMILY HEALTH SURVEY)

- NFHS is done every 5 years. *(DNB PATTERN JUNE 2009)*
  - NFHS-1 1992-93
  - NFHS-2 1997-98
  - NFHS-3 2005-06
  - NFHS-4 2014-15
- Conducted under Ministry of Health and Family Welfare.
- Nodal Agency: International Institute of Population Sciences, Mumbai.

CHLORINE

- Disinfecting action of chlorine is due to hypochlorous acid (major) and hypochlorous ion. *(DNB PATTERN DEC 2011)*
- Minimum chlorine content of water required after chlorination is 0.5 mg/L. *(DNB PATTERN DEC 2011)*
- Sterilisation and disinfection of blood spills is done by Sodium Hypochlorite (Bleach). *(DNB PATTERN DEC 2010)*
- Concentration of sodium hypochlorite in home-made bleaching powder is: 5.25–6.15%. *(DNB PATTERN NOV 2013)*

COMMITTEES

- Rural Health Scheme: Shrivastava Committee. *(DNB PATTERN 2011)*
- Manpower and planning: Bajaj Committee. *(DNB PATTERN 2010)*
- Integration of Health Services: Jungalwalla committee. *(DNB PATTERN 2009)*
- The concept of Female Health guide was given by Kartar Singh Committee. *(DNB PATTERN JUNE 2008)*
- Multipurpose Worker concept introduced by Kartar Singh Committee. *(NEET PATTERN 2015)*
- Millennium Development Goals was started in: 2000. *(DNB PATTERN NOV 2015)*

> - Sustainable Development Goals (SDGs)
> - SDG–17 goals to be met by 2030. Will replace the Millennium Development Goals which expire by 2015. Formed at Rio in 2012.

- Chairman of ESI program: Union Minister for Labour, Government of India *(FMGE PATTERN JUNE 2014)*

INDICES

- Corpulence index used in: Obesity. *(DNB PATTERN JUNE 2008)*
- Efficiency of Malaria elimination programme is evaluated using: Annual Blood Examination Rate. *(DNB PATTERN JUNE 2008)*
- Different communities best compared by: Age specific death rate. *(DNB PATTERN JUNE 2008)*
- Age independent anthropomorphic measure of malnutrition: is Mid-arm Circumference. *(DNB PATTERN 2009)*
- Poverty index does not include income. *(DNB PATTERN JUNE 2010)*
- Index of obesity that does not include height: Corpulence Index. *(DNB PATTERN JUNE 2010)*

> - OBESITY INDICES
> - Quetelet's Index: Weight/(Height)2
> - Ponderal Index: Weight/(Height)3
> - Broca's Index: Height -100
> - Corpulence Index: Actual Weight/Desirable Weight.

- Perinatal mortality includes deaths after 28 weeks to 1st 7 days after birth from a period of viability. *(DNB PATTERN JUNE 2010)*

- Extended definition of Perinatal Mortality includes crown heel length of >35 cm at birth.
  (DNB PATTERN JUNE 2010)
- Normal range of Body Mass Index (BMI) in Asian individual is 18.5 - 22.9. *(DNB PATTERN DEC 2010)*
  - Low BMI - < 18.5
  - Overweight - 23–24.9
  - Obese Type 1 - 25–30
  - Obese Type 2 – >30
- Pearl index is failures of contraception per 100 woman years of exposure. *(DNB PATTERN DEC 2011)*
- PQLI does not include: Per capita income.
  (NEET PATTERN 2013)
- NOT a component of PQLI: Per capita income
  (DNB PATTERN JUNE 2014)
- Not a scale used for assessing socioeconomic status: Likert Scale. *(DNB PATTERN JULY 2016)*
- The Child Pugh score for Chronic Liver Disease classified patients into three categories Category A(5-6), Category B(7-9), Category C (10-15). This is an example of: Ordinal Scale.
  (AIIMS PATTERN 2017)

INFECTIOUS DISEASES

- Man is a dead end host for Tetanus/Measles.
  (DNB PATTERN 2003)
- Prophylaxis to person with Malaria not on medication coming to Bihar: Mefloquine.
  (DNB PATTERN JUNE 2008)
- AFP is confirmed as Polio after surveillance after 60 days.
  (DNB PATTERN DEC 2011)
- Generation time for leprosy is 12–15 days.
  (DNB PATTERN DEC 2011)
- Endemic typhus is transmitted by flea.
  (DNB PATTERN DEC 2011)
- Regarding Poliovirus, true is type 3 most common in India, Type 1 is responsible for most epidemics, Type 2 is eradicated worldwide. *(DNB PATTERN DEC 2011)*
- Rickettsial pox is caused by Rickettsia akari.
  (DNB PATTERN DEC 2011)
- Isolation period of Hepatitis A is 2 weeks.
  (DNB PATTERN DEC 2011)
- To prevent Yellow fever, Aedes aegypti index should be less than 1%. *(DNB PATTERN DEC 2011)*

- Epidemic relapsing fever is transmitted by louse. *(DNB PATTERN DEC 2011)*
- Prevalence of Leprosy in India per 10,000 is 0.69. *(DNB PATTERN DEC 2011)*
- James Lind discovered Scurvy. *(DNB PATTERN DEC 2011)*
- Pig in H1N1 influenza acts as vector. *(DNB PATTERN DEC 2011)*
- Herd Immunity of over 70% is considered necessary to prevent the epidemic spread of Diphtheria. *(DNB PATTERN 2000)*
- National Tuberculosis Institute is located at Bangalore. *(DNB PATTERN 2003)*
- Chandler's index is for Ancylostoma Duodenale. *(DNB PATTERN JUNE 2008)*
- Dracunculiasis transmitted by drinking contaminated water. *(DNB PATTERN JUNE 2008)*
- Multibacillary Leprosy is followed up to: 5 Years. *(DNB PATTERN JUNE 2008)*
- To eradicate Measles, the percentage of children to be vaccinated is 95%. *(DNB PATTERN 2001)*
- Guinea Worm infestation is common in workers in Step wells. *(DNB PATTERN 2000)*
- Cutaneous larva migrans: Ancylostoma braziliense. *(FMGE PATTERN SEP 2012)*
- Chicken pox infective period: 1 day before and 4 days after appearance of rash. *(FMGE PATTERN SEP 2012)*
- Natural host of herpes: man. *(FMGE PATTERN SEP 2012)*
- Last case of small pox was in Somalia. *(DNB PATTERN AUG 2013)*
- Secondary Attack Rate of chicken pox: 90%. *(NEET PATTERN 2013)*
- Ty21A is a vaccine for Typhoid. *(NEET PATTERN 2015)*
- Dukoral vaccine is used for Cholera. *(NEET PATTERN 2015)*
- WHO declared global eradication of small pox on 8th May 1980. *(DNB PATTERN JULY 2016)*
- Epidemic Marker of TB: Sputum AFB positivity rate. *(DNB PATTERN JULY 2016)*
- Annual case detection rate of Leprosy: 10.17/100000. *(AIIMS PATTERN 2017)*
- Mass chemoprophylaxis for Meningococcal Meningitis is: Rifampicin. *(NEET PATTERN 2018)*

- New RNTCP software to monitor the TB Programme is called: NIKSHAY. *(NEET PATTERN 2018)*
- Kala Azar is NOT endemic in: Assam. *(NEET PATTERN 2018)*
- Kala Azar was earlier called Assam Fever but is currently NOT endemic in Assam.

VACCINATION

- Zero dose of Polio vaccine is given at birth. *(DNB PATTERN 2000, 2001)*
- Which is a live vaccine? BCG. *(DNB PATTERN 2000, 2005)*
- Vaccine can be stored at sub-centre for 1 day. *(DNB PATTERN 2000)*

> - National Switch Day
> - 25 April 2016
> - topv to bopv

- Influenza is NOT a live attenuated vaccine. *(DNB PATTERN 2000, 2006)*
- MMR is live attenuated vaccine. *(DNB PATTERN 2009)*
- Measles vaccine is NOT given before 9 months. *(DNB PATTERN 2003)*
- To eradicate Measles, the percentage of population to be vaccinated is at least 95%. *(DNB PATTERN 2006)*
- Use of Yellow Fever vaccine is absolutely contraindicated in pregnancy. *(DNB PATTERN 2007)*
- Adjuvant used in DPT vaccine is Aluminium. *(DNB PATTERN 2009)*
- Rabies vaccine pre-exposure prophylaxis is 0, 7, 28 days. *(DNB PATTERN 2009)*
- Small pox vaccine was discovered by Edward Jenner. *(DNB PATTERN 2010)*
- At PHC level, vaccine storage is by IRL. *(DNB PATTERN 2009)*
- Yellow Fever vaccination is valid for 10 years, beginning from 6 days of certification. *(DNB PATTERN 2011)*
- Day carriers can carry how many vaccine vials? 6–8. *(DNB PATTERN NOV 2013)*
- MMR vaccine is a type of Live attenuated vaccine. *(FMGE PATTERN MAR 2013)*
- Pioneer in Specific Protection by Vaccines was: Chinese. *(DNB PATTERN JULY 2016)*

- In recent reports, cases of Diphtheria are reducing. This is due to Vaccination. *(DNB PATTERN JULY 2016)*
- Surveillance every fortnight is according to which Malaria programme? Modified Plan of Operation. *(DNB PATTERN NOV 2015)*
- Mission Indradhanush was founded in December 2014. *(DNB PATTERN NOV 2015)*
- NOT passive immunity: DPT vaccine *(DNB PATTERN JUNE 2014)*
- Live attenuated vaccine is indicated in polio. *(FMGE PATTERN JUNE 2014)*
- Eradicated disease: Small pox. *(DNB PATTERN JUNE 2014)*
- Ideal interval between administration of two live vaccines is: 4 weeks. *(NEET PATTERN 2018)*

MISCELLANEOUS

- Triage is used for–victims of disaster. *(DNB PATTERN JUNE 2008)*
- Percentage of para isomer in DDT: 70–80%. *(DNB PATTERN JUNE 2008)*
- Spermicide used in contraceptive Today: Non-oxynol. *(DNB PATTERN 2003)*
- Burden of disease formula–(Positives/Tested) * Population. *(DNB PATTERN JUNE 2008)*
- Comfortable temperature range–77–80°F. *(DNB PATTERN JUNE 2008)*
- Mother to be labelled high risk: Height less than 140 cm. *(DNB PATTERN JUNE 2008)*
- The contraceptive method of choice for well-educated 37-year-old woman: Intra uterine Device. *(DNB PATTERN 2002)*
- Upper line in road to health chart corresponds to 50%. *(DNB PATTERN 2001)*
- Commonest cause of Blindness in India: Cataract. *(DNB PATTERN 2001)*
- Randomised controlled trials are clinical trials. *(DNB PATTERN 2002)*
- Extended Sickness Benefit is given for 309 days. *(DNB PATTERN 2002)*
- Best parameter for measuring air pollution is: SO_2. *(DNB PATTERN 2002)*
- Biological value is maximum in Egg. *(DNB PATTERN 2000)*
- Iodine deficient population of the world is 20 million. *(DNB PATTERN 2000)*

- ORS should be discarded after 24 hours.
  (DNB PATTERN 2011)
- Sputum positive TB-1/2 samples positive.
  (DNB PATTERN 2011)
- Highest level of integration of health service: PHC.
  (DNB PATTERN 2009)
- Pulse proteins are poor in Methionine.
  (DNB PATTERN 2009)
- Acculturation is cultural change due to socialisation.
  (DNB PATTERN 2009)
- NOT a principle of primary health care: Decentralised approach. *(DNB PATTERN 2009)*
- Desk for students is Minus desk. *(DNB PATTERN 2009)*
- Daylight factor in living room: 8%. *(DNB PATTERN 2009)*
- Not a goal for 2010 as per National Health Policy 2002: Eradicate Polio. *(DNB PATTERN 2009)*
- Poor man's iron source: Jaggery. *(DNB PATTERN 2009)*
- Reference weight of Indian men and women is 60 kg and 50 kg respectively. *(DNB PATTERN 2009)*
- ICD 10 has 21 chapters. *(DNB PATTERN 2009)*
- Prophylaxis of Meningococcal Meningitis is Rifampicin.
  (DNB PATTERN 2009)
- Desks provided with tabletops in schools to prevent basic neck problems is an example of: Primary Prevention.
  (DNB PATTERN JULY 2010)
- Egg protein biological value: 120.
  (FMGE PATTERN SEP 2012)
- Lactation period-extra energy required: 500–550 kcal.
  (FMGE PATTERN SEP 2012)
- Recommended dietary intake of Zinc at 4 months: 2 mg.
  (DNB PATTERN AUG 2013)
- For Asians, waist hip ratio >0.9 in males and >0.8 in females are indicative of Abdominal Fat accumulation.
  (DNB PATTERN AUG 2013)
- World Health Day: 7 April. *(DNB PATTERN AUG 2013)*
- Headquarters of United Nations: New York.
  (DNB PATTERN AUG 2013)
- Most common cause of Blindness in India: Cataract.
  (DNB PATTERN AUG 2013)
- Pregnant lady with moderate work needs 2600 kcal/day.
  (DNB PATTERN AUG 2013)
- pH of swimming pool water is: 7.4–7.8.
  (DNB PATTERN NOV 2013)

- Osteolathyrism is caused by: Lathyrus odoratus. *(DNB PATTERN NOV 2013)*
- Pandemic of 2003 was caused by: SARS. *(DNB PATTERN NOV 2013)*
- In ICD terminology, signs and symptoms of unknown etiology are classified as: R category. *(DNB PATTERN NOV 2013)*
- South-East Asian Regional Office of WHO (SEARO) is in: New Delhi. *(DNB PATTERN NOV 2013)*
- Recommended daily allowance of Vitamin D is: 400 IU/day. *(DNB PATTERN NOV 2013)*
- Health promotion comes under: primary prevention. *(FMGE PATTERN MAR 2013)*
- Lifestyle modification for children is: Primordial prevention. *(FMGE PATTERN MAR 2013)*
- Disease which shows changes in occurrence over a long period of time is: Secular trend. *(FMGE PATTERN MAR 2013)*
- At the top of the food pyramid: Fats and oils. *(FMGE PATTERN MAR 2013)*
- How many gram of protein is given in Mid-Day Meal? 8–12 gm. *(FMGE PATTERN MAR 2013)*
- False about BFHI: Initiates breast feeding within 4 hrs after delivery. *(NEET PATTERN 2013)*
- False about ASHA: caters to 5,000 population. *(NEET PATTERN 2013)*
- Egg is deficient in: Vitamin D. *(FMGE PATTERN JUNE 2014)*
- Epidemic dropsy is caused by: Sanguinarine *(DNB PATTERN JUNE 2014)*
- Strength of sewage is assessed by: Biological oxygen demand *(DNB PATTERN JUNE 2014)*
- Epidemiological triad consists of: Agent, host, environment *(FMGE PATTERN JUNE 2014)*
- Primary prevention is: Prevention before onset of disease *(FMGE PATTERN JUNE 2014)*
- True about ASHA: Resident of village. *(DNB PATTERN NOV 2015)*
- Function of ASHA: Mobilisation of Institutional Deliveries. *(DNB PATTERN NOV 2015)*
- Population covered by ASHA :1000. *(NEET PATTERN 2015)*
- Vision 2020 does NOT include Measles Induced Blindness. *(NEET PATTERN 2015)*
- Vanaspati Ghee is fortified with Vitamin A. *(NEET PATTERN 2015)*
- Village Nutrition Day (VHND) is observed EVERY MONTH. *(NEET PATTERN 2015)*

- Rule of Halves is related to Hypertension. *(NEET PATTERN 2015)*
- Year of Big Divide in Indian History: 1921. *(DNB PATTERN NOV 2015, NEET PATTERN 2015)*
- The Big Divide is also called Demographic Divide.
- Concept of Social Medicine was introduced by: JULES GUERIN. *(DNB PATTERN JULY 2016)*
- Emporiatrics is a science dealing with: The health of travellers. *(DNB PATTERN JULY 2016)*
- Fibers are maximum in: Corn. *(DNB PATTERN NOV 2015)*
- Iron Plus Initiative is an example of Primary Prevention. *(DNB PATTERN NOV 2015)*
- Limiting Amino Acid in Wheat: Lysine. *(DNB PATTERN NOV 2015)*
- Maximum protein in pulses is found in: Soya bean. *(DNB PATTERN NOV 2015)*
- Headquarter of UNICEF: New York *(DNB PATTERN NOV 2015)*
- Recommended fat in Prudent diet: <20-30%. *(DNB PATTERN JULY 2016)*
- If hardness of water is 50–150 mg/litre, the water is defined as Moderately Hard. *(DNB PATTERN JULY 2016)*
- Mid Day Meal includes provision of: 1/3 rd calories, 1/2 protein. *(AIIMS PATTERN 2017)*
- Pasteurisation is done at: 63 degree celsius for 30 min. *(NEET PATTERN 2018)*

LEVEL 2: HIGH YIELD FACTORS

Table 7.1: Central government committees

Comprehensive health care	Bhore Committee
Primary Health Centre	Bhore Committee
Three months SPM training for developing social physicians	Bhore Committee
Health Survey and Planning Committee	Mudaliar Committee
Basic Health worker	Chadha Committee
Multipurpose worker	Kartar Singh Committee

Table 7.2: Statistics

Line diagrams	Trend of events with passage of time
Line diagram	Secular trend is best demonstrated
Secular trend	When disease frequency is measured over a period of several years or decades

Scatter diagram	Best way to study relationship between two variables
Histogram	Discrete/continuous data in ordered columns
Bar graph	Discrete data in separate columns
Pie chart	Categorical data as a percentage of the whole
Line graph	Continuous data as points and joining as a line
Frequency Polygon	Shading in area beneath Line graph

Table 7.3: Health personnel distribution

1 Anganwadi for 1,000 population

1 Anganwadi for 700 population in tribal areas

1 Doctor for 3,500 population

1 Nurse for 5,000 population

1 ASHA (Accredited Social Health Activist) for 1,000 population

1 Pharmacist per 10,000 population

1 Lab technician per 10,000 population

1 Health worker per 5,000 population

1 Health worker per 3,000 population in tribal and hilly areas

Table 7.4: Environmental conditions—lighting and noise

Basic minimum lighting for satisfactory vision	15–20 foot candles
Daylight factor	Instantaneous illumination indoors/Simultaneous illumination outdoors* 1000
Daylight factor in living rooms	8 percent
Daylight factor in kitchens	10 percent
Recommended illumination for casual reading	100 lux
Recommended illumination for general office work	400 lux
Noise limit people can tolerate without substantial damage to hearing	85 Decibels
Acceptable noise level in class room	30–40 Decibels
Acceptable noise level in hospital wards	20–35 Decibels
Exposure producing rupture of tympanic membrane/permanent hearing loss	160 Decibels

Table 7.5: Waste disposal

Sullage	Waste water from kitchen, which does not contain human excreta
Sewage	Waste water containing solid and liquid excreta derived from houses
Garbage	Waste matter arising from preparation/cooking of food
Controlled tipping/Sanitary land fill	Most satisfactory method of refuse disposal where suitable land is available
Incineration	Hospital refuse disposal
Composting	Method of combined disposal of refuse and night soil or sludge

Table 7.6: Sterilisation methods

Incineration	Hospital refuse is best disposed
Hot air oven	Sharp instruments are sterilised
Hot air oven temperature	160–180°C
Gamma radiation	Is used to sterilise surgical instruments
Gamma radiation	Is used to sterilise Catgut
Autoclaving	Most effective method of sterilisation of linen/dressings
Formaldehyde gas	For disinfection of rooms
Iodine	Most effective skin antiseptic
Glutaraldehyde	For disinfecting fibreoptic instruments like Endoscopes
Sodium hypochlorite	For sterilising Infant feeding bottles

Table 7.7: Communication in health education

One-way communication	Didactic Method
Two-way communication	Socratic Method
Effective group in group discussion has	6–12 members
Panel discussion	4–8 qualified members discuss a given problem
Symposium	Series of speeches on a selected subject
Best method of health education to urban slum women about ORS	Demonstration
Best way to teach students	Demonstration

Table 7.8: Chlorination

Chlorine level for destruction of Guinea worm larvae	5 ppm
Chlorine acts as disinfectant when pH of water is	7

Contd...

Contd...

Table 7.8: Chlorination

Chlorine has NO effect on	Spores/protozoan cysts/helminthic ova
Minimum recommended concentration of free chlorine is	0.5 mg/L for one hour
Bleaching powder contains about	33% of available chlorine
Emergency disinfection of water	Iodine
Most effective and cheapest method for disinfecting wells	Bleaching powder
Perchloron contains	60–70% of available chlorine
Chlorine demand is estimated by	Horrock's apparatus
0.5 gm chlorine can disinfect	20 litres of water
Orthotolidine Arsenite Test (OTA)	to estimate residual chlorine

Table 7.9: Occupational health legislations

Factories Act	1948
Minimum space for each worker as per Factories Act	500 cu ft
Factories Act prohibits the work of children below	14 yrs
Maximum stipulated working hours per week	48 hrs
ESI Act	1948
Sickness benefit is payable for	91 days
Extended Sickness Benefit is payable for	309 days
Funeral expenses according to the ESI Act	1000/- max.
Extended Sickness Benefit is applicable for	Leprosy/Mental illness/Chronic congestive cardiac failure/Parkinson's disease
ESI act covers all employees getting up to	6500/- per month

Table 7.10: Arthropod borne diseases

Most sensitive index of recent transmission of Malaria	Infant Parasite Rate
Measuring the endemicity of Malaria in a community	Spleen Rate
Transmission of Malaria by Anopheline Mosquitoes was discovered by	Ronald Ross
In Filariasis, mosquito is	Intermediate Host
Vector for Bancroftian Filariasis	Culex quinquefasciatus (Culex Fatigans)
Vector for Brugian Filariasis	Mansonia
Vector for Malaria in rural areas	Anopheles culicifacies
Vector for Malaria in urban areas	Anopheles stephensi

ASHA

Accredited Social Health Activist

1 ASHA for every 1000 population.

USHA – Urban Social Health Activist–as a part of NUHM (National Urban Health Mission)–COVERS 1000-2500 population across 250-500 households.

ASHA must be a resident of the village

ASHA must be female, 25 -40 yrs.

Should have formal education up to Class 8.

Should have good communication skills and leadership qualities.

ANGANWADI WORKERS and AUXILLARY NURSE/MIDWIFE will act as resource person for training of ASHA.

PIONEERS IN PUBLIC HEALTH

Father of Epidemiology—John Snow

Father of Surgery—Ambroise Pare

Father of Indian Surgery—Sushruta

Father of Vaccination—Jenner

Father of Public Health—Cholera

Barometer of Social Welfare—Tuberculosis

Theory of Contagion—Fracastorius

Founder of Epidemiology—Fracastorius

Theory of Web of Causation—McMohan and Pugh

Multifactorial Disease Causation—Pattenkoffer

Road to Health Chart—David Morley

Prevention of Scurvy—James Lind

Term Vaccine was coined by—Louis Pasteur in honor of Edward Jenner.

8. Forensic Medicine

"I see no more than you, but I have trained myself to notice what I see"
—Sherlock Holmes in 'The Adventure of the Blanched Soldier'

REFERENCES

- *Forensic Medicine and Toxicology, 3rd ed. by RN Karmakar*
- *Essentials of Forensic Medicine and Toxicology, 34th ed. by Narayan Reddy.*
- *Review of Forensic Medicine by Sumit Seth 6th ed.*

LEVEL I: BASIC REPEATS

ACTS, SECTIONS AND LEGAL PROCEDURES

- Section for rash and negligent driving 304 IPC. *(DNB PATTERN JUNE 2009)*
- Culpable homicide not amounting to murder comes under which section of IPC? 304 IPC. *(DNB PATTERN JUNE 2009)*
- Dowry death is covered under which section of IPC? 304 B. *(DNB PATTERN DEC 2010)*
- Grievous hurt comes under IPC Section 320. *(DNB PATTERN JUNE 2011)*
- Dying declaration comes under Section 32 Indian Evidence Act. *(DNB PATTERN DEC 2009)*
- Declaration of Oslo is related to Therapeutic Abortion. *(DNB PATTERN DEC 2010)*

International Declarations	Topic of Interest
Declaration of Geneva	Related to Respect for Human Life.
Declaration of Tokyo	Guidelines for Physicians concerning Torture and other cruel, inhuman or Degrading Treatment or Punishment in relation to detention and imprisonment.
Declaration of Malta	Is related to Hunger Strikers.
Declaration of Helsinki	Is related to ethical treatment of medical experimentation involving human subjects
Declaration of Lisbon	Is related to the rights of the patient
Declaration of Sydney	Related to the determination of Death and the recovery of organs.

- If death of a married woman occurs within 7 years of marriage, inquest is done by: Magistrate.
  (DNB PATTERN DEC 2009)
- Death sentence can be awarded by Sessions Court Magistrate.
  (DNB PATTERN DEC 2011)
- Medical etiquette is conventional way of courtesy with professional members. *(DNB PATTERN DEC 2011)*
- Impotence quad hoc means impotence towards a particular woman. *(DNB PATTERN DEC 2011)*
- Minimum age for organ donation in India: 18 years. Before 18 yrs, the consent of parent is needed.
  (DNB PATTERN DEC 2009)
- Contributory negligence is by the part of patient and doctor.
  (DNB PATTERN DEC 2009)
- Under IPC 82, a person under which age is NOT criminally responsible: 7. *(DNB PATTERN 2000)*
- Transplantation of Human organs act (HOTA act) was passed by the Govt. of India in the year 1994.
  (DNB PATTERN 2007)
- Death sentence can be given by Sessions Court.
  (DNB PATTERN 2007)
- Grievous Hurt comes under which section of IPC? Section 320 IPC. *(DNB PATTERN NOV 2013)*
- Police Inquest comes under: 174 CrPC.
  (DNB PATTERN NOV 2013)
- Subpoena comes under: Section 61-69 CrPC.
  (DNB PATTERN NOV 2013)
- Concealment of birth comes under: Section 318 IPC.
  (DNB PATTERN NOV 2013)
- Postponement of death sentence of a pregnant woman comes under: Section 416 CrPC.
  (DNB PATTERN NOV 2013)
- Dowry Death IPC: Section 304 B.
  (DNB PATTERN JUNE 2014)
- IPC 320 is for: Grievous Hurt.
  (FMGE PATTERN JUNE 2014)
- Force Feeding of prisoners on Hunger Strike is lawful under: Article 21 of the constitution. *(NEET PATTERN 2015)*
- Which section of IPC defines HURT as bodily pain, disease or infirmity? Section 319 *(NEET PATTERN 2015)*
- McNaughten Rule comes under which section of the Indian Penal Code? Section 84 IPC. *(NEET PATTERN 2018)*

POISONS

ORGANOPHOSPHORUS

- Drug given in Organophosphorus poisoning: Atropine/Cholinesterase reactivators. *(DNB PATTERN JUNE 2009)*
- Drug of choice for Organophosphorus Poisoning: Pralidoxime *(FMGE PATTERN MARCH 2013)*
- BRONCHODILATION is NOT a sign of Organophosphorus Poisoning. *(DNB PATTERN JUNE 2010)*
- NOT seen in Organophosphorus Poisoning: Dilated Pupils. *(DNB PATTERN JUNE 2014)*
- Delayed onset polyneuropathy after Organophosphorus Poisoning is seen after: 2-4 weeks. *(DNB PATTERN DEC 2011)*
- OXIME is NOT an antidote for: Baygon. *(DNB PATTERN JUNE 2010)*

CYANIDE

- Prolonged administration of Sodium Nitroprusside can cause: Cyanide poisoning *(DNB PATTERN DEC 2009)*
- Fatal dose of potassium cyanide is 200 mg. *(DNB PATTERN JUNE 2010)*
- Dicobalt EDTA or Dicobalt Edetate is used as antidote for: Cyanide poisoning. *(DNB PATTERN JUNE 2010)*
- Antidote for Cyanide Poisoning: Sodium Thiosulphate. *(FMGE PATTERN MAR 2012)*

ARSENIC

- Putrefaction is delayed in: Arsenic Poisoning. *(DNB PATTERN DEC 2010)*
- Acute Arsenic poisoning is confused with: Acute Gastroenteritis/CHOLERA. *(DNB PATTERN JUNE 2012)*
- Arsenic Poisoning mimics Cholera. *(FMGE PATTERN MARCH 2013)*
- MEE'S LINES are seen with: Arsenic Poisoning. (ALDRICH MEE'S LINES). *(DNB PATTERN DEC 2011)*
- Uterine contractions are NOT a sign of: Arsenic Poisoning. *(DNB PATTERN DEC 2011)*
- NAILS and HAIR are commonly preserved in Chronic Arsenic Poisoning. *(DNB PATTERN 2000)*

OXALIC ACID

- Choustek's and Trousseau's sign are seen in: Oxalic acid poisoning. *(DNB PATTERN JUNE 2009)*
- 10 yr old boy consumes stain remover. He presented with coffee colour vomitus and restlessness. Most likely diagnosis is: Oxalic Acid Poisoning. *(FMGE PATTERN SEP 2012)*

LEAD

- Most effective management of Acute Lead Toxicity is: Chelation therapy.
- Preferred Agent for Chelation Therapy: Calcium Disodium Versenate. *(DNB PATTERN JUNE 2012)*
- Lead poisoning in children is treated by: DMSA. *(DNB PATTERN DEC 2010)*
- Saturnism is associated with: Lead poisoning. *(DNB PATTERN AUG 2013)*

ALCOHOL

- Antidote used in methyl alcohol poisoning is: Fomepizole. *(DNB PATTERN JUNE 2011)*
- Fomepizole is an antidote used in the poisoning of: Methyl Alcohol. *(FMGE PATTERN MARCH 2013)*
- The toxic effects of methanol poisoning are primarily due to: Formic Acid. *(DNB PATTERN JUNE 2012)*
- Widmark formula is used to estimate: Alcohol content in blood. *(DNB PATTERN AUG 2013)*

MISCELLANEOUS

- Atropine is NOT an antidote for: Dhatura poisoning. *(DNB PATTERN JUNE 2010)*
- DIARRHEA is NOT a symptom of Opium Poisoning. *(DNB PATTERN JUNE 2010)*
- Antidote for Acetaminophen poisoning is: N Acetyl Cysteine. *(DNB PATTERN DEC 2009)*
- Postmortem Blue discoloration is seen in: Aniline Poisoning *(DNB PATTERN DEC 2010)*
- METHYL ISOCYANATE, The gas responsible for the Bhopal Gas Tragedy causes deaths by: Pulmonary Edema. *(NEET PATTERN 2014)*
- JAMAICAN VOMITING SICKNESS is due to: Hypoglycin. *(NEET PATTERN 2015)*
- Hypoglycin is derived from Ackee Tree.
- Phossy jaw is seen in: Yellow Phosphorus poisoning. *(DNB PATTERN JUNE 2011)*
- Yellow Phosphorus is the same as White Phosphorus. It was a content of Matchsticks previously.
- Detoxification of Benzoic acid is chiefly done by: Glycine. *(DNB PATTERN DEC 2011)*
- Post-mortem staining of carbon monoxide poisoning is: Cherry Red. *(DNB PATTERN JUNE 2011)*

- Poisoning which causes Postmortem luminescence: Armillaria. Armillaria is also known as HONEY FUNGUS.
- Photobacteria fischeri also causes Post Mortem Luminescence. *(DNB PATTERN DEC 2011)*
- Antidote of choice for Benzodiazepine poisoning is: Flumazenil. *(DNB PATTERN JUNE 2012)*
- Strychnine is a: spinal poison. *(DNB PATTERN 2001)*
- Gastric Lavage is contraindicated in: Sulphuric Acid poisoning. *(DNB PATTERN 2001)*
- ALPHA BUNGAROTOXIN acts on: Acetyl choline receptor. *(DNB PATTERN 2000)*
- Copper Sulphate poisoning manifests with: Acute Hemolysis. *(DNB PATTERN 2008)*
- A patient with history of prolonged intake of some unknown poison presents with digestive disturbances, anorexia, dilated pupils, hallucinations and blackened teeth and tongue. Most likely agent is: Cocaine. *(FMGE PATTERN SEP 2012)*
- VINEYARD POISONING is caused by: Methyl Bromide. *(DNB PATTERN NOV 2013)*
- Ophitoxemia is seen with: Snake Bite. *(DNB PATTERN JUNE 2014)*
- Metal associated with proximal tubule proteinuria: Cadmium. *(NEET PATTERN 2018)*

IMPORTANT NAMES

- **FALANGA** is defined as severe beating of soles. *(DNB PATTERN JUNE 2010)*
- **TELEFONA** is beating on both ears. *(DNB PATTERN DEC 2010)*
- **SIN OF GOMORRAH** is the other name for oral coitus. *(DNB PATTERN DEC 2011)*
- **MOLOTOV COCKTAIL** is Petrol bomb. *(DNB PATTERN JUNE 2011)*
- **DURET HAEMORRHAGES** are seen in brain. *(DNB PATTERN JUNE 2011)*
- **AGONAL ARTEFACT** is Postmortem artefact. *(DNB PATTERN JUNE 2011)*
- **THANATOLOGY** deals with death. *(DNB PATTERN DEC 2011)*
- **MCNAUGHTEN** was an accused. *(DNB PATTERN 2000)*
- **PALTAUF'S HAEMORRHAGES** are seen in Drowning. *(DNB PATTERN 2000)*
- **KUNKEL'S TEST** is used for the detection of Carbon monoxide in blood. *(DNB PATTERN 2000, 2001)*

- **FRACTURE A LA SIGNATURE** is a depressed fracture. *(DNB PATTERN 2000)*
- **EWING'S POSTULATES** refer to a relationship between trauma and Malignancy. *(DNB PATTERN 2000, 2001, 2005)*
- **McEwen's Sign sign** is seen in Alcoholism. *(DNB PATTERN 2001)*
- **DEFLORATION** means Loss of virginity. *(DNB PATTERN 2002)*
- **MAGNAN'S PHENOMENON** occurs with addiction of Cocaine. *(DNB PATTERN 2003)*
- **BOXER'S ATTITUDE** in seen in Burns death. *(DNB PATTERN 2003)*
- **CHILOTIC LINE** is line on hip bone for sex determination. *(DNB PATTERN 2008)*
- Active agent in Sodomy when passive agent is a child is known as: **PEDERAST**. *(NEET PATTERN 2016)*
- **CORPUS DELICTI** deals with the: Body of Offence. *(NEET PATTERN 2015)*
- **COLD TURKEY**: Withdrawal symptoms of OPIOID WITHDRAWAL. *(NEET PATTERN 2015)*
- Casper Dictum is calculation of time since death. *(DNB PATTERN 2008)*
- Spalding's sign occurs because of Maceration. *(DNB PATTERN 2007)*
- Calibre of a firearm is distance between two diagonally opposite lands. *(DNB PATTERN JUNE 2009)*
- Gordon's classification deals with: Pathological Hypoxia. *(DNB PATTERN AUG 2013)*
- Poroscopy was discovered by: Edmond Locard. *(DNB PATTERN AUG 2013)*
- Honeycomb appearance is seen in: Heat hematoma of skull. *(DNB PATTERN AUG 2013)*
- Puppe's rule: determines the sequence of bullets fired from a firearm. *(DNB PATTERN AUG 2013)*
- Puppe's rule is **NOT VALUABLE** in cases of: Multiple bullet injuries occurring **SIMULTANEOUSLY**. *(NEET PATTERN 2014)*
- Magnan's symptom is associated with: Cocaine. *(DNB PATTERN AUG 2013)*
- Suppositious child is: Fictitious child. (SUPPOSED TO BE TRUE CHILD)
- Fraudulent Child: NOT the real heir of the father. *(FMGE PATTERN MARCH 2013)*

- Posthumous child is: Child born after death of his/her father. *(FMGE PATTERN MARCH 2003)*
- Posthumous Child is: Child born after death of his/her biological father. *(NEET PATTERN 2018)*
- Atavism is resemblance of child to his: Grandfather. *(FMGE PATTERN MARCH 2013)*
- Lynching is: Homicidal hanging. *(FMGE PATTERN MARCH 2013)*
- Throttling is: Compression of neck by human hand. *(FMGE PATTERN MARCH 2013)*
- Duret hemorrhages are seen in: Brain. (Pontine Hemorrhages) *(DNB PATTERN OCT 2013)*
- Vibices is another name for: Postmortem staining. *(DNB PATTERN NOV2013)*
- Other names: Livor Mortis/Hypostasis/Suggilations.
- Spanish Windlass is a form of: Strangulation. (Garroting would be the exact answer if available in the choice.) *(DNB PATTERN NOV 2013)*

PRESERVATIVES AND FIXATIVES

- Blood samples for DNA fingerprinting should be transported in EDTA. *(DNB PATTERN JUNE 2009)*
- Brain is stored in which preservative for autopsy? 10% formalin. *(DNB PATTERN JUNE 2009)*
- Substance commonly used for organ/tissue preservation for histopathological examination is Formalin. *(DNB PATTERN DEC 2009)*
- NOT a component of Embalming fluid: Ethanol. *(DNB PATTERN 2008)*
- Putrefaction is retarded by Phenol. *(DNB PATTERN 2007)*
- Florence test is done for: Seminal stains. *(FMGE PATTERN MARCH 2013)*
- Mesentery is preserved in what kind of death? – Anesthetic death. *(NEET PATTERN 2013)*
- Test to detect species of blood: Precipitin test. *(DNB PATTERN JUNE 2014)*
- VIRCHOW METHOD of Dissection is: Individual organ removal and dissection. *(NEET PATTERN 2016)*

WOUNDS

- Blackening around entry wound of a firearm injury is due to smoke. *(DNB PATTERN JUNE 2009)*

Forensic Medicine

- Tissue bridging is characteristic of: Lacerations. *(DNB PATTERN JUNE 2010)*
- Which of the following is seen in exit wound? Bevelled outer table. *(DNB PATTERN JUNE 2010)*
- Tentative cuts are seen in Suicide. *(DNB PATTERN JUNE 2009)*
- Hesitation cuts are seen in Suicide. *(DNB PATTERN 2002)*
- Gun powder residues on forearms can be detected by Dermal Nitrate test. *(DNB PATTERN DEC 2010)*
- Fish tailing of margins in stab wound is seen with single edged knife. *(DNB PATTERN DEC 2011)*
- Split laceration is seen with blunt perpendicular impact. *(DNB PATTERN JUNE 2009)*
- Contusion can be differentiated from postmortem staining by Incision test. *(DNB PATTERN 2000)*
- DIRT COLLAR is seen in: Fire Arm Entry Wound. *(DNB PATTERN 2000)*
- Tail of the wound tells about direction of wound. *(DNB PATTERN 2002)*
- In the case of bullet wound, the presence of singeing of hair and charring of skin indicates a distance of 6 inches. *(DNB PATTERN 2006)*
- True for Contrecoup brain injury: Occurs more in moving head. *(FMGE PATTERN SEP 2012)*
- Irregular margin is seen in: Heat rupture. *(NEET PATTERN 2016)*
- Hide and Die Reaction with terminal burrowing is seen in: Hypothermia. *(NEET PATTERN 2016)*

OTHER KEY FINDINGS IN HYPOTHERMIA:

- Erythema pernio.(Chilblain)
- Paradoxical Undressing

POSTMORTEM CHANGES

- Sign of antemortem hanging: Dribbling of saliva. *(DNB PATTERN JUNE 2009)*
- Underwater biopsy of the heart is done in Air embolism. *(DNB PATTERN JUNE 2009)*
- First structure to be opened/dissected in autopsy of air embolism case is Thoracic cavity. *(DNB PATTERN DEC 2010)*

- Venous bleeding is NOT a sign of AnteMortem injury. *(DNB PATTERN JUNE 2011)*
- Psychological autopsy is assessment of mental state of deceased person before death. *(DNB PATTERN JUNE 2011)*
- Cephalic index is used for the determination of Race. *(DNB PATTERN DEC 2010)*
- Immediate sign of death is cessation of respiration and circulation. *(DNB PATTERN DEC 2010)*
- Cutis anserina is seen in drowning. *(DNB PATTERN 2000)*
- Exhumation is usually done in the early morning.
- Exhumation is done in natural light. *(DNB PATTERN 2000)*
- Postmortem rigidity first starts in eyelids. *(DNB PATTERN 2008)*
- In normal conditions of temperature and atmosphere, the rate of cooling of dead body is 1.5 degree Fahrenheit per hour. *(DNB PATTERN 2007)*
- The order of onset of rigor mortis is Eyelids – thorax – lower limbs. *(DNB PATTERN 2007)*
- First organ to putrefy in the body: Brain. *(NEET PATTERN 2018)*
- Actually, the first organ to putrefy is the Larynx.
- Last organ to putrefy in the female is: Uterus.
- Last to putrefy in male is Prostate. *(DNB PATTERN 2007)*
- Rigor mortis appears last in: Toes. *(FMGE PATTERN MARCH 2012)*
- NOT TRUE about Prinsloo Gordon artefact is: Definitive sign of death due to manual strangulation. *(NEET PATTERN 2014)*

> **PRINSLOO AND GORDON ARTEFACT**
> - Artefact that is caused by leakage of blood from venous plexus after death.
> - Represents an artefactual postmortem hemorrhage on the posterior surface of the esophagus that may cause the doubt of manual strangulation.
> - It is NOT A DEFINITIVE SIGN OF DEATH DUE TO MANUAL STRANGULATION.

- Soft and friable extradural hematoma with HONEYCOMB APPEARANCE on autopsy is suggestive of: Heat hematoma. *(NEET PATTERN 2014)*
- Bluish Discolouration of gastric mucosa is seen in: Sodium Amytal Poisoning. *(NEET PATTERN 2018)*
- Bluish Discolouration of Gastric mucosa occurs in Copper Sulfate/Copper Subacetate/Methylene Blue/Dextropropoxyphene poisoning.

- La Facies Sympathique is seen in cases of: Hanging.
  (NEET PATTERN 2014)
- Greenish discoloration of the right caecal area during putrefaction is seen in: Sulphmethemoglobin.
  (NEET PATTERN 2015)
- Fencing posture is caused by: Coagulation of proteins.
  (NEET PATTERN 2016)
- "Streaming of Nuclei" on histopathology is seen in death due to: Electrocution. *(NEET PATTERN 2016)*
- LADDER TEARS are Transverse tears of Aortic Intima.
  (NEET PATTERN 2016)
- Smell of Mummified body: Odourless.
  (NEET PATTERN 2018)

IDENTIFICATION

- Disease causing modification of finger prints is: Leprosy.
  (DNB PATTERN 2008)
- Among the secondary changes in tooth the most useful for age determination is: Root Translucency.
  (DNB PATTERN 2008)
- Ossification of proximal end of ulna takes place at what age? 16 years. *(DNB PATTERN DEC 2010)*
- Xiphoid process fuses to the body of sternum by 40 years.
  (DNB PATTERN DEC 2009)
- Four carpal bones are present at what age? 4 years.
  (DNB PATTERN JUNE 2009)
- At the age of 12, the number of teeth is 24.
  (DNB PATTERN 2006)
- Sex can be established by examining hair root cells for the presence of Barr body. *(DNB PATTERN 2008)*
- Most common type of finger impression is Loop.
  (DNB PATTERN 2006)
- Ossification centre of clavicle that is used to confirm their bone age for legal consent to marriage: Sternal end.
  (NEET PATTERN 2014)
- Basioccipital fuses with basisphenoid at the age of: 22–25 years. *(NEET PATTERN 2018) Ref: Last Anatomy - puts it at 25 years.*

MISCELLANEOUS

- Which is not a sexual perversion? Transvestism. Transvestism is not a sexual perversion, but a gender identitiy disorder.
  (DNB PATTERN DEC 2010)
- Which is a sexual perversion? Sadism.
  (DNB PATTERN JUNE 2014)

- Sweating is not seen in Heat stroke. Sweating is seen in Heat Exhaustion. *(DNB PATTERN DEC 2010)*
- Spermin in semen is detected by Barberio test. *(DNB PATTERN 2007)*
- During first sexual intercourse, rupture of hymen occurs at 5 O' clock position. *(DNB PATTERN 2000)*
- Rupture of Hymen occurs at POSTEROLATERAL position. (5 or 6 o' clock position)
- General moral principles in medical practice is Medical Ethics. *(DNB PATTERN 2001)*
- In deaths due to starvation, gall bladder is: Distended. *(FMGE PATTERN MARCH 2013)*
- Diatoms are suggestive of death due to: Antemortem Drowning. *(FMGE PATTERN MARCH 2012)*
- Burking is a type of: Smothering. *(DNB PATTERN JUNE 2014)*
- *Burking includes Smothering and Traumatic Asphyxia.*
- Constriction pressure required to block trachea: 15 kg. *(FMGE PATTERN JUNE 2014)*
- PIQUERISM is related to: Paraphilia. *(NEET PATTERN 2014)*
- Taking off one's clothes and running naked in public is called as: Streaking. *(NEET PATTERN 2014)*
- Locard is famous for: Theory of Exchange. *(NEET PATTERN 2018)*

LEVEL II: HIGH YIELD FACTORS

- For Anthropometry, the **Bertillon** system is used.
- Fingerprinting or Dactylography uses the **Galton** system.
- Study of dental changes for identification utilises the **Gustaff son** method.
- Identification by lip print is called **Cheiloscopy**.
- Identification by matching photographs with skull is called **Superimposition**.
- Poroscopy utilises the **Locard** method.
- **Ischiopubic index** is used for determination of sex.
- **Cephalic index** is for determination of race.
- **Ponderal index** is for determination of IUGR.
- **Rule of Hasse** is for calculation of fetal age corresponding to fetal length.
- **Hydrostatic test** is for Infanticide.
- **Hydrostatic test cannot be used when** fetus is macerated or mummified.

STAINS

- **Florence test** detects Choline in seminal stains.
- **Barberio test** detects Spermine in seminal stains.
- **Precipitin test** is for differentiating between human and animal fresh blood.
- **Hemochromogen test/Takayama test** is for identification of old blood stains.
- Most reliable test for identification of blood stains: **Spectroscopy**.

PRESERVATIVES

- Preservative for blood for grouping: 25% formalin and sodium citrate
- Preservative for viscera: 10% formalin.
- Preservative for Cerebrospinal fluid: Sodium fluoride
- Preservative for transportation of urine sample to the laboratory: Thymol.

FIRE ARM INJURIES

- Composition of gunpowder (black): 15% charcoal + 10% sulphur + 75% KNO_3
- Composition of smokeless powder: Nitrocellulose + Nitroglycerine.
- In fire arm entry wound, outer table has a punched in lesion where as inner table is bevelled.
- In fire arm exit wound, outer table is bevelled and inner table has a punched out lesion.
- Abrasion collar or contusion collar is seen with rifle bullet and surrounds the dirt collar.
- Bullet which causes maximum injury: Hollow point bullet.
  (DNB PATTERN AUG 2013)
- Least injured in Blast injury: Liver.
  (DNB PATTERN AUG 2013)
- Bevelling of skull is seen in: Firearm injury.
  (FMGE PATTERN MARCH 2013)

POSTMORTEM CHANGES

- Adipocere or saponification occurs in warm watery environment.
- Mummification occurs in dry sandy environment where rapid evaporation takes place.
- Putrefaction is delayed in Strychnine, Carbolic acid, Arsenic poisoning.
- Rigor mortis is delayed in Apoplexy, Pneumonia and Asphyxia.
- Sturner's equation: Postmortem Interval (hrs) = 7.14 (Intravitreal Potassium) − 39.1. *(DNB PATTERN AUG 2013)*

- Virchow method of Autopsy includes: Organs are removed one by one. *(DNB PATTERN NOV 2013)*
- Ist Medico-Legal Autopsy was done by: Ambroise Pare. *(NEET PATTERN 2013)*

POISONING

- Smoky green urine is seen in Carbolic acid poisoning.
- Artificial Bruise is seen in Semecarpus anacardium.
- Important Abortifacients: Calotropis, Oleander, Lead
- Chelating agent of choice in Mercury and Arsenic poisoning: BAL (Dimercaprol)
- Chelating agent of choice in Lead poisoning: Calcium Disodium edetate.
- Run amok is a feature of cannabis intoxication.
- Active principle of Cannabis is Tetrahydrocannabinol.
- Bhang is prepared from dry leaves and fruit shoots of Indian Hemp plant.
- Ganja is prepared from female efflorescence.
- Charas/Hashish is prepared from leaves and stems of the plant.
- Widmark formula is used for blood alcohol concentration.
- Alcohol disappears from blood at the rate of 10–15 ml/hr.
- Bitter almond odour is seen with Hydrocyanic acid poisoning.

PRESERVATIVES AND FIXATIVES

(Ref: Karmakar's Textbook of Forensic Medicine)

Ideal preservative for preservation of viscera for chemical examination	Rectified Spirit
Commonly used preservative for preservation of viscera for chemical examination	Saturated NaCl
Rectified Spirit is NOT used with:	Carbolic Acid Acetic Acid Alcohol Phosphorus Paraldehyde Kerosene Oil
Common salt is NOT used with:	Corrosive Acids/Vegetable poisons/Aconite/Mercuric Chloride
In Post anaesthetic death, Lungs are preserved in:	Nylon bag

Contd...

Forensic Medicine

In Post anaesthetic death, Alveolar air is taken:	Using a syringe
In Post anaesthetic death	Lung/Liver/Kidney/Brain/Skeletal Muscle and Fat from Mesentery/Blood/Urine is preserved.

(Ref: Karmakar's Textbook of Forensic Medicine)

Blumen back classification	Classification of race
As per Blumen Back, Yellow represents	Mongoloid
Brown	Malayan
Red	American
Black	Ethiopian
White	Caucasian
Moritz classification	Classification of Hair
In MORITZ Classification:	Free margin and shape of scales are used
COPRA Act was passed in 1986 amended in 1993.	
1st Medicolegal Autopsy was performed by	Ambroise Pare
1st Medicolegal Autopsy in India was performed by	Buckeley
System of Dactylography was first started in	India
Dactylography is known as	Galton's system
First Fingerprint bureau was established in	Writer's building, Calcutta, 1897.
Majority of fingerprints in Indians are	Loops
Most accurate term for investigative examination of dead body	Necropsy NOT Autopsy
ADOLESCENT is defined as having age between:	12–18 yrs
Child is defined as having age between:	1–12 yrs
Infant	0–1 yrs
Birth length of a newborn is doubled at	4 yrs
Birth weight of a newborn is doubled at	6 months
Birth weight of a newborn is tripled at	1 year
Formula for Stature	Max Foot Length/0.15

Contd...

Contd...

Sturner's equation for Post-mortem Interval	Postmortem Interval (hrs) = 7.14 (Intravitreal Potassium) – 39.1
Best method for Postmortem Interval	Intravitreal Potassium estimation
Pomum Adami	Latin for Adam's apple, characteristic of mature adult men, Caused by angulation of thyroid cartilage

NAMED PARAPHILIAS

TELEPHONE SCATOLOGIA	Obscene Phone Calls for deriving Sexual pleasure
PARTIALISM	Sexual interest with exclusive focus on specific part of the body. Classified as a Fetishistic disorder under DSM 5.
COPROPHILIA	Sexual pleasure derived from FAECES.
KLISMAPHILIA	Paraphilia involving sexual pleasure from ENEMAs.
UROPHILIA	Paraphilia involving sexual pleasure from sight of URINE. Also called GOLDEN SHOWER.
NECROPHILIA (THANATOPHILIA)	Sexual Attraction involving CORPSES.
PICQUERISM	Paraphilia involving sexual pleasure from PENETRATING OR PRICKING THE SKIN OF ANOTHER PERSON. *Jack The Ripper's Murders of 1888 in London has been attributed to Picquerism.*
CUCKOLDISM	Sexual Interest derived from a partner's infidelity.
PICTOPHILIA	Sexual Interest derived from Pornography or pictures.
HYBRISTOPHILIA (BONNIE and CLYDE Syndrome.)	Sexual Interest derived from partners with criminal backgrounds.
GERONTOPHILIA	Sexual preferences for the elderly.

Contd...

Contd...
TOXICOLOGY RAPID SCAN

ALCOHOL	*McEwan's Sign (Coma)* *Jellinek's Classification (alpha/beta/gamma/delta/epsilon)* *Widmark's Formula* *Hine and Kozelka Method.* *Cavett's Test* *Breath Analyser based on Henry's Gas Law.* *Hemodialysis TOC Methanol Poisoning.* *DOC Fomepizole(Four Methyl Pyrazole)*
ERGOT	*ST. ANTHONY'S FIRE – Burning sensation of limbs on consumption of Ergot contaminated Ryebread.* *Formication – In Chronic Ergot Poisoning.*
ORGANOPHOSPHORUS	*Malathion – Alkyl Phosphate* *Parathion –Aryl Phosphate* *Chromolachyorrhoea – passage of red tears due to PORPHYRINEMIA.* *Most sensitive test: RBC Cholinesterase Test.* *Resembles BRONCHIAL ASTHMA.*
ARSENIC	*Metallic Arsenic Non poisonous* *RICE WATER Stools* *RED VELVET appearance of stomach mucosa.* *FADING MEASLES Rash.* *ALDRICH MEE'S lines.* *Black foot Disease* *MARSH and REINSCH Tests.* *Napoleon was killed by ARSENIC Posioning.* *Addison's Disease.*
MERCURY	*Minamata* *Acrodynia* *PINK'S Disease* *Hydrargyrism* *Hatter's Shakes* *Danbury Tremors* *Glass Blower's Shakes* *Brown Malt Reflex*

Contd...

Contd...

LEAD	*Saturnism – Chronic* *Punctate Basophilia* *BURTONIAN Line* *Facial Pallor – Most consistent and earliest sign* *Status Epilepticus.* *Most effective treatment – Calcium disodium versenate.*
COPPER	*PTYSALISM – copious saliva* *Clapton's Line* *Resembles WILSON'S Disease.*
ZINC	*METAL FUME FEVER* *Resembles MALARIAL CHILLS.*

9 ENT

"I believe things cannot make themselves impossible."
Stephen Hawking

REFERENCES

- *Diseases of Ear, Nose and Throat by PL Dhingra 6th ed.*
- *Essentials of Ear, Nose and Throat by Mohan Bansal 1st ed.*

LEVEL I: BASIC REPEATS

EAR

- Maximum audible tolerance is 85 db for 8 hrs. *(DNB PATTERN JUNE 2012)*
- Loudness discomfort level: 90–105 db. Stapedial Reflex is elicited at 70 -100 dB sensation level.
- **Hennebert's Sign** is a false positive fistula test seen in Congenital Syphilis. *(DNB PATTERN DEC 2011)*
- Otolith organs are concerned with function of Linear Acceleration. *(DNB PATTERN DEC 2011)*
- Carhart's notch is found in Otospongiosis. *(DNB PATTERN 2005, 2001)*
- Earliest symptom of Acoustic Neuroma: Deafness. *(DNB PATTERN 2006)*
- Malignant otitis externa is caused by: Pseudomonas aeruginosa. *(DNB PATTERN DEC 2009)*
- Length of external auditory canal is: 24 mm. *(DNB PATTERN DEC 2009)*
- Most common site of perforation of tympanic membrane in ASOM is: Anterior inferior quadrant. *(DNB PATTERN DEC 2009)*
- Quadrant for a myringotomy is: Anteroinferior. *(DNB PATTERN 2000, 2004)*
- Epley Manouevre is used for: Benign paroxysmal vertigo. *(DNB PATTERN DEC 2009)*
- Telephonist's ear is External otitis. *(DNB PATTERN 2003)*

- Semicircular canal perceives: Angular acceleration. *(DNB PATTERN JUNE 2010)*
- Otoacoustic emissions arise from: Outer hair cells. *(DNB PATTERN DEC 2009, JUNE 2010)*
- Noise Induced Hearing Loss involves damage to : Outer Hair Cells. *(AIIMS 2017 PATTERN)*
- Ototoxicity (eg : Drug Induced) also generally affects the Outer Hair Cells.
- True about Glomus tumor: Invades epitympanum. *(DNB PATTERN JUNE 2011)*
- Referred otalgia can be due to: carcinoma larynx, tongue and oral cavity. *(DNB PATTERN JUNE 2011)*
- Adenoidectomy with Grommet insertion is the treatment of choice for: Serous otitis media in children. *(DNB PATTERN JUNE 2011)*
- Attenuation reflex is lost in case of: Stapedial palsy. *(DNB PATTERN JUNE 2011)*
- 40 db sound compared to 20 db sound is 10 times. *(DNB PATTERN 2001)*
- Radical Mastoidectomy is done for Atticoantral cholesteatoma. *(DNB PATTERN 2000)*
- Otosclerosis mostly affects Stapes. *(DNB PATTERN 2000)*
- Otosclerosis most commonly starts at: Fissula Ante Fenestram. *(NEET PATTERN 2014)*
- Commonest cranial nerve involved in Acoustic Neuroma? Trigeminal. *(DNB PATTERN 2000)*
- Which of the following attains adult size before birth? Ear ossicles. *(DNB PATTERN DEC 2009)*
- Movement of stapes causes vibration in Scala vestibuli. *(DNB PATTERN 2002)*
- Dix Hallpike test for benign paroxysmal positional vertigo (BPPV)
- Hallpike test is done for assessing vestibular function. *(DNB PATTERN 2002)*
- Mass in ear, on touch bleeding heavily the cause is: Glomus jugulare. *(DNB PATTERN 2001)*
- 7th nerve involvement is NOT a feature of Gradenigo syndrome. *(DNB PATTERN 2000, 2004)*
- NOT a cause of referred pain in ear is due to: Furunculosis. *(DNB PATTERN JUNE 2009)*
- Rinne's test is positive in normals. *(DNB PATTERN 2000)*
- Ear pinna develops from: Ectoderm. *(DNB PATTERN JUNE 2010)*

- Triad of Tinnitus, Progressive deafness and vertigo along with facial weakness is seen in Acoustic Neuroma.
  (DNB PATTERN JUNE 2010)
- Investigation of choice of audiometric evaluation of an infant is: BERA. *(DNB PATTERN DEC 2010)*
- Schuller's view and Law's view is for? Mastoid air cells.
  (DNB PATTERN JUNE 2011)
- Law's view is Schuller's view with 15 degree caudal angulation.
- SADE classification is used for: Pars Tensa retraction.
  (DNB PATTERN AUG 2013)
- Korner's septum: Petrosquamosal lamina or bony plate dividing the mastoid air cells at the level of Antrum.
  (DNB PATTERN AUG 2013)
- Frequency range in normal hearing is: 20-20000 Hz.
  (DNB PATTERN NOV 2013)
- Normal frequency of Adult male voice is: 120 Hz.
  (DNB PATTERN NOV 2013)
- Normal frequency of Adult female voice: 160–250 Hz. Average - 200 Hz.
- As per Factory Act in India, maximum audible tolerance is: 90 db for 8 hrs for 5 days in a week.
  (DNB PATTERN NOV 2013)
- Maximum audible tolerance recommended by WHO is: 85 db for 8 hrs. *(DNB PATTERN NOV 2013)*
- Maximum hearing loss is seen with: Closure of oval window (60 db) > Disruption of ossicles with intact Tympanic Membrane (54 db) *(DNB PATTERN NOV 2013)*
- In Gradenigo's syndrome, cranial nerve affected by inflammation in Dorello's canal is: 6th nerve.
  (DNB PATTERN NOV 2013)
- Site of Glomus Tumor: Hypotympanum.
  (NEET PATTERN DEC 2013)
- Glomus tumors arise either in the middle ear (glomus tympanicum) or in the jugular bulb with upward erosion into the hypotympanum (glomus jugulare). *(CMDT 2013/2015)*
- Length of External Auditory canal is: 24 mm.
  (DNB PATTERN NOV 2013)
- Most likely involved semicircular canal in positive Fistula Test: Horizontal SCC. *(DNB PATTERN NOV 2013)*
- Otosclerosis presents with: Bilateral conductive deafness.
  (DNB PATTERN NOV 2013)
- Tuning fork ideal for clinical practice: 512 Hz.
  (FMGE PATTERN SEP 2012)

- Preferred method to remove insect from Ear Canal: Oil. *(FMGE PATTERN 2011)*
- Noise induced Hearing Loss can result from extended exposure to over: 85 db of sound. *(FMGE PATTERN SEP 2012)*
- Recruitment Test is used for: Cochlear Lesions. *(FMGE PATTERN JUNE 2014)*
- Length of External Auditary Canal in adult is: 24 mm. *(NEET PATTERN 2014)*
- Phenomenon of Loud sounds producing Vertigo is: Tulio Phenomenon. *(NEET PATTERN 2014)*
- Retraction of Tympanic Membrane touching the promontory is classified as SADE grade: 3. *(NEET PATTERN 2014)*
- Fowler's test is NOT used for Non Organic Hearing Loss. *(NEET PATTERN 2014)*
- Facial Palsy as a result of Herpes infection affecting Geniculate Ganglion is known as: Ramsay Hunt Syndrome. *(NEET PATTERN 2015)*
- Damage to which region will lead to inability to hear high frequency sound? Basilar Membrane near Oval Window. *(NEET PATTERN 2016)*
- Triad of Gradenigo Does NOT include Superior Oblique Palsy. *(NEET PATTERN 2016)*
- SOUND BAFFLE Operation refers to Type 4 Tympanoplasty. *(NEET PATTERN 2015)*
- Auditary Fatigue at 4000 Hz usually appears at: 90 db *(NEET PATTERN 2015)*
- BOXER'S EAR refers to Crumpled Pinna; also called Cauliflower Ear. *(NEET PATTERN 2015)*
- BILL BAR in internal auditory meatus is a vertical ridge separating: Facial Nerve and Superior Vestibular Nerve. *(NEET PATTERN 2016)*

NOSE AND PARANASAL SINUSES

- Roomy nasal cavity with thick crust formation and woody hard external nose is seen in Rhinoscleroma. *(DNB PATTERN DEC 2011)*
- Treatment of septal hematoma is Incision and drainage. *(DNB PATTERN DEC 2011)*
- Which artery is responsible for epistaxis after ligating of external carotid artery? Ethmoidal artery. *(DNB PATTERN DEC 2011)*
- Griesinger's sign is seen in Lateral sinus thrombosis. *(DNB PATTERN DEC 2011)*

- Most common site of osteomas among the paranasal sinuses is: Frontal. *(DNB PATTERN DEC 2011)*
- Ohngren's Line that divides the maxillary sinus into superolateral and inferomedial zone is related to: Maxillary Carcinoma. *(DNB PATTERN DEC 2011)*
- People working in the wood industry are exposed to increased risk of: Adenocarcinoma of PNS. *(DNB PATTERN DEC 2011)*
- Odour receptor is present in: Neurons of olfactory epithelium. *(DNB PATTERN DEC 2011)*
- Orbital cellulitis most commonly occurs after which sinus infection? Ethmoidal. *(DNB PATTERN JUNE 2011)*
- Quadrilateral cartilage is located in—Anterior part of nasal septum. *(DNB PATTERN JUNE 2008)*
- Quadrilateral cartilage is NOT attached to the sphenoid. *(DNB PATTERN 2001, 2005)*
- Young's syndrome—Nasal polyp, bronchiectasis, azoospermia. *(DNB PATTERN JUNE 2008)*
- True about Anterochoanal polyp—usually Single. *(DNB PATTERN JUNE 2008)*
- Sphenoid sinus drains into—Sphenoethmoidal recess. *(DNB PATTERN JUNE 2008)*
- Drainage of nasal mucus is by Ciliary action of Mucosa. *(DNB PATTERN JUNE 2008)*
- Caldwell-Luc's operation—For Maxillary sinus. *(DNB PATTERN JUNE 2008)*
- Nasal bone fracture is corrected by-Walsham's forceps. *(DNB PATTERN JUNE 2008)*
- Aspirin use is associated with—Nasal polyps. *(DNB PATTERN JUNE 2008)*
- Nerve coming out of Stylomastoid foramen—Facial. *(DNB PATTERN JUNE 2008)*
- In Dacryocystorhinostomy, opening is into the middle meatus. *(DNB PATTERN 2005)*
- Posterior Ethmoid sinus does NOT open into middle meatus. *(DNB PATTERN 2003)*
- Most common malignancy in maxillary antrum is: Squamous cell carcinoma. *(DNB PATTERN 2000)*
- In Dacryocystorhinostomy, opening is done into middle meatus. *(DNB PATTERN 2000)*
- Mikulicz cells and Russell Bodies are seen in: Rhinoscleroma. *(DNB PATTERN DEC 2009)*
- Nasal bone fracture is corrected by: Walsham's forceps. *(DNB PATTERN JUNE 2009)*

- Ohngren's classification of Maxillary sinus carcinoma is based on: Imaginary plane between medial canthus of eye and angle of mandible. *(DNB PATTERN JUNE 2011)*
- Vidian neurectomy is done in: Vasomotor rhinitis. *(DNB PATTERN DEC 2010)*
- Strawberry skin appearance of nasal mucosa is seen in: Sarcoidosis. *(DNB PATTERN DEC 2010)*
- Commonest Site of Nasopharyngeal carcinoma: Lateral wall. *(DNB PATTERN 2000)*
- A roomy nasal cavity with thick crust formation and woody hard external nose is seen in: Rhinoscleroma. *(DNB PATTERN JUNE 2009)*
- Most common site of CSF rhinorrhoea is: Cribriform plate. *(DNB PATTERN DEC 2010)*
- Mucocele is commonest in which among the following sinuses? Frontal. *(DNB PATTERN DEC 2010, NEET PATTERN 2014)*
- Tobey Ayer test is positive in Lateral sinus thrombosis. *(DNB PATTERN 2001)*
- Lacrimal duct does NOT drain into Middle Meatus. *(DNB PATTERN 2002)*
- NOT true about Anterochoanal polyp: Avulsion is the treatment of choice. *(DNB PATTERN DEC 2009)*
- Branches of the Kisselbach's plexus which are not derived from External Carotid Artery: Anterior Ethmoidal Arteries. *(NEET PATTERN 2018)*
- Kiesselbach's area (Little's area) does not involve: Posterior ethmoidal artery. *(DNB PATTERN JUNE 2011)*
- Septal perforation is NOT seen in Rhinophyma. *(DNB PATTERN 2002)*
- Transnasal approach is NOT used in Lateral orbitotomy. *(DNB PATTERN 2002)*
- Kiesselbach's plexus is located on the Anteroinferior part of the nasal cavity. *(DNB PATTERN 2000)*
- Woodruff's Plexus responsible for Posterior Epistaxis is located on the Lateral wall of the nasal cavity.
- NOT a feature of Trotter's Triad: 7th nerve palsy. *(DNB PATTERN 2000)*
- NOT true about Anterochoanal polyp: Avulsion is the treatment of choice. *(DNB PATTERN JUNE 2009)*
- Which is an independent bone? Inferior turbinate. *(DNB PATTERN JUNE 2009)*
- Kiesselbach's area does not involve Posterior ethmoidal artery. *(DNB PATTERN JUNE 2009)*

- Weber Ferguson Approach is used for: Maxillectomy.
  (DNB PATTERN JUNE 2009)
- Mucormycosis of paranasal sinus is most common in: Diabetes. *(DNB PATTERN JUNE 2009)*
- Angiofibroma bleeds excessively because it lacks a contractile component. *(DNB PATTERN 2001)*
- Posterior Ethmoidal sinus does NOT open in the Middle Meatus. *(DNB PATTERN 2001)*
- Paranasal sinuses are NOT absent in skull of newborn.
  (DNB PATTERN 2001)
- Sinus which continues to grow even in Adulthood: Sphenoid Sinus. *(AIIMS PATTERN 2017)*
- Alternative for Smooth Muscle Resection: Septoplasty.
  (DNB PATTERN 2001)
- Commonest presentation of Nasopharyngeal carcinoma: Nasal mass. *(DNB PATTERN 2000)*
- Which of the following is seen in Young's syndrome? Azoospermia, Infertility and Bronchiectasis.
  (DNB PATTERN JUNE 2009)
- Agammaglobulinemia can present with: Rhinitis, Giardia infections and Bronchiectasis. *(DNB PATTERN JUNE 2009)*
- A man using nasal drops continuously for a long period of time. Possible adverse effect is: Rhinitis Mediamentosa.
  (DNB PATTERN JUNE 2010)
- Treatment of choice of Nasopharyngeal carcinoma is: Radiotherapy. *(DNB PATTERN DEC 2010)*
- NOT a cause of epistaxis from anterior nasal septum: Allergic Rhinitis. *(DNB PATTERN JUNE 2010)*
- What is the cause of sudden death in a patient who recently underwent maxillary sinus irrigation? Air embolism.
  (DNB PATTERN JUNE 2010)
- Most common site of Inverted papilloma of nose: Lateral wall of nose. *(DNB PATTERN AUG 2013)*
- Pneumatised middle turbinate is called: Concha bullosa.
  (DNB PATTERN AUG 2013)
- Imaging study of choice for paranasal sinuses: CT scan.
  (DNB PATTERN NOV 2013)
- Most common site of carcinoma of paranasal sinuses is: Maxillary sinus. *(DNB PATTERN NOV 2013)*
- Age group of Angiofibroma: Adolescent male (10-20 yrs).
  (NEET PATTERN DEC 2013)
- Crooked Nose is due to: Deviated dorsum and septum.
  (DNB PATTERN NOV 2013)

- Saddle Nose—depression of nasal dorsum.
  (DNB PATTERN 2008 PATTERN)
- Rhinitis Medicamentosa is due to: chronic use of nasal drops.
  (FMGE PATTERN 2008)
- Young's operation is performed for: Atrophic Rhinitis.
  (FMGE PATTERN 2011)
- 1st sign of CP angle tumor: 5th nerve involvement.
  (DNB PATTERN JUNE 2014)
- Nerve damaged in Caldwell Luc surgery: Infraorbital nerve.
  (DNB PATTERN JUNE 2014)
- Rhinoscleroma is caused by: Klebsiella Rhinoscleromatis.
  (FMGE PATTERN JUNE 2014)
- Which is the nerve thickened shown in the picture?
  (NEET PATTERN 2018)

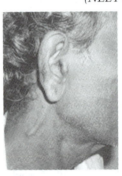

Ans: Greater Auricular Nerve.

- Which is the line shown below? *(AIIMS PATTERN 2017)*

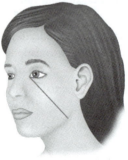

Ans: Ohngren's Line.

- Ohngren's Classification and Ohngren's Line are related to: Maxillary Sinus Carcinoma. *(NEET PATTERN 2014)*
- Laugier's Sign is NOT a feature of Lateral Sinus Thrombosis.
  (NEET PATTERN 2014)
- Water's view (Occipitomental view) is used for visualisation of: Maxillary Sinuses. *(NEET PATTERN 2018)*

- Caldwell's view (Occipitofrontal View) is used for the visualisation of: Frontal Sinuses. *(NEET PATTERN 2018)*
- Patient presents with ulcer on the side of nose which bleeds on scratching. The probable diagnosis is: Basal Cell Carcinoma. *(AIIMS PATTERN 2017)*

- Laugier's sign is a sign of basilar skull fracture
- Signs and tests a/w lateral sinus thrombosis
- Greisinger's sign
- Queckenstedt's test or Tobey Ayer's test
- Crowe beck test

RHINOSCLEROMA FACTFILE

- Caused by Klebsiella rhinoscleromatis.
- Klebsiella rhinoscleromatis is also known as: Frisch Bacillus.
- Also known as Mikulicz Disease.
- Histology shows Russell Bodies and Mikulicz Cells (Foamy Histiocytes).
- Tapir Nose (or Hebra Nose or Hippopotamus Nose)— Infiltrative stage of Rhinoscleroma. *(DNB PATTERN NOV 2013)*
- Tapir Nose is also described in Espundia (Internet Reference) caused by Leishmania Brasiliensis. So it may be a general term for chronic granulomatous deformation of the nose.
- Treatment of Rhinoscleroma: Third generation Cephalosporins/Ciprofloxacin.

- Syndrome caused by Nasopharyngeal Tumor characterised by pain similar to Trigeminal Neuralgia manifested in Lower Jaw and tongue and also middle ear deafness ?—Trotter's Syndrome. *(NEET PATTERN 2016)*
- Modified Cottle's Test is used for the assessment of: Nasal Valve Collapse. *(NEET PATTERN 2015)*
- Proof puncture (Antral Lavage) is done through: Inferior Meatus. *(NEET PATTERN 2016)*
- Juvenile Papilloma is NOT a name for Inverted Papilloma of Nose. *(NEET PATTERN 2015)*
- Double Target Sign or Double Ring Sign is seen in: Traumatic CSF Leak. *(AIIMS PATTERN 2017)*

THROAT

- Cotton Myer's Grading is used in Subglottic stenosis. *(DNB PATTERN DEC 2011)*

- Mid tracheostomy is done over 2nd and 3rd tracheal rings. *(DNB PATTERN DEC 2011)*
- Abductor of vocal cord is Posterior cricoarytenoid. *(DNB PATTERN DEC 2011)*
- Tensors of vocal cord are: Cricothyroid and internal thyroarytenoid. Internal Thyroarytenoid is also called Vocalis muscle. *(DNB PATTERN JUNE 2011)*
- Laryngocoele arises after herniation of: Thyrohyoid Membrane. *(DNB PATTERN JUNE 2011)*
- Laryngocoele is abnormal dilatation of laryngeal saccule.
- Quinsy is also known as: Peritonsillar Abscess. *(DNB PATTERN JUNE 2011)*
- In fracture maxilla, most common nerve involved is: Infraorbital nerve. *(DNB PATTERN JUNE 2011)*
- Woman with B12 deficiency, dysphagia and anemia-likely syndrome associated is: Plummer Vinson Syndrome.
- Plummer Vinson Syndrome. *(DNB PATTERN JUNE 2011)*
- True about double lumen tracheostomy tube: No inner cannula. *(DNB PATTERN JUNE 2011)*
- Supranuclear lesion of facial nerve affects: Lower part of face. *(DNB PATTERN DEC 2010)*
- NOT a cause of epistaxis: Allergic Rhinitis. *(DNB PATTERN DEC 2010)*
- Abductors of vocal cord are: Posterior cricoarytenoid. *(DNB PATTERN DEC 2009, DEC 2010)*
- During Tonsillitis, pain in the ear is due to involvement of: Glossopharyngeal nerve. *(DNB PATTERN DEC 2010)*
- In complete cleft, the hard palate is totally separated from: Vomer. *(DNB PATTERN DEC 2009)*
- Dangerous area of face is so called because: infection there can lead to cavernous sinus thrombosis and can be life threatening. *(DNB PATTERN JUNE 2009)*
- Omega shaped epiglottitis is seen in: Laryngomalacia. *(DNB PATTERN JUNE 2009)*
- Cadaveric position of vocal cords is seen in: Bilateral recurrent and superior laryngeal nerve palsy. *(DNB PATTERN JUNE 2009)*
- Acute laryngeal spasm during indirect laryngoscopy is seen in: Acute epiglottitis. So Indirect Laryngoscopy is avoided if indicated in Acute Epiglottitis. *(DNB PATTERN JUNE 2009)*
- Most common cause of acute epiglottitis is: Hemophilus Influenza. *(DNB PATTERN JUNE 2009)*

- In FESS surgery, structure preserved is: Maxillary sinus. *(DNB PATTERN JUNE 2009)*
- Tonsillectomy is contraindicated in Poliomyelitis epidemic. *(DNB PATTERN 2000)*
- Abductor of larynx is: Posterior cricoarytenoids. *(DNB PATTERN 2000)*
- Position of vocal cord in cadaver is: Intermediate. *(DNB PATTERN 2000)*
- Laryngeal nerve paralysis is seen in: Anaplastic thyroid cancer. *(DNB PATTERN 2001)*
- Taste sensation from posterior 1/3rd is carried by Glossopharyngeal nerve. *(DNB PATTERN 2001)*
- Heimlich's manoeuver is for relieving airway obstruction. *(DNB PATTERN 2001)*
- Singer's nodule is found between junction of anterior 1/3 and posterior 2/3 vocal cords. *(DNB PATTERN 2004)*
- Epulis is swelling from—Gums. *(DNB PATTERN JUNE 2008)*
- Most Common cause of Fungal Oesophagitis—Candida. *(DNB PATTERN JUNE 2008)*
- Thumb sign is seen in: Acute epiglottitis. *(DNB PATTERN DEC 2009)*
- Narrowest part of larynx: Rima Glottidis. *(DNB PATTERN AUG 2013)*
- When a patient is unable to vocalize, it is called: Aphonia. *(DNB PATTERN AUG 2013)*
- Chronic sclerosing sialadenitis is known as: Kuttner's tumour. *(DNB PATTERN NOV 2013)*
- Sialography is contraindicated in: Acute parotitis. *(DNB PATTERN NOV 2013)*
- Patulous Eustachian Tube is seen in: Pregnancy. *(DNB PATTERN NOV 2013)*
- Most common cause of Inspiratory Stridor in the neonatal period and early infancy: Laryngomalacia. *(FMGE PATTERN SEP 2012)*
- Most common congenital abnormality of the Larynx: Laryngomalacia.
- Inner cannula of Tracheostomy tube should be changed every 3rd day. *(FMGE PATTERN SEP 2012)*
- Turban Epiglottis is *Pathognomonic* of Tuberculosis. *(NEET PATTERN 2014)*
- Indication for Tracheostomy: Foreign Body obstructing Airway. *(NEET PATTERN 2018)*

LEVEL II: HIGH YIELD FACTORS

Table 9.1: Development of ear.

Pinna develops from	2nd branchial arch
Tragus (exception)	1st branchial arch
Tympanic membrane develops from	All three germinal layers
Defective fusion between 1st and IInd branchial arch structures	Preauricular sinus
Malleus and Incus	1st arch cartilage (Meckel's cartilage)
Stapes	2nd arch (Reichert's cartilage)
Mondini malformation	Cochlea with one and a half turns
Eustachian tube develops from	Tubotympanic recess

Table 9.2: Named structures of ear

Arnold's nerve	Auricular branch of vagus
Jacobsen's nerve	Tympanic branch of glossopharyngeal nerve.
Prussak's space	Shallow space between pars flaccida and neck of malleus
MacEwen's triangle	Surface landmark for mastoid antrum during mastoidectomy
Citelli's angle	Sinodural angle
Heschl gyrus	Primary auditory cortex
Toynbee's muscle	Tensor tympani
Shrapnell's membrane	Pars flaccida
Trautmann's triangle	Superior petrosal sinus/bony labyrinth/ Sigmoid sinus are boundaries.

Table 9.3: Tests/signs/phenomena in ear.

Hennebert's sign	False positive fistula sign seen in Meniere's disease, Congenital syphilis.
Tullio phenomenon	Dizziness on exposure to loud sounds seen in Labyrinthine fistula
Unterberger's test	Test for detection of pure vestibular lesions
Brun's nystagmus	Cerebello pontine lesions
Stenger's test, Chimani Moo test, Teal test	Non organic hearing loss

Table 9.4: Frequently asked investigations in the ear.

Carhart's notch	Notch at 2000 Hz in audiogram, suggests otosclerosis

Contd...

Contd...

Table 9.4: Frequently asked investigations in the ear.

Boilermaker's notch	Dip at 4000 Hz in audiogram suggesting acoustic trauma
U shaped audiogram	Congenital deafness
Roll over curve	Retrocochlear lesion
Recruitment phenomenon	For cochlear lesion ex: Meniere's disease, Presbycusis
Threshold Tone Decay test	For retrocochlear lesions

NOSE

Table 9.5: FAQ Paranasal sinuses.

1st sinus to develop:	Mastoid sinus
Ivory osteoma commonly occurs in	Frontal sinus
Most common acute sinusitis in children	Ethmoidal sinusitis
Least common sinusitis	Sphenoidal sinusitis
Nickel workers are predisposed to	Squamous cell carcinoma
Wood workers are predisposed to	Adenocarcinoma
Commonest organism causing acute bacterial sinusitis	Strep pneumoniae
Major cause of cavernous sinus thrombophlebitis	Sphenoid sinusitis

Table 9.6: FAQ Named bodies in nose.

Frisch bacillus (Klebsiella)	Rhinoscleroma
Mikulicz cells, Russell bodies	Rhinoscleroma
Saddle nose	Syphilis
Young's operation	Atrophic rhinitis
Apple Jelly nodules	TB nose
Charcot Leyden crystals	Fungal sinusitis
Mulberry like polypoidal mass	Rhinosporidiosis
Nasal maggots	Chrysomia

Table 9.7: Treatment modalities—nose.

Caldwell Luc surgery	Recurrent anterochoanal polyp
FESS	Treatment of choice for Antrochoanal polyp
Instillation of chloroform water with oil	Treatment of nasal maggots
Dapsone	Treatment of rhinosporidium seeberi

Contd...

Contd...

Table 9.7: Treatment modalities—nose.

Conservative management	Usual line of management of ethmoidal polyp
Avulsion	Single antrochoanal polyp

THROAT

Table 9.8:

Most common site of nasopharyngeal carcinoma	Fossa of Rosenmuller
Most common site of angiofibroma	Posterior part of nasal cavity
Frog face deformity	Angiofibroma
Space of Gillette	Retropharyngeal space
Most common nerve involved in Nasopharyngeal carcinoma	Abducens nerve
Hourglass sign/steeple sign	Acute laryngotracheobronchitis
Thumb sign	Acute epiglottitis
Screamer's nodes	Vocal nodules
Reinke's edema	Bilateral diffuse vocal cord polyposis

SADE CLASSIFICATION TABLE 9.9

Classification of Retraction of Tympanic Membrane – Pars Tensa

Grade 1 – Slight Retraction of Ear Drum

Grade 2 – Retracted Ear Drum touching the Incus or Stapes

Grade 3 – Tympanic Membrane touching the Promontory

Grade 4 – Tympanic Membrane adherent to the promontory.

10. Ophthalmology

"When people throw stones at you, you turn them into milestones."
—*Sachin Tendulkar*

REFERENCE

- *Comprehensive Ophthalmology by A K Khurana, 6th ed.*

LEVEL I: BASIC REPEATS

ORBIT AND EYEBALL

- Squint which can be corrected by spectacles: Accomodation squint. *(DNB PATTERN 2005)*
- Intermittent proptosis–orbital varices. *(DNB PATTERN JUNE 2008)*
- Intermittent proptosis is seen in Orbital varices. *(DNB PATTERN JUNE 2009)*
- Xanthelasma NOT true: dots occurring on lateral side of eye. *(DNB PATTERN DEC 2009)*
- Beaded margin of eyelid is seen in: Lipoid Proteinosis. *(DNB PATTERN DEC 2010)*
- The operation for placation of lower lid retractors is done for: Senile entropion. *(DNB PATTERN JUNE 2011)*
- Alkali injury to eye causes Symblepharon. *(DNB PATTERN JUNE 2011)*
- Most common intracranial tumor encroaching the orbit is: Sphenoid wing meningioma. *(DNB PATTERN JUNE 2011)*
- A patient comes with recent onset paralytic squint. Which is true of Paralytic squint? Diplopia. *(DNB PATTERN DEC 2011)*
- Miotics are used in: Convergent squints. *(DNB PATTERN DEC 2011)*
- Angle kappa is formed between which axes? Anatomical and visual axes. *(DNB PATTERN OCT 2013)*
- Most common ocular feature in Rheumatoid Arthritis: Episcleritis. *(DNB PATTERN OCT 2013)*
- Patient having difficulty in going down stairs. Muscle likely to be involved—Superior oblique palsy. *(FMGE PATTERN SEP 2012)*

- Lateral rectus—is supplied by Abducens nerve.
  (FMGE PATTERN SEP 2012)
- Secondary function of superior rectus—Adduction, Intorsion. *(FMGE PATTERN SEP 2012)*
- Retractors of upper eye lid—Levator palpebrae superioris, Muller's muscle. *(FMGE PATTERN SEP 2012)*
- Plication of lower eye lid is done for: Senile entropion.
  (FMGE PATTERN MAR 2013)
- Valve of Rosenmuller: A fold of mucus membrane found at the junction between common canaliculus and lacrimal sac.
  (DNB PATTERN JUNE 2014)
- Common canaliculus is guarded by the Valve of Rosenmuller.
- Valve of Hasner is at the opening of Nasolacrimal Duct into the inferior meatus of nose.
- OCULAR DEXTER refers to: Right Eye.
  (NEET PATTERN 2014)
- IMBERT FICK LAW Principle of Tonometry is used for: Applanation Tonometry. *(NEET PATTERN 2014)*
- Association of Intraocular Hemorrhage with Subarachnoid hemorrhage is known as: TERSON'S SYNDROME.
  (NEET PATTERN 2014)
- Lacrimal Gland Tumor moves the eyeball in which direction? INFERONASAL. *(NEET PATTERN 2014)*
- Most common primary intraorbital malignant neoplasm in children: RHABDOMYOSARCOMA.
  (NEET PATTERN 2014)
- Negative Jones 1 and Jones 2 Dye Tests indicate: Partial obstruction of Distal Nasolacrimal Duct.
  (NEET PATTERN 2015)
- BETTS Classification is used for: Ocular Trauma.
  (NEET PATTERN 2015)
- Normal Intraocular Pressure is: 16 mm.
  (NEET PATTERN 2016)
- Yoke Muscle of Right Lateral Rectus: Left Medial Rectus.
  (NEET 2018 PATTERN)
- Blow Out Fracture of Orbit involves: Floor.
  (NEET 2018 PATTERN)

SCLERA AND CONJUNCTIVA

- Maxwell Lyon sign is seen in Spring Catarrh.
  (DNB PATTERN 2007)
- Trantas nodules are seen in Vernal conjunctivitis.
  (DNB PATTERN 2005)
- Horner-Trantas spot is seen in Vernal keratoconjunctivitis.
  (DNB PATTERN DEC 2010)

Ophthalmology

- NOT true about Spring Catarrh: occurs in spring months. *(DNB PATTERN 2001)*
- Content of cobblestone in vernal conjunctivitis is Eosinophils. *(DNB PATTERN JUNE 2009)*
- Seasonal allergic conjunctivitis is: bilateral and recurrent. *(DNB PATTERN 2003)*
- Earliest feature of Vitamin A deficiency: Nyctalopia. *(DNB PATTERN 2002)*
- Percentage of Atropine seen in Atropine drops: 1%. *(DNB PATTERN 2002)*
- Herbert pits are seen in Trachoma. *(DNB PATTERN 2002)*
- Hemorrhagic conjunctivitis is caused by: Enterovirus 70. *(DNB PATTERN JUNE 2009)*
- Which is not a sequelae of Trachoma? Proptosis. *(DNB PATTERN JUNE 2009)*
- Arlt's line is seen in Trachoma. *(DNB PATTERN JUNE 2009)*
- Sclera is thinnest at: Insertion of Rectus Muscles. *(DNB PATTERN JUNE 2009)*
- Blue sclera is characteristic of Osteogenesis imperfecta. *(DNB PATTERN JUNE 2012)*
- Membranous conjunctivitis is NOT Easy to peel. *(DNB PATTERN JUNE 2011)*
- Cobble Stone Appearance is seen in: Vernal Keratoconjunctivitis. *(FMGE PATTERN JUNE 2014)*
- Organism causing acute bacterial conjunctivitis NOT associated with a polymorphonuclear response: MORAXELLA. *(NEET PATTERN 2014)*
- HEMORRHAGIC CONJUNCTIVITIS is NOT caused by: Influenza. *(NEET PATTERN 2014)*
- PINGUECULA is best characterized by: ELASTOTIC DEGENERATION. *(NEET PATTERN 2016)*
- Angular Conjunctivitis is caused by: Moraxella. *(NEET PATTERN 2016)*
- Circumcorneal congestion is not seen in: Scleritis. *(DNB PATTERN JUNE 2011)*
- Treatment of Phlyctenular Conjunctivitis is: Topical steroids. *(DNB PATTERN DEC 2011)*
- Physiological blue sclera is seen in: Premature newborn. *(DNB PATTERN OCT 2013)*
- Adrenochrome conjunctiva is due to: Topical Adrenaline use. *(DNB PATTERN AUG 2013)*
- Drug therapy for Pterygium: Mitomycin C. *(FMGE PATTERN SEP 2012)*

- Most common condition associated with Uveitis: Ankylosing Spondylitis. *(DNB PATTERN JUNE 2014)*
- Episclretis can be differentiated from Scleritis by: Blanching of vessels with 10% phenylephrine. *(NEET PATTERN 2014)*

CORNEA

- Refractive power of cornea is 30. *(DNB PATTERN 2006)*
- Drugs of choice for corneal herpes: Acyclovir. *(DNB PATTERN 2002)*
- Corticosteroids are contraindicated in Corneal Ulcer. *(DNB PATTERN JUNE 2008)*
- Keratoconus is not associated with–Hypermetropia. *(DNB PATTERN JUNE 2008)*
- Corneal ectasia with inflammation–Anterior Staphyloma. *(DNB PATTERN JUNE 2008)*
- Treatment of Mooren's ulcer is Topical steroids, immunosuppresants, soft contact lens, lamellar or full thickness corneal grafts. *(DNB PATTERN JUNE 2009)*
- Kayser-Fleischer Ring is seen in Wilson's Disease. *(DNB PATTERN JUNE 2009)*
- Satellite lesion is seen in which corneal ulcer? Fungal. *(DNB PATTERN DEC 2009)*
- Steroids are contraindicated in: Herpetic corneal ulcer. *(DNB PATTERN JUNE 2010)*
- Neuroparalytic keratitis is due to which cranial nerve? 5th nerve. *(DNB PATTERN JUNE 2010)*
- Waves present in Electroretinogram are: D wave. *(DNB PATTERN JUNE 2010)*
- Which organism can penetrate the intact cornea? Gonococcus. *(DNB PATTERN DEC 2010)*
- NOT seen in Keratoconus: KF ring. *(DNB PATTERN DEC 2010)*
- When water enters eyes, blurring of vision is due to Elimination of Refraction through cornea. *(DNB PATTERN JUNE 2009)*
- Maximum refraction takes place between: Tear film and cornea. *(DNB PATTERN JUNE 2011)*
- Pigmented neurosensory epithelium of cornea is a continuation of: Non-pigmented epithelium of choroid. *(DNB PATTERN JUNE 2011)*
- Epidemic Keratoconjunctivitis is caused by: Adenovirus Type 8. *(DNB PATTERN DEC 2011)*

- Kayser-Fleischer Ring is seen in Wilson's disease.
  (DNB PATTERN JUNE 2012)
- Amsler's sign is seen in: Fuch's Heterochromic Iridocyclitis.
  (DNB PATTERN OCT 2013)
- Most common complication of corneal transplant: Post-transplant astigmatism. *(DNB PATTERN OCT 2013)*
- Which layer of cornea plays an important role in maintaining corneal transparency? Endothelium.
  (DNB PATTERN AUG 2013)
- Nummular keratitis is caused by: Herpes Zoster.
  (FMGE PATTERN SEP 2012)
- Keratometer measures: Curvature of cornea.
  (FMGE PATTERN SEP 2012)
- Vitamin A deficiency Secondary sign is: Bitot Spot.
  (FMGE PATTERN JUNE 2014)
- Herpes infection of corneal ulcer is called: Dendritic Ulcer.
  (FMGE PATTERN JUNE 2014)
- Stroma of Cornea develops from: NEURAL CREST.
  (NEET PATTERN 2014)
- Scarpa's Staphyloma is seen in: Myopia.
  (NEET PATTERN 2014)
- Corneal sensation is measured by: AESTHESIOMETER
  (NEET PATTERN 2016)

ANTERIOR CHAMBER

- Commonest parasitic cause of Uveitis: Toxocara.
  (DNB PATTERN 2000)
- Uveoparotitis is seen in: Sarcoidosis.
  (DNB PATTERN DEC 2009)
- Behcet's disease is characterized by: Hypopyon
  (DNB PATTERN JUNE 2010)
- Iris pearl is seen in: Hansen's disease.
  (DNB PATTERN DEC 2011)
- Lisch nodules on Iris is a feature of: Neurofibromatosis.
  (DNB PATTERN DEC 2010)
- Neuroectodermal origin is of: Iris epithelium.
  (DNB PATTERN JUNE 2010)
- Most common intraocular malignancy in adults is: Melanoma choroid. *(DNB PATTERN DEC 2010)*
- Laser used in Iridotomy is: CO_2 laser.
  (DNB PATTERN DEC 2011)
- Argyll Robertson Pupil is seen in: Neurosyphilis.
  (DNB PATTERN JUNE 2012)

- Drug of choice of Iridocyclitis is: Atropine.
 (DNB PATTERN DEC 2011)
- Drug of choice of Anterior Uveitis is: Topical Steroids.
 (DNB PATTERN DEC 2011)
- Most common cause of Anterior Uveitis: Idiopathic.
 (DNB PATTERN OCT 2013)
- Junction between ciliary body and choroid—Ora serrata.
 (FMGE PATTERN SEP 2012)
- Recurrent mobile hypopyon is seen from Acute Anterior Uveitis with: Behcet's Syndrome. *(NEET PATTERN 2015)*

LENS

- Polychromatic luster is seen in Complicated Cataract.
 (DNB PATTERN 2006)
- Thickest part of Lens is: Pre Equator.
- Thinnest part of lens capsule is Posterior part.
 (DNB PATTERN 2005)
- Commonest congenital cataract is Zonular.
 (DNB PATTERN 2005)
- Commonest cause of uniocular diplopia: Cataract.
 (DNB PATTERN 2004)
- Marfan's syndrome is associated with: Ectopia lentis.
 (DNB PATTERN JUNE 2009, DNB PATTERN JUNE 2010)
- After cataract refers to opacity following extracapsular lens extraction. *(DNB PATTERN 2003)*
- Sunflower cataract is due to Chalcosis. *(DNB PATTERN 2003)*
- Most common type of Staphyloma in myopia is: Posterior.
 (DNB PATTERN 2001)
- Which Lenticonus is more common in males? Anterior lenticonus. *(DNB PATTERN JUNE 2009)*
- Second sight is seen in–Presbyopia with improved near vision. *(DNB PATTERN JUNE 2008)*
- Most common cause of blindness in India–Cataract.
 (DNB PATTERN JUNE 2008, JUNE 2009)
- Lens of eye develops from: Surface ectoderm.
 (DNB PATTERN DEC 2010)
- Thinnest part of lens is: posterior pole.
 (DNB PATTERN JUNE 2009)
- Lens contains which antigen? Sequestered Antigens.
- *(DNB PATTERN JUNE 2010)*
- Typical appearance of Diabetic cataract is: Snow flake appearance. *(DNB PATTERN DEC 2010)*
- Site of bleeding after cataract surgery is: Posterior ciliary vessels. *(DNB PATTERN DEC 2010)*

Ophthalmology

- NOT a cause of Ectopia Lentis: Cogan Reese Syndrome. *(DNB DEC 2010 PATTERN)*
- Chronic systemic steroid use causes Cataract. *(DNB PATTERN DEC 2011)*
- What is the treatment of congenital cataract involving visual axis? Immediately operate. This is to prevent Stimulus Deprivation Amblyopia. *(DNB PATTERN DEC 2011)*
- Posterior staphyloma is associated with Pathological myopia. *(DNB PATTERN DEC 2011)*
- Lens is derived from: Surface Ectoderm. *(DNB PATTERN NOV 2013)*
- Snowflake Cataract is seen in: Diabetes Mellitus. *(DNB PATTERN AUG 2013)*
- Treatment of Posterior Capsular Opacity: YAG Laser Capsulotomy. *(DNB PATTERN AUG 2013)*
- Person with low vision at day, better at night: Nuclear cataract. *(DNB PATTERN JUNE 2014)*
- Which type of antigen is Lens antigen? Heterophile Antigen. *(DNB PATTERN JUNE 2014)*
- A 6-month-old baby presenting with Bilateral Cataract, condition to be suspected is: Galactosemia. *(NEET PATTERN 2014)*
- Ring of Soemmering is seen in: Lens Capsule. *(NEET PATTERN 2014)*
- Lens of the Eye develops from: Surface Ectoderm. *(NEET PATTERN 2015)*
- Blue Dot Cataract is NOT seen in Galactosemia. *(NEET PATTERN 2016)*
- Astigmatism in emmetropic eye of Elderly person contribute to: + 3 dioptres. *(NEET 2018 PATTERN)*

VITREOUS

- Secondary Vitreous develops from: Ectoderm. *(DNB PATTERN DEC 2009)*
- Eale's disease is: Recurrent vitreous hemorrhage. *(DNB PATTERN JUNE 2011)*
- Synchysis Scintillans: occurs in Cholesterolosis Bulbi characterized by cholesterol deposits in the vitreous. *(DNB PATTERN AUG 2013)*

RETINA

- Ring scotoma is seen in Retinitis Pigmentosa. This is also called Annular Scotoma. *(DNB PATTERN 2004)*

- Macula lies at 2 disc diameters from the temporal margin of the optic disc.
- Macula lies from disc at a distance of 3 mm.
  (DNB PATTERN 2003)
- Cotton Wool spots in diabetic retinopathy are due to Retinal Nerve Fibre Infarcts. *(DNB PATTERN 2002)*
- Keith-Wagener classification is for Hypertensive Retinopathy.
  (DNB PATTERN 2001)
- Another classification system for Hypertensive Retinopathy: Wong and McIntosh Classification.
- Cherry red spot is NOT seen in Retinopathy of Prematurity.
  (DNB PATTERN 2001)
- Diabetic retinopathy is related to duration of disease.
  (DNB PATTERN 2000)
- Most important determining factor in Diabetic Retinopathy is: Duration of Diabetes.
- Salt and pepper fundus occurs in Rubella.
  (DNB PATTERN 2000)
- Panretinal photocoagulation is done in Proliferative retinopathy. *(DNB PATTERN 2000)*
- Pars planitis visual loss due to—Cystoid Macular Edema.
  (DNB PATTERN JUNE 2008)
- Rees-Elworth classification–Retinoblastoma.
  (DNB PATTERN JUNE 2008)
- Earliest feature of Diabetic Retinopathy is Microaneurysms.
  (DNB PATTERN JUNE 2009)
- Regarding Retinoblastoma TRUE Statement: 25% bilateral.
  (DNB PATTERN DEC 2009)
- Which of the following is NOT an ophthalmic emergency? Macular Hole. *(DNB PATTERN JUNE 2010)*
- Retinal detachment occurs in which layer? Sensory Retina.
  (DNB PATTERN JUNE 2010)
- Treatment of choice for clinically significant macular edema in a diabetic is Focal photocoagulation.
  (DNB PATTERN DEC 2010)
- Cattle track appearance on Fundoscopy is due to CRAO.
  (DNB PATTERN DEC 2010)
- In Retinitis Pigmentosa, there is NO early loss of central vision. *(DNB PATTERN JUNE 2011)*
- In Retinitis Pigmentosa, there is early ROD involvement and CONES are involved later.
- Extraretinal fibrovascular proliferation at ridge between normal and avascular retina is of stage 3 Retinopathy of Prematurity. *(DNB PATTERN JUNE 2011)*

Ophthalmology

- Abnormal dilatation and tortuosity of the blood vessels in ROP that may go on to Retinal Detachment is referred to as: PLUS Disease.
- Second common malignancy in patients of retinoblastoma is Osteosarcoma. *(DNB PATTERN DEC 2011)*
- Candle wax Drippings on Retinoscopy: Sarcoidosis. *(DNB PATTERN NOV 2013)*
- Most common cause of Retinal Detachment: Rhegmatogenous. *(DNB PATTERN AUG 2013)*
- Roth Spots are seen in: Acute Leukaemia. *(NEET 2018 PATTERN)*
- Roth Spots are typically described in Infective Endocarditis but can also be seen in Acute Leukemia, Anemia etc.
- A child is diagnosed to have Retinitis Pigmentosa. Examination shows Bird Beaked Facies and Normal Pressure Hydrocephalus. Probable Diagnosis is: Cockayne's Syndrome. *(AIIMS 2017 PATTERN)*

OPTIC NERVE

- Anterior ischemic optic neuritis is seen in a case of Giant Cell Arteritis. *(DNB PATTERN 2004)*
- Most dangerous injury for vision–Fracture Optic nerve canal. *(DNB PATTERN JUNE 2008)*
- Disc Edema is NOT seen in: Retrobulbar Neuritis. *(DNB DEC 2010 PATTERN)*
- Neuroretinal rim of optic nerve is thickest at Inferior portion. *(DNB PATTERN OCT 2013)*
- Derivative of Optic cup: Retina. *(DNB PATTERN AUG 2013)*
- Site of lesion of Crocodile tear syndrome: Geniculate Ganglion. *(DNB PATTERN AUG 2013)*
- Altitudinal field defect is seen in: Anterior Ischemic Optic Neuropathy. *(FMGE PATTERN SEP 2012)*

VISUAL PATHWAY

- Methyl alcohol causes blindness by acting on: Ganglion cells. *(DNB PATTERN JUNE 2011)*
- A hectic bout of fever with bilateral proptosis in a 25-year-old diabetic following an injury to face is most diagnostic of: Cavernous sinus thrombosis. *(DNB PATTERN JUNE 2011)*
- Homonymous Hemianopia is caused by lesion of: Optic tract. *(DNB PATTERN DEC 2011)*
- All of the following causes visual loss in hypertension NOT Occipital infarct. *(DNB PATTERN DEC 2011)*

- Achromatopsia is related to which area of the occipital cortex? Area V8. *(DNB PATTERN OCT 2013)*
- Humphrey Field Analyzer is a type of: Automated Static Perimeter. *(NEET PATTERN 2016)*

MISCELLANEOUS

- Photophthalmia is caused by Ultraviolet rays. *(DNB PATTERN 2006)*
- Ultraviolet Rays with a wavelength of 311–290 microns usually cause Photophthalmia.
- Snow Blindness is caused by the effect of reflected UV rays from snow.
- For Tonometry, used is 4% xylocaine. *(DNB PATTERN 2004)*
- Campimetry is used to measure Field charting. *(DNB PATTERN 2004)*
- Campimetry is used to assess the CENTRAL PART of the visual field.
- Cause of unilateral amblyopia: High anisometropia. *(DNB PATTERN 2003)*
- Dalen-Fuchs nodules are seen in Sympathetic Ophthalmitis. *(DNB PATTERN 2001)*
- Vossius ring occurs in Concussion injury. *(DNB PATTERN 2000)*
- Thyroid ophthalmopathy MRI finding swelling of: Muscle Bellies. *(DNB PATTERN JUNE 2008)*
- Muscle Insertions are spared.
- Most common muscle involved in Thyroid Ophthalmopathy: Inferior Rectus.
- Eye involvement is seen in Seronegative JRA. *(DNB PATTERN JUNE 2009)*
- Which of the following is seen in Horner's syndrome? Anhidrosis. *(DNB PATTERN JUNE 2009)*
- NOT true about Chalazion: Horizontal incision to be made to squeeze out contents. *(DNB PATTERN DEC 2009)*
- True about amplitude of accommodation is: about 10 diopters in emmetropic eye. *(DNB PATTERN DEC 2009)*
- Earliest ocular sign in Acoustic Neuroma: Loss of corneal sensation. *(DNB PATTERN DEC 2009)*
- Definition of blindness according to WHO: 3/60. *(DNB PATTERN DEC 2009)*
  - Clinically, this is taken as an inability to count fingers in daylight at a distance of 3 metres.

Ophthalmology

- In Acute Angle Closure Glaucoma, NOT seen: Snow banking. *(DNB PATTERN JUNE 2010)*
- During DCR surgery, an osteotomy was done in the anterior and superior region. Which area does it accidentally open into? Anterior ethmoidal sinus. *(DNB PATTERN JUNE 2010)*
- Structure associated with horizontal movement of eye is: Pons. *(DNB PATTERN JUNE 2010)*
- Dalen-Fuchs nodules is pathognomonic of Sympathetic Ophthalmitis. *(DNB PATTERN JUNE 2010)*
- Anticholinergic is NOT used in Glaucoma. *(DNB PATTERN DEC 2010)*
- TRUE regarding Herpes Zoster Ophthalmicus: Vesicles appear before pain. *(DNB PATTERN DEC 2010)*
- In Herpes Zoster Ophthalmicus, the least involved nerve is: Facial. *(DNB PATTERN JUNE 2011)*
- Shortest acting mydriatic is: Tropicamide. *(DNB PATTERN JUNE 2011)*
- Visual Acuity of 6/60 is classified as Low vision. *(DNB PATTERN JUNE 2011)*
- Vitamin A supplementation in a 10-month-old child with Xerophthalmia is three doses of 1 lakh units. *(DNB PATTERN DEC 2011)*
- NOT a cause of night blindness: Devic's disease. *(DNB PATTERN DEC 2011)*
- After a leisure trip, a patient comes with gritty pain in the eye and joint pain. The most probable diagnosis is Reiter's syndrome. *(DNB PATTERN DEC 2011)*
- Painless loss of vision is NOT attributed to Angle Closure Glaucoma. *(DNB PATTERN DEC 2011)*
- Horner's syndrome component? Anhidrosis. *(DNB PATTERN DEC 2011)*
- Ciliary muscle is derived from: Mesoderm. *(DNB PATTERN NOV 2013)*
- Eye donation fortnight: August 25–September 8. *(DNB PATTERN NOV 2013)*
- Most common cause of visual impairment in Diabetic Retinopathy: Diabetic Maculopathy. *(DNB PATTERN OCT 2013)*
- More specific answer to this question would be Diabetic Macular Edema.
- Barkan's membrane is seen in: Congenital Glaucoma. *(DNB PATTERN AUG 2013)*
- Glaucoma Flecken is seen in: Acute Angle closure Glaucoma. *(DNB PATTERN AUG 2013)*

- Wave length of CO_2 Laser: 9400–10600 nanometer.
  (DNB PATTERN AUG 2013)
- First nerve to be affected in cavernous sinus thrombosis: 6th nerve. *(FMGE PATTERN SEP 2012)*
- Silent Choroid on Fluoroscein angiography is a feature of: Stargardt's Disease. *(JIPMER 2017 PATTERN)*
- 100 Day Glaucoma is seen in: Central Retinal Vein Occlusion (CRVO). *(NEET PATTERN 2018)*

LEVEL II: HIGH YIELD FACTORS

Table 10.1: Devices in ophthalmology

Ishihara charts	Color vision
Perimetry	Field of vision
Keratometry	Central corneal curvature
Pachymeter	Thickness of cornea
Bjerrum screen	Field of vision
Campimetry	Central field of vision/Blind Spot
Goldmann 3 mirror lens	Visualization of Retina
Jaeger cards	Near vision acuity
Snellen's charts	Visual Acuity
Broken Landolt's Rings	Visual Acuity in Illiterate patients
Slit lamp	Diagnosis of vitreous opacities
Distant Direct Ophthalmoscopy	Done at 22 cm
Direct Ophthalmoscopy	Magnified/Virtual/Erect image
Indirect Ophthalmoscopy	Real/Inverted/Magnified (RIM) image
Indirect Ophthalmoscopy	Best for visualizing the periphery of retina/ideal for examining Vitreous
Gonioscopy	Angle of anterior chamber
Shaffer's grading	Grading of angle of Anterior chamber
Schiotz Tonometer	Most commonly used for determination of Intraocular Pressure
Tonography	Method for determining aqueous flow
Maddox Rod test	Macular function
Amsler's grid test	Macular function
Purkinje image 1	Formed by anterior surface of cornea/erect image
Purkinje image 2	Formed by posterior surface of cornea/erect image
Purkinje image 3	Formed by anterior surface of Lens/erect image
Purkinje image 4	Formed by Posterior surface of Lens/inverted image

Contd...

Contd...

Table 10.2: Frequently asked features in ophthalmology

Iris Nodules	Tuberculoma
Cherry Red spots	CRAO/Berlin's edema/Tay Sach's disease/Niemann-Pick disease
Salt and Pepper fundus	Rubella/Syphilis
Roth's spots	Infective Endocarditis
White Reflex in Pupil	Retinoblastoma/Pseudoglioma
Follicles	Trachoma/Spring Catarrh
Argyll Robertson pupil	Syphilis/Diabetes Mellitus
Adie's Tonic pupil	Diabetes Mellitus/Shy-Drager syndrome
Dendritic Ulcer	Herpes Simplex virus
Numular keratitis	Herpes Zoster Ophthalmicus
Ulcer serpens	Pneumococcal hypopyon ulcer
Horner-Trantas spots	Vernal Keratoconjunctivitis
Munson's sign	Keratoconus
Vogt's striae	Keratoconus
Fleischer's ring	Keratoconus
Sunflower cataract	Wilson's disease
Brushfield's spots	Down's syndrome
Soemmering ring	After cataract
Elschnig's pearls	After cataract
Snow flake opacities in Lens	Diabetes Mellitus
Christmas Tree pattern of lens opacities	Myotonia Dystrophica
Ectopia Lentis	Commonly in Marfan's syndrome; also Weill Marchesani syndrome
Photophthalmia (Snow Blindness)	Ultraviolet rays
Photoretinitis (Eclipse Burn)	Infrared rays

Table 10.3: Lens and cataract

Lens is thinnest	Posteriorly (3 microns)
Lens is thickest	Near Equitorial region (20 microns)
Lens is developed from	Surface Ectoderm
Only structure in eye which continues to grow through out life	Lens
85% glucose metabolism in Lens is by	Anaerobic Glycolysis
Oil droplet cataract	Galactosemia
Most common form of cataract	Age related Cataract

Contd...

Contd...

Anterior Lenticonus/Anterior Polar Cataract	Alport syndrome
Most common type of Congenital cataract	Zonular/Lamellar cataract
Lens subluxation upwards and outwards	Marfan's syndrome
Lens subluxation downwards and inwards	Homocystinuria
Lens subluxation downwards	Weill-Marchesani syndrome
Most common systemic disorder associated with Ectopia Lentis	Marfan's syndrome

Table 10.4: Visual development

Visual Acuity at birth	6/60
Newborn eye is	Hypermetropic
Optic nerve and differentiation continues up to	1 month after birth
Conjunctival and Corneal epithelium develops from	Surface ectoderm
Lacrimal gland develops from	Surface ectoderm
Lens develops from	Surface ectoderm
Corneal stroma and Endothelium develops from	Cranial neural crest cells
Sclera develops from	Cranial neural crest cells
Ciliary muscles develop from	Cranial neural crest cells
Sphincter and dilator papillae develops from	Neuroectoderm

Table 10.5: Ocular pharmacology

Drug associated with Follicular conjunctivitis	Brimonidine
Drug causing macular toxicity	Intravitreal Gentamicin
Orange colored tears	Rifampicin
Drug contraindicated in Sulfonamide allergy	Acetazolamide
Iris cysts are a side effect of	Echothiophate

Table 10.6: Optics and refraction

Refractive index of Cornea	1.37
Power of a reduced eye	58D
Most important factor affecting convergence of light rays on Retina	Refractive index of cornea
Soft Contact Lens	HEMA
Hard Contact Lens	PMMA
Gas permeable Lens	Cellulose Acetate
Maximum visual acuity	Rigid Gas permeable Lens

Contd...

Contd...

Table 10.7: Cornea and conjunctiva

Termination of cornea at Limbus is formed by	Schwalbe's line
Cornea is avascular and derives nutrition mainly from	Aqueous Humor
Most important layer maintaining the transparency of the cornea	Endothelium
Megalocornea and epibulbar dermoids are a feature of	Goldenhar syndrome

Table 10.8: Spring catarrh

Type 1 Hypersensitivity

More common in summer NOT in spring!

Giant papillae

Cobble Stone Appearance of Conjunctiva

Pavement stone Appearance of Conjunctiva

Horner-Trantas Spots – composed of Eosinophils

Shield Ulcers

Punctate Keratopathy

Pseudogerontoxon or Cupid's Bow

Table 10.9: Acanthamoeba keratitis

Acanthamoeba does NOT require any host to complete its life cycle (AI 05)

More common in immunocompromised patients (AI 05)

Swimming in pool with contact lens/ocular trauma with vegetative matter – predisposing factors

Severe pain is typical due to Keratoneuritis

Cultured on Non-Nutrient Agar with an overlay of E. coli

Medications: Polyhexamethylene Biguanide/Propamidine/Chlorhexidine

Table 10.10: Retinoblastoma and other ocular tumors

Trilateral Retinoblastoma	Bilateral Retinoblastoma with Pinealoblastoma
Retinoblastoma is bilateral in	35–40% cases
Most common presentation	Leukocoria
Most common non-ocular malignancy associated with Retinoblastoma	Osteosarcoma
Most specific histopathological feature of Retinoblastoma	Fleurettes
Retinoblastoma is inherited as	Autosomal Dominant

Contd...

Contd...

Knudson's 2 hit hypothesis	Hypothesis in which two alleles should be knocked off for development of Retinoblastoma
Retinoblastoma gene	13q14

COMMUNITY OPHTHALMOLOGY

Most Common cause of ocular morbidity in the community	Refractive Error
Most common cause of Low vision in India	Cataract
Most common cause of Blindness in the world	Cataract > Glaucoma > Trachoma
Most common cause of Blindness in the developing countries	Cataract
Most common cause of Blindness in the developed countries in individuals more than 60 years of age	ARMD
Most common cause of blindness in children in India	Vitamin A Deficiency
Most common cause of avoidable or preventable blindness in children in India	Vitamin A Deficiency
Most common cause of treatable blindness in children in India	Cataract
Highest prevalence of Blindness in India is in (NPCB survey 1986–1989)	Jammu and Kashmir
Cut off value for differentiating normal from abnormal in School vision screening program in India	6/9
Initial screening personnel for detection of refractive errors in school children	School teachers preferably females
Eye Donation Fortnight	August 25–September 8

VISUAL DEVELOPMENT

Visual acuity at birth	6/60
New born eye is	Hypermetropic (AIIMS 93, PGI 96)
Optic nerve myelination and differentiation continues up to	1 month after birth (AI 93)
Critical period for the development of fixation reflex	2–3 months of age (AI 1995)
Lens develops from	Surface Ectoderm (AIIMS 2003, 2006)
Conjunctival and corneal epithelium develops from	Surface Ectoderm (AIIMS 2006)
Lacrimal gland develops from	Surface Ectoderm (AIIMS 2006)

Contd...

Contd...

Corneal stroma and endothelium develops from	Cranial Neural crest (AIIMS 2009)
Sclera develops from	Cranial Neural crest cells (AIIMS 2006)
Sphincter papillae and Dilator papillae develops from	Neuroectoderm (NEET PATTERN 2013)
Vitreous develops from	Neuroectoderm, Surface Ectoderm and mesoderm
Ciliary muscles develop from	Cranial Neural Crest cells
Cornea develops from	Both surface ectoderm and cranial neural crest cells

EMBRYOLOGY OF EYE

Neuroectoderm	Surface Ectoderm	Mesoderm	Cranial Neural Crest
Neurosensory Retina	Lens	Extraocular muscles	Corneal stroma and endothelium
Retinal pigment epithelium	Epithelial glands	Vitreous	Sclera
Ciliary Epithelium	Conjunctival and corneal epithelium	Temporal part of sclera	Ciliary muscles
Iris epithelium	Lacrimal gland	Endothelial lining of orbital vessels	Ciliary ganglion
Optic Nerve, axons and glial cells	Vitreous	Bony orbit	
Vitreous	Eyelids		
Sphincter papillae and dilator pupillae			

OCULAR PHARMACOLOGY

Antiglaucoma drug causing Depression	Timolol (AIIMS 2003)
Antiglaucoma drug causing altered lipid profile	Timolol (AIIMS 2003)
Contraindication for Timolol	COPD/Bronchospasm (PGI 2004)
Ocular agent most likely to cause Follicular conjunctivitis	Brimonidine
Xerostomia is a side effect of	Brimonidine (AI 2006)
Ocular agent contraindicated in patients allergic to sulfonamides	Acetazolamide (AI 2005)

Mechanism of action of Latanoprost	Acts by increasing aqueous outflow through uveoscleral pathway (AI 2004)
Advantage of Dorzolamide over Acetazolamide	Good intraocular penetration due to better lipid permeability (AI 2006)
Bull's eye Keratopathy is a side effect of	Chloroquine
Intravitreal Gentamicin causes	Macular toxicity
Corneal punctuate erosions are a side effect of	Idoxuridine
Cherry Red Spot is a side effect of	Quinine
Central Scotoma and Xanthopsia are side effects of	Digitalis
Pigmentary Retinopathy is a side effect of	Chlorpromazine

LENS

Equitorial diameter of Lens	10–11 mm (TN 2001)
Thickness of Lens	3.5–5 mm thick
Lens is thinnest	Posteriorly (UP 2008)
Lens is thickest	Near equatorial region
Refractive Power of Lens	15 dioptres
Lens accounts for	25% of total refractive power of eye
Lens is formed from	Surface Ectoderm
Only structure in eye which continues to grow throughout life	Lens
Glucose enters the lens by	Simple Diffusion and also Facilitated diffusion from Aqueous Humor
Major mode of metabolism in Lens is by	Anaerobic Glycolysis

EPONYMOUS SIGNS IN OPHTHALMOLOGY

Purtscher's Retinopathy	Retinopathy of bilateral peripapillary patches and retinal whitening and hemorrhages after compression injury to the head.

Wyburn Mason Syndrome	Dilated and tortuous retinal vascular abnormalities and AV malformations in the Mid Brain.
Stargardt Disease	Hereditary Retinal Disorder involving ABCA4 mutations.
Cogan Reese Syndrome	Unilateral Glaucoma with Nodules and extension to Endothelium and Descemet's Membrane.
Dua's Layer	New anatomic layer of the cornea (Pre Descemet Layer) first described by Harminder Dua in 2013.
Charles Bonnet Syndrome	Vivid Complex Visual Hallucinations in a a psychologically intact person.

11. Orthopaedics

"To succeed in life, you need three bones. A wish bone, a back bone and a funny bone."
—*Reba McEntire*

REFERENCES
- *Essential Orthopaedics by Maheshwari, 5th ed.*
- *Apley's System of Orthopaedics and Fractures, 9th ed.*

LEVEL I: BASIC REPEATS

TUBERCULOSIS

- First sign of Tuberculous Arthritis—Reduced joint space. *(DNB PATTERN JUNE 2008)*
- Most common site of Tuberculous spine—T12/L1. *(DNB PATTERN JUNE 2008)*
- TB spine most commonly affects: Thoracic. *(DNB PATTERN JUNE 2009)*
- Spina ventosa is the name given to radiographic picture of Tubercular Dactylitis. *(DNB PATTERN DEC 2011)*
- Carpel Tunnel syndrome is NOT caused by Tuberculosis. *(DNB PATTERN DEC 2010)*
- Pott's spine is commonest at which spine? Thoracolumbar. *(DNB PATTERN DEC 2010)*
- Poncet's disease: Polyarthralgia associated with TB. *(DNB PATTERN AUG 2013)*
- In TB Hip, during the stage of synovitis, there is Apparent Lengthening. *(NEET PATTERN 2016)*

OTHER INFECTIOUS BONE DISEASES

- Periosteal reaction in a case of Acute Osteomyelitis can be seen earliest at: 7-10 days. *(FMGE PATTERN MAR 2012)*
- Indication for using systemic steroids in a case of Rheumatoid Arthritis: Mononeuritis Multiplex. *(FMGE PATTERN MAR 2012)*
- Crystals deposited in Pseudogout: Sodium Pyrophosphate. *(FMGE PATTERN MAR 2013)*
- Primary Hematogenous Osteomyelitis of children primarily involves: Metaphysis. *(NEET PATTERN 2014)*

Orthopaedics

- Avascular Necrosis of Lunate is known as: Kienbock's Disease. *(NEET PATTERN 2015)*

FRACTURES

- Tardy ulnar nerve palsy is seen in Malunited lateral condylar fracture. *(DNB PATTERN DEC 2011)*
- Most common complication of Colles' fracture is stiffness of fingers. *(DNB PATTERN 2000)*
- Cubitus varus is the most common complication of supra condylar fracture of Humerus. *(DNB PATTERN 2004)*
- Monteggia fracture is the fracture of proximal 1/3rd of Ulna. *(DNB PATTERN 2003)*
- Gunstock deformity is seen in: Supracondylar fracture humerus. *(DNB PATTERN JUNE 2009)*
- Jones' fracture is Avulsion fracture of base of fifth metatarsal. *(DNB PATTERN JUNE 2009)*
- Diaphysis fracture involves: Long bones. *(DNB PATTERN JUNE 2010)*
- Fracture of distal tibial epiphysis with anterolateral displacement is called as: Tillaux fracture. *(DNB PATTERN JUNE 2010)*
- A 10-year-old sustained an elbow injury about 4 yrs back. He now complains of deformity at the elbow and numbness of the ulnar two fingers of the ipsilateral two fingers of the ipsilateral hand. Most probably the injury sustained was Fracture of the lateral condyle of the Humerus. *(DNB PATTERN 2006)*
- Stress fracture of 2nd metatarsal is known as March fracture. *(DNB PATTERN JUNE 2008)*
- Most common site of March fracture is: shaft of 2nd and 3rd metatarsals. *(DNB PATTERN JUNE 2009)*
- Attitude of the lower limb in fracture Neck of femur—External rotation and adduction. *(DNB PATTERN JUNE 2008)*
- Commonest cause of Anterior compartment syndrome is: Fracture. *(DNB PATTERN 2000)*
- Best way to treat a fracture neck of femur in a child is: Hip Spica in abduction and internal rotation. *(DNB PATTERN JUNE 2010)*
- Avascular Necrosis occurs commonly in intracapsular fracture Neck of Femur. *(DNB PATTERN JUNE 2008)*
- Fracture shaft of Humerus causes damage to Radial nerve. *(DNB PATTERN JUNE 2009, JUNE 2010)*

- Cotton's fracture involves: Ankle.
  (DNB PATTERN DEC 2010)
- Tension Band wiring is used for: Olecranon fracture.
  (DNB PATTERN JUNE 2011)
- Ideal treatment of a 3 day old fracture neck of femur in a 50-year-old male would be Compression screw fixation.
  (DNB PATTERN 2004)
- Hawkins' sign denotes: Retained vascularity.
  (DNB PATTERN OCT 2013)
- Motor cyclist's fracture is Skull base breaks into two: Anterior and Posterior. *(DNB PATTERN OCT 2013)*
- Charlie Chaplin Gait: Tibial Torsion.
  (DNB PATTERN AUG 2013)
- Cozen's Test: Tennis Elbow. *(DNB PATTERN AUG 2013)*
- Gallow's Traction is used for: Fracture Shaft of Femur.
  (NEET PATTERN 2016)
- Bone that most commonly fractures when a person falls on outstretched hand: Radius. *(NEET 2018 PATTERN)*
- Perilunate Dislocation is: Lower radius, Scaphoid and Lunate in alignment, Capitate out of plane. *(NEET 2018 PATTERN)*

PERILUNATE DISLOCATION

- 'PIECE OF PIE' Appearance.
- Triangular Appearance of Lunate.
- Associated with Scaphoid Fracture in 60% cases.

BONE TUMOURS

- Which isotope is used for treating bone cancer? Strontium 90. *(DNB PATTERN JUNE 2012)*
- Commonest benign bone tumor is: Osteochondroma.
  (DNB PATTERN 2004)
- Chemotherapeutic agent of choice for Osteogenic sarcoma: Methotrexate. *(DNB PATTERN 2001)*
- Radiotherapy is the treatment of choice in Ewing's sarcoma.
  (DNB PATTERN 2001)
- Sun ray Appearance is suggestive of Osteosarcoma.
  (DNB PATTERN 2003)
- Predominantly osteoblastic metastasis is seen in Prostate carcinoma. *(DNB PATTERN DEC 2009)*
- The bone tumor seen in children with characteristic Onion Peel periosteal reaction is: Ewing's sarcoma.
  (DNB PATTERN DEC 2010)

- Snowstorm appearance of knee joint with multiple loose bodies are seen in Synovial chondromatosis.
 (DNB PATTERN JUNE 2011)
- Most common malignancy of bone is secondary.
 (DNB PATTERN DEC 2011)
- Which of the following arises in the medullary canal of diaphysis? Ewing's sarcoma. *(DNB PATTERN 2001)*
- Bone tumor arising from epiphysis is Chondroblastoma.
 (DNB PATTERN JUNE 2011)
- Most common primary malignancy of bone: Multiple Myeloma. *(DNB PATTERN OCT 2013)*
- Osteosarcoma is most common at which site? Near the knee.
 (DNB PATTERN JUNE 2014)
- Bone Tumor which closely resembles Osteomyelitis: Ewing's Sarcoma. *(NEET PATTERN 2014)*
- Tumor arising from the Epiphysis in Children: Chondroblastoma. *(NEET PATTERN 2015)*
- Fallen Fragment Sign: Simple Bone Cyst.
 (NEET 2018 PATTERN)

OSTEOPOROSIS AND OSTEOMALACIA

- Looser's zone is characteristic of Osteomalacia.
 (DNB PATTERN 2003)
- Intranasal calcitonin is given for the treatment of Osteoporosis.
 (DNB PATTERN DEC 2010)
- Treatment of choice for postmenopausal osteoporosis-Raloxifene.
 (DNB PATTERN JUNE 2008)

DISLOCATIONS

- Attitude of lower limb seen in posterior dislocation of hip is Flexion, adduction and Internal Rotation.
 (DNB PATTERN 2002, DEC 2011)
- In congenital dislocation of hip, clinical sign which shows that the affected thigh is at a higher level when the knees and hips are flexed to 90 degrees is known as Galeazzi's sign.
 (DNB PATTERN 2006)
- In inferior shoulder dislocation, nerve most commonly injured is: Axillary N. *(DNB PATTERN DEC 2010)*
- Most common type of Elbow dislocation is: Posterior.
 (DNB PATTERN DEC 2010)
- Hill Sach lesion is seen in: Anterior dislocation of shoulder joint. *(DNB PATTERN JUNE 2010)*

- Vascular sign of Narath is seen in: Posterior dislocation of Hip. *(DNB PATTERN JUNE 2009)*
- A 4-year-old boy is complaining of pain around elbow held in pronation with extension and normal X ray. What is the possible diagnosis? Pulled elbow. *(DNB PATTERN DEC 2011)*
- Position of shoulder in posterior dislocation of shoulder: Adducted and internally rotated. *(NEET PATTERN 2014)*
- Unhappy Triad of O'Donoghue Does not involve PCL tear. *(NEET PATTERN 2015)*
- Subluxation of Proximal Radioulnar Joint is known as: Nursemaid's Joint. *(NEET PATTERN 2015)*

SIGNS AND TESTS

- Allen's test for integrity of Palmar arch tests both radial and ulnar arteries. *(DNB PATTERN JUNE 2012)*
- In Froment's sign, adductor pollicis is tested. *(DNB PATTERN 2003)*
- Cozen test is done for Tennis Elbow. *(DNB PATTERN JUNE 2011)*
- Thomas test is used for testing Hip flexion. *(DNB PATTERN DEC 2010)*
- Card test is for testing the Ulnar nerve. *(DNB PATTERN 2007)*
- Lachman's sign is positive in Anterior cruciate ligament injury. *(DNB PATTERN 2003)*
- True about slipped capital femoral epiphysis is: Trethowan sign is seen. *(DNB PATTERN JUNE 2010)*
- Siffert Katz sign is seen in: Blount's disease. *(DNB PATTERN DEC 2009)*
- Kanavel's sign does not include Pain on passive flexion of the fingers. *(NEET PATTERN 2016)*

MUSCLES, LIGAMENTS AND JOINTS

- Type of cells predominantly present in Rheumatoid Arthritis: Macrophages. *(NEET 2018 PATTERN)*
- Rheumatoid Arthritis affects which part of axial skeleton?— Cervical vertebra. *(DNB PATTERN JUNE 2008)*
- Arthritis Mutilans is seen in: Psoriatic Arthropathy. *(DNB PATTERN JUNE 2011)*
- Joints NOT involved in Rheumatoid arthritis are DIP joints. *(DNB PATTERN DEC 2011)*
- Most common cause of Neuropathic joints: Diabetes. *(DNB PATTERN 2001)*

- Most common cause of Clutton joints-Diabetes Mellitus. *(DNB PATTERN JUNE 2008)*
- Neuropathic joint NOT seen in—Sarcoidosis. *(DNB PATTERN JUNE 2008)*
- Trigger finger is stenosing tenovaginitis of flexor tendon of affected finger. *(DNB PATTERN 2000)*
- Mallet finger is avulsion of terminal slip of extensor tendon to terminal phalanx. *(DNB PATTERN 2000)*
- Fibrosis is most commonly seen in Sternocleidomastoid. *(DNB PATTERN 2007)*
- NOT true about Klippel Feil syndrome—Bilateral shortening of Sternocleidomastoid. *(DNB PATTERN DEC 2011)*
- Myositis ossificans is: Post-traumatic ossification. *(DNB PATTERN JUNE 2012)*
- Myositis Ossificans is most commonly seen in Elbow joint. *(DNB PATTERN 2000)*
- Osteoarthritis does not involve Ankle joint. *(DNB PATTERN DEC 2011)*
- In gout, tophi are NOT seen in Muscles. *(DNB PATTERN DEC 2011)*
- Volkmann's Ischaemia most commonly involves the flexor digitorum profundus. *(DNB PATTERN 2000)*
- First sign of Volkmann's ischaemia: Pain on passive movements. *(DNB PATTERN 2001)*
- Standing on toes is NOT possible in paralysis of-Gastrocnemius. *(DNB PATTERN JUNE 2008)*
- Duputyren's contracture most often involves Ring finger. *(DNB PATTERN 2001)*
- Nerve closely related to shoulder joint capsule: Axillary Nerve. *(DNB PATTERN 2002)*
- Management of congenital pseudoarthrosis of knee: Vascularised fibular graft. *(DNB PATTERN 2002)*
- Which is not a fibrous joint? First costochondral joint. *(DNB PATTERN JUNE 2011)*
- Pseudoflexion deformity of hip is seen in: Iliopsoas abscess. *(DNB PATTERN JUNE 2009)*
- Indication of surgical compartment release in compartment syndrome in any compartment is absolute pressure greater than 30 mm Hg. *(DNB PATTERN DEC 2010)*
- Adventitious bursa is abnormal bursa occuring over friction site. *(DNB PATTERN 2004)*
- Triple arthrodesis involves fusion of talocalcaneal, talonavicular and calcaneocuboid joints. *(DNB PATTERN 2005*

- Musculocutaneous Nerve does NOT lie in close proximity with the Humerus. *(NEET PATTERN 2015)*
- Structure which is intracapsular extrasynovial: Long Biceps Tendon. *(NEET PATTERN 2016)*
- Tendons affected in DeQuervain's Tenosynovytis: Extensor Pollicis Brevis and Abductor Pollicis Longus. *(NEET 2018 PATTERN)*
- Mnemonic: DeQuervain is a rich man i.e APL(above poverty line) !!!
- Which kind of joint does 8th and 9th rib costal cartilage form? Synovial Joint. *(NEET 2018 PATTERN)*

METABOLIC BONE DISEASE

- In renal osteodystrophy, skeletal abnormality is most commonly due to: Hyperphosphatemia. *(DNB PATTERN DEC 2011)*
- Characteristic sub periosteal bone resorption in Hyperparathyroidism is best seen in: Radial border of middle phalanx. *(DNB PATTERN DEC 2011)*
- Marble Bone disease is better known as: Osteopetrosis. *(DNB PATTERN DEC 2009)*
- Disease caused by osteoclast dysfunction: Osteopetrosis. *(DNB PATTERN 2007)*
- Shepherd Crook Deformity is seen in: Fibrous Dysplasia. *(DNB PATTERN JUNE 2010)*

CTEV

- Early CTEV is treated by: Manipulation and Corrective splint both. *(DNB PATTERN DEC 2010)*
- Treatment of club foot should begin as soon as possible after birth. *(DNB PATTERN 2000)*
- Which is not true about CTEV shoe? Straight outer border. *(DNB PATTERN JUNE 2009)*

MISCELLANEOUS

- Rate of Nerve regeneration–1 mm/day. *(DNB PATTERN JUNE 2008)*
- Claw hand is seen in Ulnar nerve injury. *(DNB PATTERN 2001)*
- Also called Spinster's Claw.
- Meralgia paresthetica involves Lateral cutaneous nerve of thigh. *(DNB PATTERN DEC 2009)*

Orthopaedics

- Genu valgus deformity is seen when long axis of tibia and fibula moves lateral to the long axis of femur. *(DNB PATTERN DEC 2011)*
- Which of the following is a fenestrated Hip prosthesis? Austin Moore Prosthesis. *(DNB PATTERN DEC 2010)*
- Charlie Chaplin Gait is seen in Tibial torsion. *(DNB PATTERN DEC 2010)*
- Salmonella Osteomyelitis is common in Sickle cell Disease. *(DNB PATTERN DEC 2010)*
- Non traumatic amputation is seen in Sickle cell Anemia, Diabetes Mellitus and Leprosy. *(DNB PATTERN DEC 2009)*
- Avascular necrosis can be retarded by 1500 mg of calcium daily. *(DNB PATTERN JUNE 2009)*
- The deformity of tibia in triple deformity of the knee is: Flexion, posterior subluxation and external rotation. *(DNB PATTERN JUNE 2009)*
- Forced inversion in plantar flexed foot injuries is due to: Talofibular ligament. *(DNB PATTERN JUNE 2009)*
- Avascular necrosis of head of femur occurs commonly at subcapital region. *(DNB PATTERN 2000)*
- Commonest site of acute osteomyelitis in infant is: Femur. *(DNB PATTERN 2003)*
- Dactylitis NOT seen in—Sarcoidosis. *(DNB PATTERN JUNE 2008)*
- Hill Sachs lesion is seen in: Posterolateral part of humeral head. *(DNB PATTERN OCT 2013)*
- Idiopathic scoliosis is most commonly: Dextroscoliosis of Thoracic spine. *(DNB PATTERN OCT 2013)*
- Agnes Hunt Traction is used for: Correction of hip deformity. *(DNB PATTERN OCT 2013)*
- Bone cement setting time is: 8-10 minutes. *(DNB PATTERN OCT 2013)*
- Flip Test is: SLR Test which is positive in both sitting and lying down position. *(DNB PATTERN AUG 2013)*
- Panner's disease: Osteochondritis of the capitulum of the distal humerus. *(DNB PATTERN AUG 2013)*
- Osgood Schlatter's disease involves: Tibial Tuberosity. *(DNB PATTERN OCT 2013)*
- Diagnostic manoeuvre for Medial meniscus injury: McMurray's Test. *(FMGE PATTERN MAR 2013)*
- Hand Knee Gait is seen in: Polio. *(FMGE PATTERN MAR 2013)*
- Most common joint involved in Osteoarthritis in India: Knee *(FMGE PATTERN 2009)*

- Hip is the mosy commonly involved joint in Osteoarthritis in the Western countries.
- While using Axillary crutches, the elbow should be flexed to: 30 degrees. *(FMGE PATTERN MAR 2013)*
- Joint least involved in Primary Osteoarthritis: Coracoclavicular joint. *(FMGE PATTERN MAR 2013)*
- Total claw hand is caused by injury to: Ulnar and Median Nerve. *(FMGE PATTERN 2005)*
- Partial claw hand is caused by injury to: Ulnar Nerve. *(FMGE PATTERN 2009)*
- Bone Multicellular Unit consists of: Osteoblast and Osteoclast. *(DNB PATTERN JUNE 2014)*
- Injury to Supraspinatus muscle causes: Rotator Cuff Injury. *(FMGE PATTERN JUNE 2014)*
- Most common site of Osteochondritis: Lateral Part of Medial femoral condyle. *(NEET PATTERN 2014)*
- Thurstan Holland's Sign is seen in Salter Harris Type 11 fractures. It is also called Shiny Corner Sign. *(NEET PATTERN 2014)*
- Fracture involving Physis, Epiphysis and Metaphysis is Salter Harris Type IV. *(NEET PATTERN 2015)*
- Most common type of acute knee injuries seen in athletes comprise: ACL, MCL and Lateral Meniscus Tear. *(NEET PATTERN 2014)*
- Injury to Ulnar Nerve at the wrist causes paralysis of: Adduction of the Thumb. *(NEET PATTERN 2014)*
- In Holstein Lewis Fracture, the nerve most commonly involved is: Radial Nerve. *(NEET PATTERN 2014)*
- Malgaigne's fracture refers to Supracondylar fracture Humerus. *(NEET PATTERN 2014)*
- Tom Smith Arthritis is: Septic Arthritis of Infancy. *(NEET 2018 PATTERN)*
- As an Intern, 1st priority to pass on to Orthopaedics Post Graduate would be: Patient's finger is blackening.
- Other options:
- 10 cm abrasion
- Inability to extend arm
- Intra-articular fracture of elbow joint. *(NEET 2018 PATTERN)*

Orthopaedics

LEVEL II: HIGH YIELD FACTORS

Table 11.1: Splints

Von Rosen splint	Congenital dysplasia of hip
Dennis Brown splint	Congenital talipes equino varus
Aeroplane splint	Brachial plexus injury
Milwaukee brace	Scoliosis
Volkmann's splint	Volkmann's ischaemic contracture
Cock up splint	Radial nerve palsy
Thomas splint	Fracture femur
Knuckle Bender splint	Ulnar nerve palsy

Table 11.2: Skeletal tuberculosis

Commonest site of skeletal TB	Spine
Commonest complication of skeletal TB	Cold abscess
Earliest sign of TB spine	Reduction in disc space
Investigation of choice of spine TB	MRI
Most significant sign of Pott's paraplegia	Ankle clonus
Spina ventosa	TB dactylitis
Caries sicca	TB shoulder joint
Wandering acetabulum	TB hip
Stage 1 TB hip	Flexion/Abduction/External Rotation (FABER)
Stage 2 TB hip	Flexion/Adduction/Internal Rotation (FADIR)
Stage 3 TB hip	Flexion/Adduction/Internal Rotation (FADIR)

Table 11.3: Named bursitic diseases

Bunion	Chronic bursitis of great toe
Morrant Baker's cyst	Posteromedial bursitis of popliteal fossa
Tailor's ankle	Chronic lateral malleolar bursitis
Student's elbow	Olecranon bursitis
Brodie's bursa	Medial head of gastrocnemius bursa
Clergyman's knee	Infrapatellar bursitis
Tennis elbow	Lateral epicondylitis of humerus
Golfer's elbow	Medial epicondylitis of humerus

IMPORTANT CLINICAL TESTS AND SIGNS IN ORTHOPAEDICS

SHOULDER JOINT

Apprehension test	Look of apprehension as the patient resists any attempt made to dislocate the shoulder joint.
Bryant's sign	Lowering of the axillary folds suggests shoulder dislocation
Callaway's test	Girth of the affected shoulder is increased in shoulder dislocation
Duga's test	Inability to touch the chest with the elbow when the hand of the affected shoulder is placed on the opposite shoulder in subluxation/dislocation of shoulder
Hamilton's test	Shoulder dislocation
Painful Arc test	Subacromial bursitis

ELBOW JOINT

Cozen's test	Lateral epicondylitis
Reverse Cozen's test (Golfer's Elbow test)	Medial epicondylitis (Golfer's elbow)

WRIST JOINT

Finkelstein's test	De Quervain's disease
Finsterer's sign	Pain on percussion of 3rd metacarpal in Keinbock's disease of lunate
Maisonneuve's sign	Malunited Colle's fracture
Phalen's sign (Dorsal) – Prayer sign	Carpel Tunnel syndrome (Median nerve paraesthesia)
Carpal lift test	Earliest sign of carpal bone fracture.
Bracelet test	Rheumatoid arthritis
Bunnel littler's test	Osteoarthritis of DCP joint
Allen's test	Entrapment of vessels at the wrist

HIP JOINT

Thomas test	Unilateral fixed flexion deformity of hip
Kothari's method	Method to measure fixed adduction Deformity of hip
Trendelenburg's test	Test for abductor mechanism of the Hip in standing up position.
Important causes of Trendelenberg's positive:	1. Gluteal weakness/paralysis as in Polio
	2. Gluteal inhibition as in hip pain
	3. Gluteal insufficiency due to: Coxa vara.
	4. CDH

Contd.

Contd...

Telescopy test	Test for hip stability in lying down position
Telescoping is also seen in: Also in old and neglected posterior dislocation of hip, nonunion fracture neck of femur	CDH
Other special tests of the hip	Fabere test, Stinchfield test

KNEE JOINT

Patellar tap test	Moderate knee joint effusion
Fluctuation test	Large knee joint effusion
Q angle (Quadriceps angle)	Angle between quadriceps tendon (Rectus femoris) and patellar tendon
Q angle < 13 degree	Patella alta
Q angle > 18 degree	Tibial torsion/Subluxating patella/Genu valgum
Valgus stress test	Medial collateral ligament injury
Varus stress test	Lateral collateral ligament injury
Anterior Drawer test	Anterior instability of knee (Anteromedial bundle)
Posterior Drawer test	Posterior instability of knee
Mc Murray's test	Meniscal injury
Apley's compression and distraction tests	Meniscal injuries
Lachman's test	Anterior cruciate ligament injury (Posterolateral bundle)

SACROILIAC JOINT

Gapping test (Sacroiliac stretch test)	Sprain of anterior sacroiliac ligament
SQUISH test	Sprain of posterior sacroiliac ligament
Iliac compression test	Sacroiliac sprain/fracture of wing of the ileum
Gaenselen's test	Sacroiliac joint disease
Sacral Apex test	Sacroiliac joint arthritis
Erichsen's test	Sacroiliac joint disease
Passive SLRT and Braggard's Sign	To differentiate between disc prolapse sciatica and sacroiliac joint involvement

SPINE

Straight leg raising test (SLRT)	Nerve root irritation
Lasegue test (Flexing hip and knee to 90 degree)	Nerve root compression or irritation
Braggard's sign positive	Ask the patient to passively dorsiflex the foot after passive SLRT, If pain increases, indicative of Sciatica, if pain does NOT increase, it is suggestive of Sacroiliac or Lumbosacral joint involvement.

Table 11.4: Common orthopaedic instruments

Thomson's prosthesis	Non fenestrated femoral head prosthesis
Austin Moore prosthesis	Femoral head prosthesis with two fenestrations
Smith Peterson's nail	Used for internal fixation of fracture of femoral neck
Kuntscher nail	Clover leaf shaped-used for internal fixation of fracture of femoral shaft
Dynamic hip screw	Used for internal fixation of trochanteric fractures

Table 11.5: FAQ bone tumours

Gardner's syndrome	Multiple osteomas
Osteoid osteoma	Nocturnal pains relieved by Aspirin and appearing as radiolucent nidus
Osteosarcoma	Syndromes associated: Li Fraumeni syndrome, Werner syndrome, Bloom syndrome, Rothmund Thomson syndrome
Ollier's syndrome	Non familial multiple enchondromatosis
Maffucci's syndrome	Familial multiple enchondromatosis
McCune Albright syndrome	Precocious puberty associated with Polyostotic fibrous dysplasia
Multiple myeloma	Most common primary bone tumour
Most common site of chordoma	Sacro coccygeal
Physaliferous cells	Chordoma
Osteoblastic metastases	Most frequently produced by prostate and breast
Ewing's sarcoma	Homer Wright pseudorosettes
Ewing's sarcoma	Arises in the medullary cavity of the diaphysis of long bones

Table 11.6: Named fractures

Aviator's fracture	Fracture neck of talus
Bumper fracture	Compression fracture of lateral condyle of tibia
Boxer's fracture	Fracture of distal 5th metacarpal
Bennett's fracture	Intra-articular fracture of base of first metacarpal
Bankart's fracture	Fracture of anterior glenoid associated with shoulder dislocation–Anterior type
Cotton's fracture	Trimalleolar fracture of ankle
Clay Shoveller's fracture	Stress avulsion fracture of spinous processes of C6, C7 or T1
Chauffeur's fracture	Intra articular fracture of radial styloid
Essex Lopresci fracture	Comminuted radial head fracture with distal radioulnar joint subluxation
Jones' fracture	Fracture of base of 5th metatarsal extending into intermetatarsal joint
Jefferson fracture	Burst fracture of 1st cervical vertebra
Lisfranc's fracture	Fracture dislocation of midfoot
Maissoneave's fracture	Spiral fracture of proximal fibula
Pilon fracture	Comminuted fracture of distal articular fracture with fibular fracture
Pott's fracture	Bimalleolar fracture
Runner's fracture	Stress fracture of distal fibula
Tillaux fracture	Salter Harris fracture type 3 of the tibia
Hangman's fracture	Fracture of both C2 pedicles
Hill Sach's fracture	Impacted posterior humeral head fracture occurring during anterior shoulder dislocation
Galeazzi fracture	Radius shaft fracture with dislocation of distal radioulnar joint
Gosselin fracture	V shaped distal tibia fracture

Table 11.7: CTEV

External fixators for CTEV	Joshi's external stabilising system (JESS)/Illizarov system
Sequence of correction of deformity in CTEV	Forefoot adduction/inversion/equinus
Surgery for CTEV	Calcaneocuboid fusion/Lateral wedge resection
Splint used in CTEV	Dennis Brown splint

Table 11.8: Miscellaneous

Champagne glass pelvic cavity	Achondroplasia

Contd...

Table 11.8: Miscellaneous

Marie Strumpell disease	Ankylosing spondylitis
Trident hand	Achondroplasia
Rugger Jersey spine	Osteopetrosis
Sprengel's deformity	Congenital elevation of the scapula
Erlenmeyer flask appearance	Osteopetrosis
Pseudogout	Calcium pyrophosphate crystal deposition
Joint mice	Osteoarthritis
Felty's syndrome	Rheumatoid arthritis, neutropenia and splenomegaly
Rheumatoid arthritis	Autoantibodies against Fc portion of IgG
Paget's disease	Cotton wool appearance

FAQ BONE PATHOLOGY

Basic structural unit of Lamellar bone	Osteon
Central canal in the osteon	Haversian canal
Connecting channels of Haversian canals	Volkmann' canals
Strands of fibrous tissue connecting the bone	Sharpe's fibres
Bone hypertrophy occurs the plane of stress. This is called	Wolff's law
Callus is otherwise called	Woven bone
Osteoblasts are rich in	Alkaline phosphatase
Osteocytes are rich in	Glycogen and PAS positive granules
Osteoclasts are rich in	Hydrogenases, collagenases and acid phosphatase.
Multinucleate mesenchymal cells present in	Bone osteoclasts

SALTER HARRIS CLASSIFICATION

(Ref: Dahnert's Radiology Review, 4th ed.)

Classification for **Epiphyseal Plate Injuries**

Courtesy Robert Bruce Salter and W. Robert Harris ...... orthopaedic surgeons in Toronto, Canada.

Prognosis is worse in Lower Extremities irrespective of Salter Harris Type.

Addition to Salter Harris Classification was done by **Rang and Ogden** who added Type 6,7,8,9.

Mnemonic: SALTR

Slip of Physis: Type 1 includes SCFE (Slipped capital femoral epiphysis)

Above Physis: Type 2 (Most common) – Corner Sign/Thurston Holland's Sign

Lower than Physis: Type 3 – Intraarticular fracture

Through Physis: Type 4 – involves Physis + Epiphysis + Metaphysis.

Rammed Physis: Type 5 – (Least common) – Poorest prognosis/ Growth impairment in 100%

TRIPLANE FRACTURE
Vertical fracture of epiphysis + Horizontal cleavage plane through Physis + Oblique fracture of adjacent metaphysis.

RARE NAMES OF COMMON EPONYMOUS FRACTURES

Chauffeur's fracture	Hutchinson fracture Lorry Driver's fracture Backfire fracture
Colle's fracture	Pouteau fracture Most common fracture of forearm
Galeazzi fracture	Piedmont fracture
Monteggia fracture	Classification of Monteggia type Fractures is known as Bado's classification
Smith's fracture	Reverse Colle's fracture Reverse Barton's fracture Goyrand fracture Garden spade deformity
Tibial plateau fractures	Schatzker classification
Lateral malleolar fractures	Weber's classification
Shepherd's fracture	Fracture of lateral tubercle of posterior process of talus. Described by Francis Shepherd. No high incidence in Shepherds !!!

12. Medicine

"Wear your failure as a badge of honour."
—**Sundar Pichai**
CEO, Google.

REFERENCE

- *Harrison's Textbook of Internal Medicine, 19th ed.*

LEVEL I: BASIC REPEATS

NERVE AND MUSCLE

- Myotonia congenita does NOT involve Proximal muscle groups. *(DNB PATTERN 2000)*
- Mononeuritis multiplex is a symptom of Polyarteritis nodosa, Hypertensive vasculitis, Leprosy. *(DNB PATTERN 2000)*
- HLA associated with Myasthenia Gravis: HLA B8. *(DNB PATTERN 2000, 2004)*
- Increased frequency of HLA B27 is NOT seen in Myasthenia gravis. *(DNB PATTERN 2008)*
- Acetylcholine receptors are affected in Myasthenia gravis. *(DNB PATTERN 2001)*
- Lateral medullary syndrome is due to the thrombosis of Posterior inferior cerebellar artery. *(DNB PATTERN 2000)*
- Sensation first lost in Syringomyelia is Pain and Temperature. *(DNB PATTERN 2000)*
- Carbamazepine is NOT used in the treatment of Status epilepticus. *(DNB PATTERN 2001)*
- Brain Death is defined as Isoelectric EEG for 30 min. *(DNB PATTERN 2001)*
- Albuminocytological dissociation is seen in Guillain-Barré syndrome. *(DNB PATTERN 2001)*
- Bleeding in Pons causes Coma and Pinpoint pupil. *(DNB PATTERN 2001)*
- In Foster-Kennedy syndrome, the tumor is in Subfrontal area. *(DNB PATTERN 2001)*
- Commonest cause of stroke in elderly is Thrombosis. *(DNB PATTERN 2004)*

- Lasegue's sign is seen in Nerve root pressure.
  (DNB PATTERN 2004, 2007)
- Todd's paralysis is mostly seen after Grand mal epilepsy.
  (DNB PATTERN 2003)
- Hemiparesis is NOT a feature of Vertebral artery occlusion.
  (DNB PATTERN 2008)
- Increase in protein without pleocytosis in cerebral fluid is seen with Guillain-Barré syndrome. *(DNB PATTERN 2008)*
- Thick nerves are NOT seen in Alcoholic polyneuropathy.
  (DNB PATTERN 2008)
- Myopathy is NOT a feature of Vitamin B12 deficiency.
  (DNB PATTERN 2007)
- Dystrophin gene is of great diagnostic significance in Duchenne muscular dystrophy. *(DNB PATTERN 2007)*
- Neck rigidity without fever is seen in Subarachnoid hemorrhage. *(DNB PATTERN 2006)*
- Adenoma sebaceum in Tuberous sclerosis is—Angiofibroma.
  (DNB PATTERN JUNE 2008)
- Enzyme deficient in Parkinsonism: Tyrosine hydroxylase.
  (DNB PATTERN JUNE 2012)
- Flapping tremor does NOT occur in: Parkinsonism.
  (DNB PATTERN JUNE 2012)
- Subacute combined degeneration of Spinal cord occurs in: Vitamin B12 *(DNB PATTERN JUNE 2012)*
- Drug of choice for trigeminal neuralgia: Carbamazepine.
  (DNB PATTERN JUNE 2009)
- Acetylcholine deficiency in cortex is seen in Alzheimer's disease. *(DNB PATTERN JUNE 2009)*
- NOT true about Weber's syndrome is: Contralateral facial nerve palsy. *(DNB PATTERN DEC 2009).*

In Weber's syndrome, there is ipsilateral 3rd nerve palsy.

- Wallenberg syndrome does NOT involve 12th nerve.
  (DNB PATTERN DEC 2009)
- Lateral medullary syndrome is most commonly due to involvement of vertebral artery.
  (DNB PATTERN DEC 2009)
- Posterior inferior cerebellar artery is next common. V4 segment of the ipsilateral vertebral artery is most commonly affected in Wallenberg's syndrome.
- Dysmetria is due to lesion of cerebellum.
  (DNB PATTERN JUNE 2010)
- Not true of Tabes dorsalis: Deep tendon reflexes are retained. *(DNB PATTERN JUNE 2010)*
- Hippocampus lesion affects memory transformation from short term to long term. *(DNB PATTERN JUNE 2010)*

- Diazepam poisoning is treated by Flumazenil.
  (DNB PATTERN DEC 2010)
- Nervous system is primarily affected in Tetanus.
  (DNB PATTERN DEC 2010)
- Most common false localizing sign is Diplopia.
  (DNB PATTERN DEC 2010)
- Clinical features of conus medullaris are all except late bladder involvement. *(DNB PATTERN JUNE 2011)*
- Seizures are not a manifestation of Amoebiasis.
  (DNB PATTERN JUNE 2011)
- All are true about treatment of Guillain-Barré syndrome except use of corticosteroids. Corticosteroids are usually avoided in GBS. *(DNB PATTERN JUNE 2011)*
- True about Guillain-Barré syndrome all except descending paralysis. *(DNB PATTERN DEC 2011)*
- Part of brain involved in Narcolepsy: Hypothalamus.
  (DNB PATTERN DEC 2011)
- First center that gets activated before skilled voluntary movements: Neocortex. *(DNB PATTERN DEC 2011)*
- Acute onset areflexic quadriparesis with blurred vision and absent pupillary response in 20-year-old male: Botulism.
  (DNB PATTERN JUNE 2011)
- In tuberculous meningitis, opening pressure is not low.
  (DNB PATTERN JUNE 2011)
- Drug of choice for acyclovir resistant Human herpes virus: FOSCARNET. *(DNB PATTERN JUNE 2011)*
- Commonest site for Hypertensive bleed: Putamen.
  (DNB PATTERN DEC 2010)
- Schirmer's test for facial nerve. *(DNB PATTERN DEC 2011)*
- Episodic weakness does NOT occur in Hyperglycemia.
  (DNB PATTERN DEC 2011)
- NOT true about Migraine: Sumatriptan used for chronic migraine. *(DNB PATTERN DEC 2009)*
- Facial nerve involvement in Geniculate ganglion causes Ramsay Hunt syndrome. *(DNB PATTERN DEC 2009)*
- Ramsay Hunt syndrome involves commonly 7th and 8th cranial nerves together. *(DNB PATTERN DEC 2009)*
- Recurrent facial palsy, recurrent facial edema and plication of the tongue in Melkersson-Rosenthal syndrome.
  (DNB PATTERN DEC 2009)
- Earliest feature of Multiple sclerosis: Optic neuritis.
  (DNB PATTERN JUNE 2010)
- This is not the earliest symptom, the earliest being sensory loss and the next optic neuritis.

- Multiple sclerosis not associated with Hydrocephalus. *(DNB PATTERN JUNE 2011)*
- Most common inherited peripheral neuropathy: Charcot-Marie-Tooth type 1. *(DNB PATTERN NOV 2013)*
- Tropical spastic paraparesis is caused by: HTLV 1. *(DNB PATTERN AUG 2013)*
- Useful bedside test for Myasthenia gravis: Ice pack test. *(DNB PATTERN AUG 2013)*
- Drug of choice for Acute dystonia: Central anticholinergics—Benztropine *(DNB PATTERN AUG 2013)*
- Klein-Levin syndrome: Recurrent hypersomnia/hyperphagia/hypersexuality. *(DNB PATTERN AUG 2013)*
- CSF PROTEIN 14-3-3 is elevated in Creutzfeldt-Jakob disease. *(DNB PATTERN AUG 2013)*
- Increased muscle tone is a feature of: Extrapyramidal tract involvement. *(NEET PATTERN 2016)*
- Most common cause of Intracranial hemorrhage: Intracerebral hemorrhage. *(NEET PATTERN 2016)*
- Most common etiology of Mollaret's meningitis is: Herpes simplex 2. *(NEET PATTERN 2016)*
- A patient comes with headache describing it as the worst headache of his life. There is no facial deficit. What is the next line of investigation? NCCT Head. *(AIIMS PATTERN 2017)*
- Proptosis and Hypotropia releived within 5 minutes of administering an IV drug is indicative of: Myasthenia Gravis. *(AIIMS PATTERN 2017)*
- Treatment for Intractable Sydenham's Chorea: Valproate. *(NEET PATTERN 2018)*
- NOT a feature of NF-1: Acoustic Neuroma. *(NEET PATTERN 2018)*
- Minimal Brain Dysfunction was a term used to define: ADHD. *(NEET PATTERN 2018)*

GIT

- Pseudomembranous colitis is caused by Clostridium difficile. *(DNB PATTERN 2000, 2001)*
- Osmotic diarrhea is seen in Lactase deficiency. *(DNB PATTERN 2000, 2006)*
- Poor prognostic factor in Acute pancreatitis is Increased blood sugar. *(DNB PATTERN 2000, 2006)*
- Diarrhea is NOT a feature of Hyperparathyroidism. *(DNB PATTERN 2000)*

- Gastric ulcer is caused by Helicobacter pylori.
  (DNB PATTERN 2000)
- Vitamin deficiency seen in Tropical sprue: Vitamin B12.
  (DNB PATTERN 2001)
- Splenomegaly is characteristic of Hairy cell leukemia.
  (DNB PATTERN 2001, 2004)
- Massive splenomegaly is NOT found in Acute myeloid leukemia. *(DNB PATTERN 2004)*
- Terry's nail is found in Cirrhosis.
  (DNB PATTERN 2001, 2008)
- Most common symptom of Primary biliary cirrhosis: Pruritus. *(DNB PATTERN 2004, 2006)*
- Mallory's hyaline is seen in Alcoholic hepatitis.
  (DNB PATTERN 2004)
- Clubbing of fingers is NOT seen in Cirrhosis of liver.
  (DNB PATTERN 2003)
- Most common cause of Peritonitis in a patient with cirrhosis: E. coli *(DNB PATTERN 2007)*
- Delta virus is associated with Hepatitis B virus.
  (DNB PATTERN 2007)
- Significant perinatal transmission is for Hepatitis B virus.
  (DNB PATTERN 2007)
- Indicator of active multiplication of Hepatitis B virus is HbeAg. *(DNB PATTERN 2007)*
- Gluten sensitive enteropathy is most associated with HLA DQ2. *(DNB PATTERN 2007)*
- Aflatoxin is a Hepatic carcinogen.
  (DNB PATTERN JUNE 2008)
- Wilson's disease is diagnosed in increased urinary copper.
  (DNB PATTERN DEC 2011)
- Chronic active hepatitis is differentiated from chronic persistent hepatitis by histopathology.
  (DNB PATTERN DEC 2011)
- Testicular atrophy is not a sign of Chronic liver disease.
  (DNB PATTERN DEC 2010)
- Glutathione-s-transferase is used as a hepatic prognostic marker following surgery. *(DNB PATTERN DEC 2010)*
- Diagnosis of Carcinoid tumor is by 5-HIAA (5-hydroxy-indoleacetic acid). Nicotinamide is preferred over Niacin because of flushing with Niacin.
  (DNB PATTERN JUNE 2010)
- Vitamin deficiency in Celiac disease: Vit A, D, K, B12, folic acid deficiency. *(DNB PATTERN DEC 2009)*

- Antiendomysial antibodies are seen in Coeliac disease. *(DNB PATTERN DEC 2010)*
- Specific drug for Intrahepatic cholestasis of pregnancy: Ursodeoxycholic acid. *(DNB PATTERN AUG 2013)*
- Complication of Vit. E overdose: Necrotizing enterocolitis. *(NEET PATTERN 2013)*
- Antimitochondrial antibodies are seen in: Primary sclerosing cholangitis. *(DNB PATTERN JUNE 2014)*
- Large bowel colonic diarrhea is NOT associated with large volume stool. *(NEET PATTERN 2016)*
- Alpha-1 antitrypsin deficiency is associated with Chronic liver disease. *(NEET PATTERN 2016)*
- Pancreatic lipase deficiency is NOT a part of Zieve's syndrome. *(NEET PATTERN 2016)*
- Vitamin deficiency uncommon in Celiac disease: Vitamin B12. *(NEET PATTERN 2016)*
- Most common site of chronic gastric ulcer: Pyloric Antrum. *(NEET PATTERN 2018)*
- Heller's Myotomy is done for: Achalasia Cardia *(NEET PATTERN 2018)*

RESPIRATORY SYSTEM

- Hamman-Rich syndrome is treated with Steroids. *(DNB PATTERN 2000, 2001, 2004)*
- Respiratory acidosis is seen in Emphysema. *(DNB PATTERN 2000, 2006)*
- Respiratory acidosis is NOT seen in Salicylate poisoning. *(DNB PATTERN 2000, 2001)*
- Pneumatocele is commonest in Staphylococcal pneumonia. *(DNB PATTERN 2000, 2006)*
- Deficiency of surfactant leads to Hyaline membrane disease. *(DNB PATTERN 2000)*
- ACTH producing Lung carcinoma is: Oat cell carcinoma. *(DNB PATTERN 2001)*
- Consolidation is NOT a cause of Type 2 respiratory failure. *(DNB PATTERN 2002)*
- Prolonged wheeze is NOT an indication for ICU admission for Bronchial asthma. *(DNB PATTERN 2001, 2004)*
- Hypertension is NOT a feature of Pulmonary embolism. *(DNB PATTERN 2001)*
- Minimum air required to produce Air embolism: 50 mL. *(DNB PATTERN 2004)*
- FEV1/FVC < 70 is seen in: seen in Pulmonary emphysema. *(DNB PATTERN 2003)*

- Most sensitive investigation for Bronchiectasis: HRCT. *(DNB PATTERN 2003)*
- Hamman's sign is positive in Mediastinal emphysema. *(DNB PATTERN 2003)*
- Multiple sites of narrowing of peripheral pulmonary artery occurs with Rubella. *(DNB PATTERN 2008)*
- In an asthmatic patient, FEV1 would show greater improvement on inhaling a bronchodilator. *(DNB PATTERN 2008)*
- Monoclonal antibody used in asthma: Omalizumab. *(DNB PATTERN 2008)*
- SIADH producing Lung carcinoma is: Oat cell carcinoma. *(DNB PATTERN 2006, 2008)*
- Alpha one antitrypsin deficiency causes Emphysema. *(DNB PATTERN 2007)*
- Adrenals should always be imaged in a patient with suspected bronchogenic carcinoma. *(DNB PATTERN 2007)*
- Earliest change in high altitude: increased 2,3 BPG. *(DNB PATTERN 2006)*
- Increased cardiac output is NOT a complication of Continuous positive airway pressure ventilation. *(DNB PATTERN JUNE 2008)*
- In Pneumocystis carinii pneumonia, there is intra-alveolar exudates with thickening of interalveolar septae with edema. *(DNB PATTERN JUNE 2008)*
- Prophylaxis of Pneumocystis carinii is advised for any HIV infected individual with CD4 count < 200 or CD4 percentage < 15% or presenting with oropharyngeal candidiasis. *(DNB PATTERN JUNE 2008)*
- NOT seen in ARDS: Hypercapnia. *(DNB PATTERN JUNE 2012)*
- Silent chest in Bronchial asthma indicates grave prognosis. *(DNB PATTERN DEC 2010)*
- Not a feature of Consolidation: Trachea shifted to side of consolidation. *(DNB PATTERN DEC 2010)*
- Shock lung is also known as ARDS. *(DNB PATTERN JUNE 2010)*
- In obstructive lung, all are true except Residual volume is normal. *(DNB PATTERN JUNE 2010)*
- Hyperventilation is NOT a cause of Pulmonary hypertension. *(DNB PATTERN DEC 2009)*
- Caplan's syndrome is Pneumoconiosis with Rheumatoid arthritis. *(DNB PATTERN DEC 2009)*

- Cystic fibrosis does NOT affect Endocrine system.
(DNB PATTERN JUNE 2010)
- Most common cause of pulmonary abscess in Cystic fibrosis– Pseudomonas aeruginosa. *(DNB PATTERN DEC 2010)*
- XDR TB is defined as: Resistance to at least INH and rifampicin + any quinolones + at least 1 injectable 2nd line drug. *(FMGE PATTERN MARCH 2012)*
- Paradoxical breathing is seen in: Diaphragmatic palsy. *(FMGE PATTERN MARCH 2012)*
- Which parameter is almost the same at apex and base of lung? Oxygen concentration in blood. *(FMGE PATTERN MARCH 2013)*
- Occupational exposure which is yet NOT confirmed on causing a lung problem: Lead. *(FMGE PATTERN MARCH 2013)*
- ECG pattern in Pulmonary embolism is: S1Q3T3. *(FMGE PATTERN MARCH 2013)*
- Investigation of choice for diagnosing lung sequestration: Angiography. *(FMGE PATTERN MARCH 2009)*
- Most practical assessment of severity of Pneumonia: CURB 65. *(DNB PATTERN AUG 2013)*
- Palpatory thud and auscultatory slap are seen in: Tracheal foreign body. *(DNB PATTERN AUG 2013)*
- Most common indication for Ventilator: Primary respiratory failure with Hypoxemia. *(NEET PATTERN 2013)*
- Most common cause of Type 2 Respiratory failure: Chronic obstructive pulmonary disease. *(FMGE PATTERN JUNE 2014)*
- Isolation period in TB: 2 weeks. *(FMGE PATTERN JUNE 2014)*
- Predisposing factor to Buerger's disease is: Smoking. *(FMGE PATTERN JUNE 2014)*
- Bilateral upper lobe bronchiectasis suggests a diagnosis of: Cystic fibrosis. *(NEET PATTERN 2015)*
- Brock's syndrome is: Middle lobe bronchiectasis. *(NEET PATTERN 2015)*
- Bronchiectasis sicca is seen in: Tuberculosis. *(NEET PATTERN 2015)*
- Samter's triad refers to the association between Aspirin sensitive asthma and Nasal block. *(NEET PATTERN 2015)*
- NOT seen in ABPA: Pleural Effusion. *(NEET PATTERN 2018)*
- Pleural Effusion is a rare manifestation in ABPA.
- GOLD Criteria for Very Severe COPD: FeV1/FVC<0.7 and FeV1<30%predicted. *(NEET PATTERN 2018)*

- GOLD (Global Initiative for Chronic Obstructive Lung Disease) CRITERIA FOR COPD
- FeV1/FVC < .70 is common for all grades of COPD.
  - Grade 1-Mild FeV1 >/= 80%predicted.
  - Grade 2-Moderate- FeV1 between 50% and 80% of predicted.
  - Grade 3-Severe-FeV1 between 30% and 50% of predicted.
  - Grade 4-Very Severe-FeV1 < 30% predicted.

CVS

- Most subtle symptom of decreased cardiac output is Fatigue. *(DNB PATTERN 2000, 2006)*
- Treatment of Acute cardiac tamponade: Emergency paracentesis. *(DNB PATTERN 2000)*
- ST segment elevation is NOT a sign of Digitalis toxicity. *(DNB PATTERN 2000, 2001)*
- Drug of choice of Variant angina is Calcium channel blockers. *(DNB PATTERN 2001, 2006)*
- Erythema nodosum is NOT a criteria for diagnosing Rheumatic fever. *(DNB PATTERN 2001)*
- Atherosclerosis is inversely related to HDL. *(DNB PATTERN 2002)*
- Intensity of murmur is increased in Valsalva maneuver in Hypertrophic obstructive cardiomyopathy. *(DNB PATTERN 2001)*
- Best indicator of Myocardial infarction after 48 hours: Troponin T. *(DNB PATTERN 2001)*
- Mitral regurgitation is NOT caused by Malaria. *(DNB PATTERN 2001, 2004)*
- Mitral regurgitation is NOT a feature of Endomyocardial fibroelastosis. *(DNB PATTERN 2001, 2006)*
- Asymmetric pulse is NOT seen in Supravalvular aortic stenosis. *(DNB PATTERN 2002, 2008)*
- Dressler's syndrome is characterized by Pericardial effusion. *(DNB PATTERN 2004)*
- P waves are absent in Atrial fibrillation. *(DNB PATTERN 2004, 2006)*
- Notching of ribs is seen in Coarctation of aorta. *(DNB PATTERN 2004, 2007)*
- Angina pectoris occurs most commonly in Aortic stenosis. *(DNB PATTERN 2004)*
- Earliest diagnosis of Myocardial infarction is by CPK MB. *(DNB PATTERN 2004, 2007)*

- In Myocardial infarction, the correct sequence of increase in enzyme levels is CPK/AST/LDH. *(DNB PATTERN 2003)*
- Unstable angina does NOT cause ST segment elevation. *(DNB PATTERN 2007)*
- Acute sinus bradycardia responds to Atropine. *(DNB PATTERN 2007)*
- Congenital long QT syndrome can lead to Polymorphic ventricular tachycardia. *(DNB PATTERN 2007)*
- Pulsus alternans is seen in Left ventricular failure. *(DNB PATTERN 2005)*
- Displacement of cardiac apex to: Left and Downward. *(DNB PATTERN JUNE 2008)*
- In Sinus Bradycardia, pulse rate is less than 60. *(DNB PATTERN JUNE 2008)*
- Blood culture is diagnostic in: Infective endocarditis. *(DNB PATTERN JUNE 2008)*
- Most common cause of infective endocarditis—Streptococcus viridans. *(DNB PATTERN JUNE 2008)*
- Atherosclerosis associated Infection: Chlamydia pneumonia. *(DNB PATTERN JUNE 2008)*
- Osler's nodes are associated with–Subacute bacterial endocarditis. *(DNB PATTERN JUNE 2008)*
- Physiological murmur does NOT include: Diastolic murmur. *(DNB PATTERN JUNE 2008)*
- Metabolic syndrome is NOT associated with: Increased HDL. *(DNB PATTERN JUNE 2008)*
- Loud P2 is associated with: Pulmonary hypertension. *(DNB PATTERN JUNE 2008)*
- Angina duration: 1–5 mins. *(DNB PATTERN JUNE 2008)*
- Double apical impulse is seen in: Hypertrophic obstructive cardiomyopathy. *(DNB PATTERN JUNE 2012)*
- Mid diastolic murmur with Presystolic accentuation is seen in: Mitral stenosis. *(DNB PATTERN JUNE 2012)*
- Low voltage in ECG: Pericardial effusion. *(DNB PATTERN JUNE 2009)*
- This sign is called EWART'S SIGN.
- ASD patient with murmur similar to MR and left axis deviation of 40 degree: Floppy mitral valve. *(DNB PATTERN DEC 2011)*
- Diagnostic criteria for Infective endocarditis does NOT include ESR. *(DNB PATTERN JUNE 2011)*
- Normal axis of heart: – 30 to + 90. *(DNB PATTERN JUNE 2009)*

- Roth's spots – Infective endocarditis.
  (DNB PATTERN JUNE 2010)
- NOT true about Right ventricular failure: normal JVP.
  (DNB PATTERN DEC 2011)
- Drug contraindicated in Hypertrophic obstructive cardiomyopathy: Digoxin. *(DNB PATTERN DEC 2010)*
- Drug of choice in Paroxysmal supraventricular tachycardia: Adenosine. *(DNB PATTERN DEC 2010)*
- Drug of Choice in PSVT in pregnancy: Adenosine.
- QRS interval > 0.16 seen in Bundle branch block.
  (DNB PATTERN DEC 2011)
- Drug of choice of Anaphylactic shock is intravenous adrenaline. *(DNB PATTERN JUNE 2010)*
- Cannon 'a' waves in JVP represents: Complete heart block.
  (FMGE PATTERN MARCH 2013)
- Austin flint murmur is a mid diastolic murmur.
  (FMGE PATTERN MARCH 2013)
- Following acute left ventricular failure, pulmonary edema generally begins to appear when left atrial pressure approaches: 25 mm Hg. *(FMGE PATTERN MARCH 2011)*
- Best time to administer nitrates for nocturnal angina: Evening. *(FMGE PATTERN SEP 2011)*
- Most common valvular lesion after myocardial infarction: MR. *(FMGE PATTERN SEP 2008)*
- Most common cause of mitral stenosis: Rheumatic heart disease. *(DNB PATTERN AUG 2013)*
- Carcinoid of heart produces what valvular lesion ?—Tricuspid regurgitation and pulmonary stenosis.
  (DNB PATTERN AUG 2013)
- Carcinoid Heart Disease is called Hedinger's Syndrome.
- Defibrillator energy in Joule: Monophasic 360 Joules/Biphasic 200 Joules, 150 Joules. *(DNB PATTERN JUNE 2014)*
- False about **Dressler's syndrome**: Steroids form mainstay of treatment. *(NEET PATTERN 2014)*
- **Auenbrugger's sign** is seen in Pericardial effusion.
  (NEET PATTERN 2014)
- **Rytand murmur** is seen in A-V block.
  (NEET PATTERN 2014)
- **Epsilon wave** is seen in: Arrhythmogenic right ventricular dysplasia. *(NEET PATTERN 2015)*
- **Duroziez's sign** is seen in: Aortic regurgitation.
  (NEET PATTERN 2015)
  – Duroziez Sign is seen on Femoral artery auscultation.

- **Vitum's sign** is seen in: Tricuspid regurgitation.
  (NEET PATTERN 2015)
  - In Vitum's Sign, Tricuspid Regurgitation murmur increases on Liver compression.
- **Carvallo's sign** representing a diastolic murmur that increases on inspiration is seen in: Tricuspid Regurgitation.
  (NEET PATTERN 2015)
- Rivero Carvallo's Sign has also been described in Tricuspid Stenosis.
- Dose of reteplase for management of Acute myocardial infarction: 10 IU. *(NEET PATTERN 2015)*
- Target BP before thrombolysis in ischemic stroke is below: 185/110 mm Hg. *(NEET PATTERN 2016)*
- Pseudo P Pulmonale occurs in: Hypokalemia.
  (NEET PATTERN 2018)
- Myocardial Stunning Pattern is seen in: TAKUTSUBO Cardiomyopathy. *(NEET PATTERN 2018)*
- Alternative drug in place of Adrenaline in Cardiac Arrest: High Dose Vasopressin. *(NEET PATTERN 2018)*
- Ankle Brachial Pressure Index ABPI artificially increased in: Calcified Arteries due to Atherosclerosis.
  (NEET PATTERN 2018)

RENAL SYSTEM

- Urinary pH > 8 indicates urinary tract infection.
  (DNB PATTERN 2000, 2005)
- Peptic ulcer is NOT a manifestation of Renal cell carcinoma.
  (DNB PATTERN 2000)
- Hyperkalemia is a prominent feature of Type 4 Renal tubular acidosis. *(DNB PATTERN 2000)*
- Diabetes insipidus is characterized by decreased urine and increased plasma osmolality. *(DNB PATTERN 2000)*
- Kimmelstiel-Wilson bodies are characteristic of Diabetic nephropathy. *(DNB PATTERN 2001, 2003)*
- Bence Jones protein are NOT seen in Acute glomerulonephritis. *(DNB PATTERN 2001, 2004)*
- Restless leg syndrome is caused by Chronic renal failure.
  (DNB PATTERN 2008)
- Cancer causing Polycythemia: Renal cell carcinoma.
  (DNB PATTERN 2008)
- HIV associated nephropathy is a type of Collapsing glomerulopathy. *(DNB PATTERN 2007)*
- Most common cause of nephritic syndrome in adults is: Membranous glomerulonephritis. *(DNB PATTERN 2006)*

- Chronic renal failure anemia due to—Erythropoietin deficiency. *(DNB PATTERN JUNE 2008)*
- Most common cause of Secondary hypertension–Renovascular disease. *(DNB PATTERN JUNE 2008)*
- Normal urinary protein excretion: <150 mg/dL and normal urinary albumin < 30 mg/dL. *(DNB PATTERN JUNE 2008)*
- Nephritic Syndrome is associated with Hematuria/Oliguria/Hypertension NOT Edema. Even though edema may be present, it is NOT a typical feature. *(DNB PATTERN JUNE 2008)*
- Most sensitive investigation for detecting early Diabetic nephropathy: Microalbuminuria. *(DNB PATTERN JUNE 2012)*
- False about Poststreptococcal Glomerulonephritis: Recurrence common. *(DNB PATTERN DEC 2011)*
- Erythropoietin is given as treatment of chronic renal failure. *(DNB PATTERN JUNE 2010)*
- Hypercalcemia is not seen in CRF. *(DNB PATTERN DEC 2010)*
- Fibrinogen is NOT decreased in Nephrotic syndrome. *(DNB PATTERN JUNE 2011)*
- Creatinine clearance is used to assess glomerular function. *(DNB PATTERN DEC 2011)*
- Signs and symptoms of CRF is seen when renal function deteriorates more than 60%. *(DNB PATTERN DEC 2011)*
- Nonoliguric renal failure seen in Aminoglycoside toxicity. *(DNB PATTERN DEC 2011)*
- Patient with Bronchiectasis develops nephrotic syndrome. Most probable diagnosis is Amyloidosis. *(DNB PATTERN DEC 2011)*
- True about Nephrogenic diabetes insipidus: Renal tubular unresponsiveness to ADH. *(DNB PATTERN JUNE 2011)*
- Treatment of Neurogenic diabetes insipidus is Desmopressin. *(DNB PATTERN JUNE 2011)*
- Urine of athlete becomes red in color after long race. This is due to Myoglobinuria. *(DNB PATTERN DEC 2010)*
- In a patient if administration of vasopressin does not increase urine osmolality, it indicates renal hyposensitivity to ADH. *(DNB PATTERN JUNE 2009)*
- Best test for initial stage of renal insufficiency: Serum creatinine. *(DNB PATTERN JUNE 2010)*
- Renal papillary necrosis is caused by alcohol ALSO BY Diabetes, Sickle cell anemia, Analgesics. *(DNB PATTERN JUNE 2010)*

- Microalbuminuria is urinary albumin excretion rate of 30–300 mg/day. *(FMGE PATTERN MARCH 2004)*
- Earliest sensitive test to diagnose Diabetic nephropathy: Microalbuminuria. *(FMGE PATTERN MARCH 2013)*
- NOT a component of Dialysate in Hemodialysis?—Aluminum–Sodium, Potassium, Glucose are components of Dialysate. *(FMGE PATTERN MARCH 2013)*
- This one is obvious since Aluminum from dialysis tubes have been implicated in Dialysis dementia.
- Chronic kidney disease is defined as GFR LESS THAN-ml/min/1.73 m^2. *(FMGE PATTERN MARCH 2004)*
- Nodular glomerulosclerosis is pathognomonic for: Diabetic nephropathy. *(FMGE PATTERN SEP 2009)*
- Acute kidney injury in RIFLE criteria is: Urine output < 0.5 mL/kg/hr for more than 12 hrs. *(DNB PATTERN NOV 2013)*
- Most common cause of Renal artery stenosis in people above 50 yrs: Atherosclerosis. *(DNB PATTERN NOV 2013)*
- Pathological finding in Benign nephrosclerosis: Hyaline arteriolosclerosis. *(NEET PATTERN 2013)*
- Trace element in Dialysis patients implicated in the causation of Osteomalacia: Aluminum. *(NEET PATTERN 2014)*
- ANURIA is defined as: Urine output less than 100 ml/hr. *(NEET PATTERN 2016)*
- MICROSCOPIC HEMATURIA is defined as: 3 or more RBC/HPF. *(NEET PATTERN 2016)*
- Distal renal tubular acidosis is associated with: Calcium stones. *(NEET PATTERN 2015)*
- Defect in CHLORIDE Channel is a feature of Dent's disease. *(NEET PATTERN 2015)*
- Dialysis disequilibrium occurs due to: Reverse urea effect. *(NEET PATERN 2016)*
- Best guide for Fluid administration: Urine Output. *(AIIMS PATTERN 2017)*
- BARTER'S SYNDROME is caused by a defect in: Thick Ascending Limb of Loop of Henle. *(NEET PATTERN 2018)*
- Patient presenting with Cutaneous vasculitis, Glomerulonephritis and Peripheral neuropathy. Next investigation is: ANCA. *(NEET PATTERN 2018)*

HEMATOPOIETIC SYSTEM

- In Von Willebrand Disease, Prothrombin time is normal. *(DNB PATTERN 2000, 2005)*
- Patient with cyanosis shows normal arterial PO$_2$. Diagnosis is Anemic hypoxia. *(DNB PATTERN 2000)*

- Increased ESR is NOT a feature of Sickle cell anemia. *(DNB PATTERN 2001)*
- Photosensitivity is seen in Congenital erythropoietic porphyria. *(DNB PATTERN 2001)*
- Increased IgM is NOT found in Henoch-Schonlein purpura. *(DNB PATTERN 2002)*
- Sickle cell anemia is NOT an Autosomal dominant disorder. *(DNB PATTERN 2001)*
- Streptolysin is a fibrinolytic agent. *(DNB PATTERN 2001)*
- Mycosis fungoides is a T cell tumor. *(DNB PATTERN 2001)*
- Male with Hemophilia A married a normal female, regarding children: All females are carriers. *(DNB PATTERN 2001)*
- Diagnosis of Beta thalassemia is established by Hb electrophoresis. *(DNB PATTERN 2001, 2007)*
- Beta thalassemia is NOT an Autosomal dominant condition. *(DNB PATTERN JUNE 2008)*
- Hemolytic anemia due to intrinsic red cell defect is seen in Hereditary spherocytosis. *(DNB PATTERN 2001)*
- CRP is NOT raised in Sickle cell anemia. *(DNB PATTERN 2004)*
- Methemoglobinemia can occur due to exposure to Aniline. *(DNB PATTERN 2004)*
- Philadelphia chromosome is NOT involved in CLL. *(DNB PATTERN 2004)*
- Vit. K dependent clotting factors are 2, 7, 9, 10. *(DNB PATTERN 2003)*
- Splenectomy is best indicated in Hereditary spherocytosis. *(DNB PATTERN 2003)*
- Blood loss of 40–60% is termed severe in Hemorrhagic Shock. *(DNB PATTERN 2008)*
- Palpable purpura does NOT occur in Thrombocytopenia. *(DNB PATTERN 2007)*
- Pure red cell aplasia is associated with—Thymoma. *(DNB PATTERN JUNE 2008)*
- Low erythropoietin level is seen in: Renal failure. *(DNB PATTERN JUNE 2012)*
- Polycythemia is seen in: Cor pulmonale. *(DNB PATTERN JUNE 2008)*
- Bevacizumab is Anti VEGF antibody. *(DNB PATTERN AUG 2013)*
- Increased thrombin time is seen in: Fibrinogen deficiency. *(DNB PATTERN AUG 2013)*

- Cryoprecipitate is used for: Hypofibrinogenemia/DIC/Hemophilia. *(DNB PATTERN AUG 2013)*
- Initial investigation of choice in DVT: Duplex USG. *(NEET PATTERN 2013)*
- Gold standard investigation in DVT: Contrast venography. *(NEET PATTERN 2013)*
- NOT a feature of Pulmonary thromboembolism: Virchow's sign. *(NEET PATTERN 2013)*
- Patient on Unfractionated heparin develops Thrombocytopenia. Management is with: Lepirudin/Argatroban/Bivalirudin/Fondaparinux. (Alternate anticoagulant). Platelet transfusion is NOT indicated. *(NEET PATTERN 2013)*
- Specific test for Heparin Induced Thrombocytopenia (HIT): Serotonin release assay. *(Harrison 18th ed.)*
- Hyperfibrinogenemia is not seen in DIC. *(NEET PATTERN 2014)*
- T cell Lymphoma is caused by: HTLV 1. *(FMGE PATTERN JUNE 2014)*
- APLASTIC ANEMIA with skeletal abnormalities, short stature and pancreatic exocrine failure suggest a diagnosis of: SHWACHMAN DIAMOND SYNDROME. *(NEET PATTERN 2014)*
- Gold standard test for the diagnosis of Paroxysmal nocturnal hemoglobinuria (PNH) is: Flow cytometry. *(NEET PATTERN 2015)*
- Shelf life of blood in a blood bank in CPDA buffer: 35 days. *(NEET PATTERN 2015)*
- Endogenous Pyrogen: PG E2. *(NEET PATTERN 2018)*

CONNECTIVE TISSUE DISORDERS AND STORAGE DISORDERS

- Blue sclera disease is Osteogenesis imperfecta. *(DNB PATTERN 2000)*
- Shrinking lung syndrome is seen in SLE. *(DNB PATTERN 2000, 2005)*
- Libman-Sacks endocarditis is seen in: SLE. *(DNB PATTERN JUNE 2012)*
- Coffee does NOT precipitate an acute attack of Gout. *(DNB PATTERN 2001)*
- Glycogen storage type 2 is a lysosomal disorder. *(DNB PATTERN 2001)*
- Caplan's syndrome is a manifestation of Rheumatoid arthritis. *(DNB PATTERN 2004, 2007)*

- Mucin clot test is done to detect Hyaluronate in Synovial fluid. *(DNB PATTERN 2008)*
- Drug induced lupus is associated with Antihistone antibodies. *(DNB PATTERN JUNE 2008)*
- C1 esterase inhibitor deficiency is seen in: Hereditary angioedema. *(DNB PATTERN AUG 2013)*
- Immunosuppressant acting on T lymphocytes: Tacrolimus. Also Cyclosporine, Sirolimus. *(NEET PATTERN 2013)*
- Bilateral upper limb pulseless disease is: Takayasu arteritis. *(NEET PATTERN 2016)*

METABOLIC

- Anion gap is NOT increased in Renal tubular acidosis. *(DNB PATTERN 2000)*
- Normal Anion Gap Acidosis is seen in Renal tubular acidosis. *(DNB PATTERN 2003, 2004)*
- Increased anion gap acidosis is NOT seen in Diarrhea. *(DNB PATTERN 2008)*
- Excessive excretion of Chloride does NOT occur in Fanconi syndrome. *(DNB PATTERN 2000)*
- Hypokalemia is seen with Metabolic Alkalosis. *(DNB PATTERN 2000)*
- Cheyne-Stokes breathing associated with—Metabolic alkalosis. *(DNB PATTERN JUNE 2008)*
- Metabolic alkalosis is associated with Hypokalemia. *(DNB PATTERN 2001, 2005)*
- Electrolytes are increased in sweat in Cystic fibrosis. *(DNB PATTERN 2001)*
- Tumor lysis syndrome is NOT a cause of Hypercalcemia. *(DNB 2007, JUNE 2012)*
- Hypochloremia, hypokalemia and alkalosis are features of Congenital hypertrophic pyloric stenosis. *(DNB PATTERN 2007)*
- Granulomatous condition with Hypercalcemia—Sarcoidosis. *(DNB PATTERN JUNE 2008)*
- Tall T waves are NOT associated with Hypokalemia. They are seen with Hyperkalemia. *(DNB PATTERN JUNE 2008)*
- Chronic renal failure is associated with: Metabolic acidosis. *(DNB PATTERN JUNE 2012)*
- Paracetamol poisoning causes Metabolic acidosis. *(DNB PATTERN JUNE 2009)*
- High anion gap acidosis seen in all except renal tubular acidosis. *(DNB PATTERN JUNE 2009, DEC 2010)*

- All are seen in Sodium bicarbonate therapy except Hypercalcemia. *(DNB PATTERN JUNE 2011)*
- Normal anion gap acidosis seen in Hyperchloremic acidosis. *(DNB PATTERN DEC 2011)*
- All are seen in severe Metabolic alkalosis except Pulmonary edema. *(DNB PATTERN DEC 2010)*
- ST segment elevation not seen in Hypocalcemia. *(DNB PATTERN JUNE 2010)*
- Hypercalcemia seen in all except Acute pancreatitis. *(DNB PATTERN JUNE 2010)*
- NOT seen in Pheochromocytoma: Hypocalcemia. *(DNB PATTERN JUNE 2010)*
- Definitive treatment of Hypermagnesemia: Hemodialysis. *(DNB PATTERN JUNE 2009)*
- Hypokalemic Metabolic Acidosis with Hypertension occurs in: Liddle's Syndrome. *(NEET PATTERN 2018)*

INFECTIOUS DISEASES

- Quinolones are NOT the drug of choice for Leptospirosis. *(DNB PATTERN 2000)*
- Drug of choice of Kala Azar is Stibogluconate sodium. *(DNB PATTERN 2000)*
- Acyclovir is NOT included in HIV pinprick prophylaxis. *(DNB PATTERN 2001)*
- Drug used for Giardiasis and Amoebiasis: Metronidazole. *(DNB PATTERN 2001, 2004)*
- Drug of choice of Toxoplasmosis is Pyrimethamine. *(DNB PATTERN 2001)*
- Hematoxylin bodies of Gross are seen in SLE. *(DNB PATTERN 2008)*
- Commonest opportunistic infection in HIV is Pneumocystis carinii. *(DNB PATTERN 2008)*
- Furuncle is caused by: Staphylococcus aureus. *(DNB PATTERN JUNE 2008)*
- Disease causing orchitis: Mumps. *(DNB PATTERN JUNE 2008)*
- Best confirmatory serological test for Syphilis: FTA–ABS. *(DNB PATTERN JUNE 2012)*
- Most common primary site for Congenital tuberculosis is: Liver. *(DNB PATTERN JUNE 2012)*
- NOT true in Scrub typhus is: Icterus. *(DNB PATTERN JUNE 2012)*

- Fulminant Hepatitis E is seen in: Pregnant women.
  (DNB PATTERN JUNE 2012)
- Protective level of Antitetanus serum for Immunity: 0.15 IU/mL. *(NEET PATTERN 2013)*
- Most common subtype of Hepatitis B in India: ayw.
  (NEET PATTERN 2016)
- Serum marker indicative of HBV vaccination: Anti-HBs.
  (NEET PATTERN 2016)

HIV

- CCR 5 mutation linked to resistance to HIV infection.
  (DNB PATTERN DEC 2011)
- HIV in West Africa is HIV 2 Subtype A.
  (DNB PATTERN JUNE 2011)
- HIV seroconversion after needle prick is < 3 in 100.
  (DNB PATTERN JUNE 2011)
- Most common renal pathology in HIV is Focal segmental glomerulosclerosis. *(DNB PATTERN JUNE 2010)*
- Diagnostic test for HIV in window period: p24 antigen.
  (DNB PATTERN JUNE 2010)
- Treatment of choice for HIV and TB along with Rifampicin is Ritonavir. *(DNB PATTERN DEC 2009)*
- Most common opportunistic infection with HIV which presents as difficulty in breathing with CD4 count less than 200: Pneumocystis carinii. *(DNB PATTERN DEC 2009)*
- In asymptomatic HIV, prophylaxis for Pneumocystis carinii starts when CD4 count is less than 200.
  (DNB PATTERN JUNE 2009, DEC 2011)
- Window period in HIV infection is 3 months.
  (DNB PATTERN DEC 2011)
- NOT associated with HIV: Hypogammaglobulinemia.
  (DNB PATTERN DEC 2011)
- Least common cause of seizures in AIDS: Progressive multifocal leukoencephalopathy (PML).
  (DNB PATTERN JUNE 2011)
- Drug of choice for Diarrhea in AIDS: Octreotide.
  (DNB PATTERN JUNE 2011)
- Approximate Time Interval between HIV infection and manifestation of AIDS: 8–10 years.
  (NEET PATTERN 2018)

HEPATITIS B

- Hep. B can be transmitted through all routes except stool.
  (DNB PATTERN DEC 2011)

- Only serological marker present during window period in Hep. B infection is: Anti-HBc.
  (DNB PATTERN JUNE 2009)
- HBsAg positive, HBeAg negative, AST, ALT Normal, Next step is serial monitoring. *(DNB PATTERN JUNE 2011)*
- Marker for efficacy of Hep-B vaccination is Anti HBsAg.
  (DNB PATTERN DEC 2010)
- Worst prognosis is Hep-B and Hep-D coinfection.
  (DNB PATTERN DEC 2010)
- HBsAg negative, Anti-HBs positive, Anti-HBc positive—immunity due to infection of Hep. B.
  (DNB PATTERN DEC 2009)
- Chances due to vertical transmission of Hep. B are 25–30%.
  (DNB PATTERN DEC 2011)

ENDOCRINE

- Hyponatremia is NOT a feature of Conn's syndrome.
  (DNB PATTERN 2001)
- Anasarca is NOT a feature of Conn's syndrome.
  (DNB PATTERN 2006)
- Conn's syndrome—Hyperaldosteronism with Hypokalemia.
  (DNB PATTERN JUNE 2008)
- Commonest cause of Paroxysmal hypertension: Pheochromocytoma. *(DNB PATTERN 2001)*
- Growth hormone secretion is inhibited by Hyperglycemia.
  (DNB PATTERN 2005)
- Adrenal insufficiency does NOT cause: Increased Sodium Potassium ratio. *(DNB PATTERN JUNE 2012)*
- ACTH is produced by which carcinoma: Small cell carcinoma lung. *(DNB PATTERN JUNE 2012)*
- Acromegaly is mediated by Somatomedin.
  (DNB PATTERN DEC 2010)
- Gum hypertrophy is seen in all except Estrogen therapy.
  (DNB PATTERN DEC 2011)
- NOT seen in Gigantism: Mental retardation.
  (DNB PATTERN DEC 2010)
- Hirsutism is NOT seen in Testicular Feminization Syndrome.
  (DNB PATTERN JUNE 2010)
- Female to male ratio for Microprolactinoma is 20:1
  (DNB PATTERN AUG 2013)
- NOT seen in Primary hyperparathyroidism: Increased bone mineral density. *(DNB PATTERN JUNE 2014)*

MISCELLANEOUS

- Glycosylated hemoglobin percentage which indicates good control of Diabetes: 7%. *(DNB PATTERN 2000, 2003)*
- Exogenous insulin is differentiated from endogenous by—Presence of 'C' peptide. *(DNB PATTERN JUNE 2008)*
- Ion used in Insulin storage: Zinc. *(DNB PATTERN JUNE 2008)*
- Osteoarthritis is NOT a component of Felty's syndrome. *(DNB PATTERN 2000)*
- Metal required in synthesis of Retinol is Zinc. *(DNB PATTERN 2001)*
- Most common Malignant melanoma is Superficial spreading. *(DNB PATTERN 2001)*
- Drug of choice of Malignant melanoma is Dacarbazine. *(DNB PATTERN 2001)*
- Riboflavin deficiency causes Angular stomatitis. *(DNB PATTERN 2001)*
- Goat milk is deficient in Folate. *(DNB PATTERN 2001)*
- Major effect of damage in Galactosemia is on Liver/Eyes and Brain. *(DNB PATTERN 2001)*
- Galactosemia is associated with Liver cirrhosis. *(DNB PATTERN JUNE 2008)*
- Pendred syndrome—chromosome 7q is involved. *(DNB PATTERN 2008)*
- Difference in gene expression based on parent-of-origin is called Uniparental disomy. *(DNB PATTERN 2008)*
- Drug of choice of Refractory histiocytosis: Cladribine. *(DNB PATTERN 2008)*
- Glucose Fever is: High fever on administration of IV Glucose without Glucocorticoid administration in Addison's disease. This is due to uncorrected hypoglycemia. *(FMGE PATTERN JUNE 2014)*
- Treatment of choice for Acute Sarcoidosis is: Prednisolone. *(NEET PATTERN 2014)*
- Not true about Churg-Strauss Syndrome: Intravascular Granulomas. *(NEET PATTERN 2014)*
- Extravascular granulomas are common in Churg Strauss Syndrome though Intravascular granulomas have also been reported.
- Correct sequence of cell cycle is G0 –G1- S-G2-M. *(DNB PATTERN 2007)*
- Significant weight loss is defined as: 5% in 1–2 months. *(DNB PATTERN JUNE 2012)*

- Most effective treatment in Diabetic ketoAcidosis is: Insulin. Dawn phenomenon is: Morning Hyperglycemia due to insufficient Insulin. *(DNB PATTERN JUNE 2012)*
- Diabetic neuropathy can be mononeuritis/polyneuritis/autonomic neuropathy. *(DNB PATTERN DEC 2010)*
- Drugs given for painful Diabetic neuropathy: Gabapentin, Duloxetine, Pregabalin. *(DNB PATTERN JUNE 2011)*
- Ragged Red Fibers are seen in: MERRF syndrome. *(FMGE PATTERN MARCH 2013)*
- Most common presentation of Euthyroid sick syndrome: Low T3, normal T4, TSH. *(DNB PATTERN OCT 2013)*
- Osborne waves on ECG are indicative of: Hypothermia. *(DNB PATTERN AUG 2013)*
- Early morning hyperglycemia with decreased blood glucose at 2 A.M suggests: Somogyi effect. *(NEET PATTERN 2016)*
- Low cholesterol is not associated with Hypothyroidism. *(NEET PATTERN 2016)*
- Most common cause of Intracranial hemorrhage is: Intracerebral hemorrhage. *(NEET PATTERN 2015)*

BLEEDING DIATHESIS

- INR in warfarin therapy is 2.5. *(DNB PATTERN DEC 2011)*
- Harrison 18th ed. says for most therapeutic purposes, INR on warfarin should be between 2.0–3.0. For mechanical heart valves, INR should be 2.5–3.5.
- Henoch-Schonlein purpura is due to IgA deposition. *(DNB PATTERN DEC 2009)*
- Artery responsible for bleeding in Hemoptysis: Bronchial artery. *(DNB PATTERN DEC 2009)*
- Both PT and APTT are prolonged in Factor 2 deficiency. Factor 2 is prothrombin. In both fibrinogen and prothrombin deficiency only, PT and APTT are both increased. PT and APTT are both normal in Factor 13 deficiency. *(DNB PATTERN JUNE 2009)*
- Thrombocytopenia, recurrent infections and eczema is seen in Wiskott Aldrich syndrome. *(DNB PATTERN DEC 2010)*
- 1st sign of hepatocellular failure is increased Prothrombin time. 1st sign of hepatic encephalopathy is change in sleep pattern. *(DNB PATTERN DEC 2011)*
- Spontaneous bleeding is seen in Hemophilia. *(DNB PATTERN JUNE 2009)*

- Postcircumcision bleed/recurrent hemarthroses/retroperitoneal and rarely intracranial hemorrhages are the presentation of Hemophilia whereas Von Willebrand disease presents with mucosal bleeds/epistaxis/menorrhagia/ bleeds following dental extraction.

MULTIPLE ENDOCRINE NEOPLASIA

- MEN 1 NOT associated with Medullary carcinoma thyroid.
  (DNB PATTERN JUNE 2009, DNB PATTERN JUNE 2010)
- MEN 2B NOT associated with Hyperparathyroidism.
  (DNB PATTERN JUNE 2011)
- Most virulent form of Medullary Carcinoma Thyroid is associated with: MEN 2B. *(NEET PATTERN 2014)*
- CDK NIB mutation is associated with: MEN 4.
  (NEET PATTERN 2016)

PHEOCHROMOCYTOMA

- Vanillylmandelic acid is increased in urine in Pheochromocytoma. This is a relatively very specific, but less sensitive test for Pheochromocytoma.
  (DNB PATTERN DEC 2011)
- 40-year-lady comes with Pheochromocytoma. Characteristic symptom is Paroxysmal hypertension.
  (DNB PATTERN DEC 2011)

TUMOR SYNDROMES

- All are seen in Multiple myeloma except Dystrophic calcification. *(DNB PATTERN JUNE 2011)*
- Thymoma NOT associated with Hypergammaglobulinemia.
  (DNB PATTERN JUNE 2010)
- Thymoma associated with Hypogammaglobulinemia is called GOOD'S SYNDROME.
- Good prognosis Hodgkin's lymphoma: Lymphocyte predominant. *(DNB PATTERN DEC 2010)*
- NOT seen in Neurofibromatosis: Shagreen patches.
  (DNB PATTERN JUNE 2011)
- Chronic lymphatic leukemia is characterized by small lymphocytes in peripheral smear, hepatosplenomegaly, more than 50 years of age. *(DNB PATTERN JUNE 2011)*
- Mutation of Wilms' tumor on 11p13.
  (DNB PATTERN JUNE 2009)
- Drug not effective in Multiple myeloma: Hydroxyurea.
  (DNB PATTERN JUNE 2009)

- Drug of choice of Chronic myeloid leukemia: Imatinib. *(DNB PATTERN JUNE 2011)*
- Bad prognostic factor for Acute Lymphoblastic Leukemia (ALL): B-cell Acute Lymphoblastic Leukemia. *(DNB PATTERN JUNE 2011)*
- Adenomatous polyps of AR inheritance and CNS tumors is known as: Turcot's syndrome. *(DNB PATTERN JUNE 2014)*
- LYNCH SYNDROME is NOT associated with APC gene. *(NEET PATTERN 2014)*
- Lynch Syndrome is associated with MLH1/2, MSH6, PSM2 genes.
- Tumor syndrome associated with Congenital hypertrophy of Retinal pigment epithelium: Gardner's syndrome. *(NEET PATTERN 2016)*
- Best provocative test for the diagnosis of Gastrinoma: Secretin injection test. *(NEET PATTERN 2016)*
- KOENEN'S tumor is seen in: Tuberous sclerosis. *(NEET PATTERN 2016)*

THYROID AND PARATHYROID

- Low cholesterol is not a finding in Hypothyroidism. *(DNB PATTERN DEC 2009)*
- Rib notching is not a feature of Hypothyroidism. *(DNB PATTERN DEC 2009)*
- Superior and Inferior Rib Notching can both be seen in HYPERPARATHYROIDISM.
- Hypothyroidism is caused by Lithium/Hemochromatosis/Scleroderma. *(DNB PATTERN JUNE 2010)*
- Secondary Hyperparathyroidism is NOT seen in: Parathyroid Adenoma. *(DNB PATTERN JUNE 2011)*
- Flapping tremor is NOT seen in Thyrotoxicosis. *(DNB PATTERN DEC 2010)*
- Hypothyroidism in Sub-Himalayan regions is due to Iodine deficiency. *(DNB PATTERN DEC 2010)*
- This is referred to as the Himalayan Goitre Belt where soil and water lacks natural Iodine.

MISCELLANEOUS

- Not a criterion to assess reliability of the relative while taking history: Observational ability. *(AIIMS PATTERN 2017)*
- Reliability is assessed by factors like Time of Cohabitation, Educational Status, Blood Relation etc.

LEVEL II: HIGH YIELD FACTORS

Table 12.1: HIV

The risk of HIV transmission following infected skin puncture	0.3%
The risk of HIV transmission following mucus membrane exposure	.09%
The risk of HIV in vertical transmission in developing countries is	25–35%
The risk of HIV in vertical transmission in developed countries	15–25%
There is no evidence that HIV transmission can occur as a result of	exposure to tears, sweat and urine
Earliest detection test for HIV is	Nucleic acid amplification testing
Standard screening test for HIV is ELISA	99.5 % sensitive
Western blot test tests for detection of	2/3 HIV PROTEINS – p24, gp41, gp120/160
Gold standard for the diagnosis of HIV infection:	Positive ELISA with confirmatory Western blot
The commonest cause of needle stick injuries causing HIV is	Improper disposal of the needle- in which more than half is due to recapping of the needle.
Most common strain causing HIV across the World	HIV 1
HIV-1 evolved from	Chimpanzees (Pan troglodytes) species
HIV-2 mainly in	West Africa
HIV belongs to	Family Retroviridae and subfamily Lentivirus
HIV virus was first identified in	1986
Most common subtype of HIV	Subtype C
Most common subtype of HIV in India	Subtype C
Most common subtype of HIV in Europe	Subtype B

Table 12.2: Hepatitis B and C

The risk of Hep. B infection following a percutaneous exposure	6–30%
The risk of Hep. C infection following a percutaneous exposure	1.8%
First virologic marker in Hep. B infection is	HBsAg
Serologic marker of Hep. B during window period	IgM Anti-HBc

Contd...

Contd...

Best marker for a recent Hep. B infection	IgM Anti-HBc
Protective antibody conferring immunity to Hep. B infection	Anti-HBs
Qualitative marker of Hep. B replication and activity	HBeAg
Quantitative marker of Hep. B replicative phase	HBV DNA
Most sensitive indicator for Hep C infection	HCV RNA
Incubation period for Hep. B	30–180 days.
Papular acrodermatitis of childhood or Gianotti-Crosti syndrome is a complication of	Hep. B infection

Table 12.3: Celiac disease

Most sensitive and specific antibodies in Celiac sprue	Antiendomysial antibodies
Other antibodies in Celiac sprue	Antigliadin antibodies and Anti-transglutaminase antibodies
The Antiendomysial antibody in Celiac sprue	IgA
Definitive investigation for Celiac sprue	Small intestinal biopsy
The presence of a characteristic histopathologic appearance that revert toward normal following the initiation of a gluten free diet	Establishes the diagnosis of Celiac sprue
Celiac sprue is premalignant	Can complicate into lymphoma/other neoplasms
All patients with celiac sprue have	HLA DQ2/DQ8
Gliadin or active component of Gluten	is present in wheat, barley, rye and oats but not in rice
Vitamin deficiency in Celiac disease	Vit. A, D, K, B12, Folic acid deficiency

Table 12.4: Cystic fibrosis

First organism cultured from CF samples	H. influenzae/Staph. aureus
Mycobacterium tuberculosis	is rare association in CF
Most common fungal infection in CF	Aspergillus fumigatus
Most common cause of Pulmonary abscess in Cystic fibrosis	Pseudomonas aeruginosa

Table 12.5: Pheochromocytoma

Most common sign/manifestation of Pheochromocytoma:	Hypertension
10% of Phaeo bilateral, 10% extra adrenal, less than 10% malignant, recurrence rate < 10% after surgery	Rules of 10 in pheochromocytoma

Contd...

Contd...

2nd most common manifestation	Paroxysms occur in more than half the cases of Pheochromocytoma
Most sensitive biochemical test for Pheochromocytoma:	Plasma metanephrine > urine fractionated metanephrines and catecholamines
Most sensitive imaging for Pheochromocytoma	T2 weighted MRI with Gadolinium contrast
Drug used for the medical management of Pheochromocytoma in pregnancy	Phenoxybenzamine
Phenoxybenzamine should be administered	10–14 days prior to surgery
Other relevant manifestations of Pheochromocytoma	*Hypercalcemia*/fever/increased ESR/Impaired glucose tolerance/ Cardiomyopathy/elevated amylase/ polyuria and rhabdomyolysis
RET mutations are	Highly predictive of Pheochromocytoma
Pheochromocytoma should be excluded or removed	Before thyroid or parathyroid surgery

Table 12.6: Endocrinology–FAQ

Gynecomastia is a sign of	Thyrotoxicosis
Most common symptom of Thyrotoxicosis	Hyperactivity/irritability/dysphoria
Most common sign of Thyrotoxicosis	Tachycardia
Most common symptom of Hypothyroidism	Tiredness/weakness
Most common sign of Hypothyroidism	Cool extremities/dry coarse skin
Development of Diabetic neuropathy	Correlates with duration of diabetes and glycemic control
Most common form of Diabetic neuropathy is	Distal symmetric polyneuropathy
Most common mononeuritis in Diabetes Mellitus	3rd nerve involvement

EPONYMOUS SIGNS OF CARDIOVASCULAR SYSTEM

Wellens' syndrome or Sign in ECG	Proximal critical stenosis of the Left anterior descending artery
Brugada syndrome	Familial sodium channelopathy with RBBB with ST elevation in V1–V3
Wolff-Parkinson-White syndrome	Pre-excitation syndrome due to re-entrant bundle of AV tissue distal to AV node. (DELTA wave in ECG)
SGARBOSSA criteria	Risk assessment of patients with Chronic LBBB

Contd...

Contd...

Takotsubo cardiomyopathy	Cardiomyopathy with Hypertrophic LV Inferior wall and Hypotrophic LV Superior wall (OCTOPUS JAR HEART)
De Winter ECG	Myocardial Infarction with Proximal LAD occlusion
Osborn J waves in ECG	Hypothermia
Lown-Ganong-Levine syndrome	Pre-excitation syndrome due to re-entrant bundle of AV tissue close to AV node
Romano-Ward syndrome	Autosomal dominant Inherited Long QT syndrome. NOT associated with Deafness. Defect of Na and K channels
Jervell and Lange-Nielsen syndrome	Autosomal recessive Inherited Long QT syndrome. Associated with Sensorineural deafness, defect of Na and K channels

13. Surgery

"No matter how good you are at planning, the pressure never goes away. So I don't fight it. I feed off it. I turn pressure into motivation to do my best."

—**Dr. Benjamin Carson**
Youngest ever H.O.D of Paediatric Neurosurgery in U.S at 33 yrs.

> **REFERENCES**
> - *Sabiston's Textbook of Surgery, 20th ed.*
> - *Bailey and Love Short Practice of Surgery, 27th ed.*

LEVEL I: BASIC REPEATS

GENERAL SURGERY

- Catgut is made from intestine of Sheep. *(DNB PATTERN 2000, 2006)*
- Isograft is graft between monozygotic twins. *(DNB PATTERN 2007)*
- Best fluid for resuscitation during shock is Crystalloids. *(DNB PATTERN JUNE 2012)*
- Best fluid for burns in first 24 hours is Ringer lactate. *(DNB PATTERN JUNE 2012)*
- Ideal gas for laparoscopy is CO_2. *(DNB PATTERN JUNE 2012)*
- MC cause of septicemia gram negative bacteria. *(DNB PATTERN JUNE 2012)*
- Insufflation pressure during laparoscopy is 12-15 mm Hg. *(DNB PATTERN JUNE 2011)*
- Nonabsorbable suture among the following is polyethylene. *(DNB PATTERN JUNE 2011)*
- Operation theatre fire is most commonly due to electrosurgical equipments (68%). *(DNB PATTERN DEC 2010)*
- Relative Humidity of operation theatre should be maintained at: 55-65%. *(DNB PATTERN NOV 2013)*
- Most common CNS tumor to undergo calcification: Oligodendroglioma. *(DNB PATTERN JUNE 2014)*
- True about Catgut: Degraded by enzymatic degradation. *(NEET PATTERN 2018)*

- Colour of 22 gauge cannula used: Blue.
  (AIIMS PATTERN 2017)
- Fr in Foley's Catheter denotes: Diameter.
  (AIIMS PATTERN 2017)
- The French size is three times the diameter in millimetres.
- Diameter(mm) = French Size/3
- Modified Shock Index is a ratio of: Heart Rate by Mean Arterial Pressure. *(AIIMS PATTERN 2017)*

ORAL CAVITY

- Most common cyst of jaw is a Radicular cyst.
  (DNB PATTERN 2004)
- Tooth is fixed in its socket by periodontal membrane.
  (DNB PATTERN 2007)
- Vincent's Angina is caused by Borrelia vincenti.
  (DNB PATTERN 2001)
- Dentigerous Cyst arises from an unerupted tooth.
  (DNB PATTERN 2000)
- Locally invasive malignant odontoma: Ameloblastoma.
  (DNB PATTERN 2007)
- Treatment for squamous cell carcinoma T3N0M0 is Maxillectomy and radiotherapy. *(DNB PATTERN DEC 2011)*
- Progressive dysphagia for solids and liquids found in carcinoma of hypopharynx. *(DNB PATTERN JUNE 2011)*
- Stain used to diagnose premalignant lesion of lip is Toluidine blue. *(DNB PATTERN JUNE 2011)*

SALIVARY GLANDS

- Commonest site of Sialectasis: Submandibular gland.
  (DNB PATTERN 2003)
- TRUE regarding Mixed Parotid tumor: firm and encapsulated. *(DNB PATTERN 2005)*
- Swelling of deep parotid gland presents as swelling of the temporal region. *(DNB PATTERN 2001)*
- Commonest parotid tumor is Pleomorphic Adenoma.
  (DNB PATTERN 2000)
- Nerve in Frey syndrome is Auriculotemporal nerve.
  (DNB PATTERN DEC 2011)
- Most common site of salivary gland calculi is submandibular gland. *(DNB PATTERN JUNE 2011)*
- MC malignant tumor of parotid: Mucoepidermoid Ca.
  (DNB PATTERN DEC 2010)

- Malignant salivary gland tumor painful presents with skin ulceration, cervical lymphadenopathy present, treatment is en bloc surgical excision ± radiotherapy.
  (DNB PATTERN DEC 2010)
- Structure damaged most commonly during surgery on ranula is submandibular duct. *(DNB PATTERN DEC 2010)*
- Frey's syndrome is associated with surgery of parotid.
  (DNB PATTERN JUNE 2009)
- Perineural spread is seen in Adenoid cystic tumor.
  (DNB PATTERN JUNE 2009)
- Minor mucus retention cysts in the floor of mouth either from an obstructed minor salivary gland or from sublingual salivary gland. Treatment: Marsupialization.
  (DNB PATTERN DEC 2009)
- NOT true about ranula—they arise from submandibular gland. Ranula is a mucus retention cyst that arises from sublingual gland. *(DNB PATTERN DEC 2009)*

LARYNX

- T3N1M1 stage of Ca larynx: Stage 4.
  (DNB PATTERN 2002)

NECK

- Probable cause of sudden death in case of superficial injury to neck: Air embolism through external jugular vein.
  (DNB PATTERN 2005)
- Bezold's abscess is seen in Sternocleidomastoid.
  (DNB PATTERN 2005)
- In neck dissection surgery, the structure preserved is Phrenic Nerve. *(DNB PATTERN 2004)*
- Treatment of T4N0M0 stage of head and neck carcinoma is Chemoradiation. *(DNB PATTERN DEC 2011)*

THYROID

- Congenital sensorineural deafness with abnormal iodine metabolism and goiter in children is called Pendred syndrome. *(DNB PATTERN 2002)*
- Calcitonin secreting tumor is: Medullary carcinoma thyroid.
  (DNB PATTERN 2003)
- Hypotension is NOT a presentation of Hyperthyroidism.
  (DNB PATTERN 2001)
- Familial carcinoma thyroid is usually Medullary type.
  (DNB PATTERN 2001)

- Occult thyroid malignancies are usually papillary.
  (DNB PATTERN 2001)
- Most aggressive Medullary carcinoma thyroid is seen in MEN 2B. *(DNB PATTERN 2007)*
- Most common location of thyroglossal cyst is: Subhyoid.
  (DNB PATTERN 2007)
- Hyoid bone is related to—Thyroglossal cyst.
  (DNB PATTERN JUNE 2008)
- Most common surgically repairable cause of hyperparathyroidism is adenoma. *(DNB PATTERN JUNE 2011)*
- Thyroid nodule of 4 cm causing compressive symptoms–INV OC FNAC, FNAC cannot distinguish follicular adenoma from carcinoma, managed by subtotal thyroidectomy.
  (DNB PATTERN JUNE 2011)
- Cold nodules are not the diagnostic feature of thyroid malignancy. *(DNB PATTERN JUNE 2011)*
- Orphan Annie eye Nuclei-Papillary carcinoma thyroid.
  (DNB PATTERN DEC 2010)
- Thyroid Ca with good prognosis is papillary.
  (DNB PATTERN DEC 2010)
- MC site of thyroglossal cyst: subhyoid.
  (DNB PATTERN JUNE 2009)
- Long standing nodular goiter can change to: Follicular Carcinoma Thyroid. *(FMGE PATTERN SEP 2012)*
- RET proto oncogene is associated with the development of: Medullary Carcinoma Thyroid. *(NEET PATTERN 2018)*

ESOPHAGUS

- TNM staging of esophageal carcinoma is done by: CT Scan.
  (DNB PATTERN 2002)
- Usual site of foreign body impaction in the esophagus is above the cricopharynx. *(DNB PATTERN 2003)*
- Barrett's esophagus is example of metaplasia.
  (DNB PATTERN JUNE 2008)
- Bleeding tendency in case of esophageal varices depends upon size and site of varices. *(DNB PATTERN 2004)*
- Primary therapy for esophageal varices is sclerotherapy.
  (DNB PATTERN 2001)
- Adenocarcinoma of esophagus is most likely to be due to Barrett's Esophagus. *(DNB PATTERN 2007)*
- Heller's operation is done for Achalasia cardia.
  (DNB PATTERN JUNE 2012)
- What is giant hiatal hernia—Paraesophageal.
  (DNB PATTERN DEC 2011)

- 61-year-female presents with recurrent pneumonia, regurgitation of food and feeling of fullness. Most probable diagnosis is Hiatal hernia. *(DNB PATTERN DEC 2011)*
- Most common complication of Hiatal hernia—esophagitis. *(DNB PATTERN DEC 2011)*
- Heller's operation is done for Achalasia cardia. *(DNB PATTERN JUNE 2011)*
- 24 hours pH manometry is gold standard investigation for reflux esophagitis. *(DNB PATTERN JUNE 2011)*
- MC site of spontaneous rupture of esophagus: cardio-esophageal junction. *(DNB PATTERN JUNE 2009)*
- Most common site of Iatrogenic esophageal perforation: Killian's Triangle. *(DNB PATTERN AUG 2013)*
- Achalasia Cardia is due to: Loss of peristalsis of the esophagus. *(DNB PATTERN AUG 2013)*
- Heller's operation is done for: Achalasia Cardia. *(DNB PATTERN AUG 2013)*
- Esophageal motility is assessed by: Manometry. *(DNB PATTERN AUG 2013)*
- Most accurate information regarding T Stage of an Esophageal Carcinoma is obtained through an: Endoscopic USG. *(NEET PATTERN 2014)*

STOMACH

- True regarding gastroschisis is: A herniation of abdominal contents through the body wall. *(DNB PATTERN 2003)*
- Most common benign mesenchymal tumor of stomach: Leiomyoma. *(DNB PATTERN 2002)*
- True regarding Brunner's glands is: they are stimulated by Acetylcholine. *(DNB PATTERN 2004)*
- Linitis Plastica is a type of Carcinoma stomach. *(DNB PATTERN 2001)*
- Hypertrophic pyloric stenosis occurs after 1 month of birth. *(DNB PATTERN 2001)*
- Gastrojejunostomy without any spillage of contents is a clean contaminated wound. *(DNB PATTERN 2001)*
- Hourglass deformity of the stomach is seen in Gastric Ulcer. *(DNB PATTERN 2000)*
- NOT a feature of early gastric cancer: involvement of mucosa, submucosa and muscularis. *(DNB PATTERN 2007)*
- Most characteristic of Congenital Hypertrophic Pyloric Stenosis: Tumor is best felt during feeding. *(DNB PATTERN 2007)*

- Paradoxical aciduria is seen in Pyloric obstruction. *(DNB PATTERN JUNE 2012)*
- Vitamin deficiency in gastric cancer patients is Vitamin B_{12}. *(DNB PATTERN DEC 2011)*
- NOT a boundary of gastrinoma triangle-Junction of hepatic ducts. *(DNB PATTERN DEC 2011)*
- Omphalocele is caused by failure of gut to return to the body cavity from its physiological herniation during 6th to 10th week. *(DNB PATTERN DEC 2010)*
- Extensive ileal resection causes gastric hypersecretion, not pancreatic hypersecretion. *(DNB PATTERN DEC 2010)*
- Metabolic abnormalities associated with Congenital Hypertrophic Pyloric Stenosis in the early phase-NOT aciduria. *(DNB PATTERN DEC 2010)*
- Fistula leading to highest electrolyte imbalance: Gastric fistula. *(DNB PATTERN DEC 2009)*
- Dieulafoy's disease: Aberrant tortuous arteriole in the lesser curvature with potential for torrential bleed. *(DNB PATTERN AUG 2013)*
- Vagotomy causes: Gastric Atony. *(DNB PATTERN AUG 2013)*
- Gastrinoma Triangle is NOT bound by: Splenic Vein and Inferior Mesenteric Vein. *(NEET PATTERN 2016)*
- Abdominal mass best demonstrated in Congenital Hypertrophic Pyloric Stenosis is: During feeding. *(NEET PATTERN 2018)*

INTESTINES

- 50% intestinal resection is NOT a cause of Malnutrition. *(DNB PATTERN 2002)*
- Bishop Koop operation is done for uncomplicated Meconium Ileus. *(DNB PATTERN 2002)*
- Chemotherapy is useful in this gastrointestinal malignancy: Hodgkin's Lymphoma. *(DNB PATTERN 2002)*
- 14 C Xylose test is used for Bacterial Overgrowth. *(DNB PATTERN 2005)*
- Most common type of intussusceptions is: Ileocolic. *(DNB PATTERN 2000)*
- Intestinal perforation is NOT a complication of Round Worm infection. *(DNB PATTERN 2001)*
- Commonest complication of diverticulosis of the sigmoid colon: Bleeding per rectal. *(DNB PATTERN 2000)*
- Commonest cause of bleeding from Lower GI tract is: Diverticulosis. *(DNB PATTERN 2000)*

- Granulomas with abscess formation—ulcerative colitis/TB/Crohn's disease. *(DNB PATTERN JUNE 2008)*
- MC cause of lower GI bleed in India—Typhoid enteritis. *(DNB PATTERN JUNE 2012)*
- Commonest site of volvulus is Sigmoid colon. *(DNB PATTERN JUNE 2012)*
- All are true of Ulcerative colitis except cobblestoning. *(DNB PATTERN DEC 2011)*
- Treatment of duodenal atresia: Duodenoduodenostomy. *(DNB PATTERN JUNE 2011)*
- Least malignant potential for colorectal Ca is seen in polyps associated with Peutz Jegher's syndrome. *(DNB PATTERN DEC 2010)*
- Anomaly associated with duodenal atresia—Down's syndrome. *(DNB PATTERN JUNE 2009)*
- Patient in coma for 20 days, best way for nutrition—feeding via jejunostomy. *(DNB PATTERN 2007)*
- Premalignant polyposis is Familial Polyposis. *(DNB PATTERN 2006)*
- Pseudopolyposis is seen in Ulcerative Colitis. *(DNB PATTERN 2006)*
- Double Bubble Sign is seen in Duodenal Atresia. *(DNB PATTERN 2007)*
- Sentinel lymph node biopsy is not done in carcinoma colon. *(DNB PATTERN JUNE 2012)*
- Vitamin deficiency seen in short bowel syndrome is Vitamin B_{12}. *(DNB PATTERN DEC 2011)*
- A lady comes with polyps in intestine, melanotic pigmentation of lip and positive family history the diagnosis is Peutz Jeghers syndrome. *(DNB PATTERN DEC 2011)*
- Which screening test for colon cancer is proven effective in RCT? Colonoscopy. *(DNB PATTERN DEC 2011)*
- Colon cancer is seen in people taking High fat diet. *(DNB PATTERN DEC 2011)*
- MC cause of small intestinal obstruction is postoperative adhesion. *(DNB PATTERN DEC 2010)*
- Increase in risk of colorectal cancer is associated with—Low fiber diet. *(DNB PATTERN JUNE 2008)*
- Patient is having diarrhea and colic on and off with mass in Right Iliac Fossa. Most probable diagnosis is Carcinoma Caecum. *(DNB PATTERN DEC 2009)*
- Burst abdomen is seen how many days after surgery?—7-10 days. *(DNB PATTERN NOV 2013)*

Surgery

- NOT TRUE regarding Crohn's Disease: Continuous lesions on Endoscopy. *(NEET PATTERN 2018)*

APPENDIX

- Ochsner Sherren regime is most suitable for the management of appendicular abscess. *(DNB PATTERN 2000)*
- Appendicular stump is obtained by Ligation and inversion. *(DNB PATTERN 2007)*
- Hydrocele is a type of Exudation cyst. *(DNB PATTERN 2007)*
- Ochsner Sherren regimen is used for Appendicular lump. *(DNB PATTERN JUNE 2012)*
- Position of Appendix likely to present with SUPRAPUBIC PAIN in a patient with Acute Appendicitis: Subcecal. *(NEET PATTERN 2014)*
- Obturator Sign in Acute Appendicitis is most commonly associated with: Pelvic Appendix. *(NEET PATTERN 2016)*
- Treatment of Choice for a 0.5 mm carcinoid tumor at the tip of Appendix is: Appendectomy. *(NEET PATTERN 2016)*

RECTUM AND ANAL CANAL

- False regarding solitary rectal ulcer: It is usually malignant. *(DNB PATTERN 2002)*
- Hirschsprung's disease is best diagnosed by Full thickness rectal biopsy. *(DNB PATTERN 2000)*
- Hirschprung's disease is confirmed by Rectal Biopsy. *(DNB PATTERN 2006)*
- In villous papillomas of the rectum, Potassium loss is present. *(DNB PATTERN 2007)*
- Treatment of choice of squamous cell carcinoma of anus is chemoradiation. *(DNB PATTERN JUNE 2012)*
- Hirschsprung's disease—aganglionic segment is normal or contacted. *(DNB PATTERN DEC 2010)*
- In Hirschsprung's disease: only the contracted segment is affected. *(DNB PATTERN AUG 2013)*
- Ripstein's Procedure is done for: Rectal Prolapse. *(NEET PATTERN 2016)*

HERNIA

- Direct inguinal hernia with femoral hernia is best managed by Bassini's repair. *(DNB PATTERN 2002)*
- Howship Romberg sign is associated with obturator hernia. *(DNB PATTERN 2003)*

- Strangulation without obstruction is seen in Richter's Hernia. *(DNB PATTERN 2004, 2006)*
- Richter's hernia is seen most commonly with a femoral hernia. *(DNB PATTERN 2007)*
- NOT a treatment of femoral hernia: TRUSS. *(DNB PATTERN 2007)*
- In Nyhan classification, type 3A is Direct inguinal hernia. *(DNB PATTERN DEC 2011)*
- Hernia with highest rate of strangulation is femoral hernia. *(DNB PATTERN JUNE 2011)*
- Pascal's law is used in which repair of hernia repair—Stoppa'a preperitoneal hernia repair. *(DNB PATTERN JUNE 2010)*
- Spigelian Hernia is: Hernia occurring at the level of Arcuate line. *(FMGE PATTERN 2005)*
- Treatment of choice in Inguinal Hernia in infants is: Herniotomy. *(FMGE PATTERN MAR 2012)*
- Strangulation most commonly occurs in: Spigelian Hernia. *(FMGE PATTERN 2005)*
- Most common type of Hernia in the young: Indirect Inguinal. *(FMGE PATTERN SEP 2009)*
- Hernia which often simulates a peptic ulcer: Fatty Hernia of Linea Alba. *(FMGE PATTERN 2005)*
- Treatment of Congenital Hydrocele: Herniotomy. *(FMGE PATTERN SEP 2012)*
- Four Layer suture repair of Inguinal Hernia with double breasting of posterior wall of Inguinal Canal is known as: Shouldice's Repair. *(NEET PATTERN 2014)*
- An inguinal hernia with Acute Appendicitis occurring in the sac is known as: Amyand's Hernia. *(NEET PATTERN 2014)*
- Nerve most likely to be injured during Hernia Surgery: Lateral Femoral Cutaneous Nerve. *(NEET PATTERN 2016)*
- Inguinal Ligament does NOT bound the Triangle of Doom. *(NEET PATTERN 2016)*
- Open preperitoneal large mesh repair for Complex Inguinal Hernia: Stoppa Operation. *(NEET PATTERN 2016)*

LIVER AND GALLBLADDER

- Fatty liver is NOT an indication for Liver transplantation. *(DNB PATTERN 2002)*
- Most common primary tumor of Liver is Hemangioma. *(DNB PATTERN 2004)*
- Size of Common Bile Duct is 7.5 mm long. *(DNB PATTERN 2001)*

- Pneumobilia is NOT seen in Mirizzi's syndrome.
  (DNB PATTERN 2001)
- Commonest liver tumor is secondaries.
  (DNB PATTERN 2000)
- Cirrhosis is seen secondary to Bile duct obstruction.
  (DNB PATTERN 2006)
- Child's criteria is used in Cirrhosis.
  (DNB PATTERN 2000, 2006)
- Most common cause of Hemobilia: Trauma.
  (DNB PATTERN 2000, 2006)
- Site of portal obstruction in patients with Cirrhosis is the sinusoids. *(DNB PATTERN 2007)*
- Von Meyer Complexes seen in—Bile duct Hamartoma.
  (DNB PATTERN JUNE 2008)
- Type 2 cholangiocarcinoma involves division of both hepatic ducts and not extending outside.
  (DNB PATTERN DEC 2011)
- Mirizzi's syndrome is gallbladder stone compressing common hepatic duct. *(DNB PATTERN JUNE 2011)*
- First treatment in asymptomatic gallbladder stone is wait and watch. *(DNB PATTERN JUNE 2011)*
- Most common gallbladder stone is cholesterol.
  (DNB PATTERN JUNE 2011)
- Contraindication for laparoscopic cholecystectomy is coagulopathy, COPD-severe, end stage liver disease, congestive heart failure. *(DNB PATTERN JUNE 2011)*
- Treatment of retained CBD stone: Endoscopic sphincterotomy. *(DNB PATTERN JUNE 2011)*
- Not a feature of Hemobilia–fever.
  (DNB PATTERN DEC 2010)
- Emphysematous cholecystitis—caused by Clostridial species, E. coli and Klebsiella, Not caused by Pseudomonas.
  (DNB PATTERN DEC 2010)
- Hydatid cyst Scolicidal agent NOT used—Povidone Iodine.
  (DNB PATTERN JUNE 2008)
- Gall stones in children is NOT caused by Leptospira interrogans infection. *(DNB PATTERN JUNE 2009)*
- Murphy's sign is seen in: Acute Cholecystitis.
  (FMGE PATTERN MAR 2013)
- Cullen's sign is seen in: Acute Hemorrhagic Pancreatitis.
  (FMGE PATTERN MAR 2013)
- Number of Liver lobes as per Couinaud's classification: 8.
  (FMGE PATTERN 2005)

- Investigation of choice in gallbladder stone: Ultrasound. *(NEET PATTERN 2013)*
- Treatment of choice for Congenital Biliary Atresia: Kasai's Procedure. *(NEET PATTERN 2015)*

PANCREAS

- Commonest complication of Pseudopancreatic cyst is: Infection. *(DNB PATTERN 2003)*
- Migratory thrombophlebitis is a feature of Pancreatic Carcinoma. *(DNB PATTERN 2004)*
- Common cause of death due to Acute Pancreatitis: Shock. *(DNB PATTERN 2001)*
- Commonest pancreatic tumor: Insulinoma. *(DNB PATTERN 2007)*
- NOT used in treatment of acute pancreatitis: Antibiotics. *(DNB PATTERN DEC 2011)*
- Difference between acute and chronic pancreatitis is Acute pancreatitis has reversible changes. *(DNB PATTERN DEC 2011)*
- Whipple's triad (insulinoma) includes fasting hypoglycemia, plasma glucose levels <2.8 mmol/l, relief of symptoms on IV glucose. *(DNB PATTERN JUNE 2011)*
- Pseudocyst pancreas–is not a true cyst and its wall does not have an epithelial lining. *(DNB PATTERN JUNE 2011)*
- Greyish discoloration of flanks in Acute Pancreatitis is referred to as Grey Turner's sign. *(DNB PATTERN DEC 2010)*
- Treatment of choice for asymptomatic pseudocyst of pancreas–Conservative. *(DNB PATTERN 2007)*
- In acute pancreatitis, NOT seen: Hypercalcemia. *(DNB PATTERN 2007)*
- Most common complication of ERCP: Post ERCP Pancreatitis. *(FMGE PATTERN JUNE 2014)*
- Increase in serum pancreatic enzymes is more common after ERCP than Pancreatitis itself, if that is an option, may be the better answer.
- Cut off score for Acute Pancreatitis is defined as: Apache 11 score >8. *(NEET PATTERN 2015)*
- Hemobilia is NOT a part of Mirizzi's Syndrome. *(NEET PATTERN 2014)*
- Best investigation for Carcinoma Head of Pancreas is: Guided Biopsy. *(NEET PATTERN 2018)*

KIDNEYS

- Excessive intake of Vitamin C causes oxalate stones. *(DNB PATTERN 2002)*
- False regarding renal transplantation: Right kidney is usually preferred. *(DNB PATTERN 2003)*
- Most common predisposing factor for Pyelonephritis is vesicoureteral reflex. *(DNB PATTERN 2004)*
- Staghorn calculus is made up of Phosphate. *(DNB PATTERN 2000)*
- Cold ischemic time of the kidney is 6 hrs. *(DNB PATTERN 2000)*
- First symptom of tuberculosis of kidney is increased frequency. *(DNB PATTERN 2006)*
- Fever is NOT a part of Wilm's Tumor triad. *(DNB PATTERN 2006)*
- Whitaker test is for Hydronephrosis. *(DNB PATTERN JUNE 2012)*
- Treatment of blunt trauma of kidney is conservative. *(DNB PATTERN JUNE 2011)*
- Nephroureterectomy is indicated in Transitional Ca of pelvis extending till ureter. *(DNB PATTERN JUNE 2011)*
- One side kidney is normal, other side contracted with scar- Chronic pyelonephritis. Other DD: chronic glomerulonephritis, Benign hypertensive nephrosclerosis. *(DNB PATTERN JUNE 2011)*
- Xanthogranulomatous Pyelonephritis associated stones are due to: Proteus infection. *(DNB PATTERN JUNE 2011)*
- Renal cell carcinoma not true is—common in women. *(DNB PATTERN JUNE 2008)*
- Acute papillary tip necrosis—occurs in Diabetes Mellitus. *(DNB PATTERN JUNE 2008)*
- Middle aged man with renal failure with B/L abdominal mass— Probable diagnosis is ADPKD. *(DNB PATTERN JUNE 2008)*
- Renal Imaging of choice in patient with allergy—USG. *(DNB PATTERN JUNE 2008)*
- Renal transplant is an example of allograft. *(DNB PATTERN DEC 2009)*
- Most common carcinoma after renal transplant: Carcinoma of skin and Lips. *(NEET PATTERN 2013)*

SKIN

- Floor of a tuberculous ulcer contains Apple Jelly granulations. *(DNB PATTERN 2005)*

- Keloid formation is NOT seen over Face.
  (DNB PATTERN 2001)
- MC cause of cellulitis Streptococcus.
  (DNB PATTERN JUNE 2012)
- Most common site of Felon is Thumb.
  (DNB PATTERN DEC 2011)
- Melanoma staging—Breslow's classification/Clark's classification.
  (DNB PATTERN JUNE 2009)
- Most common site of Basal cell carcinoma is not upper lip, but nose. *(DNB PATTERN 2007)*
- Decubitus Ulcer is best classified as: Pressure Ulcer.
  (NEET PATTERN 2014)
- Most common site for a venous ulcer to develop: Medial Aspect of ankle above the malleoli. *(NEET PATTERN 2014)*
- Smallest recommended margin for wide excision of a Melanoma measuring 0.5 mm in depth should be: 1 cm.
  (NEET PATTERN 2016)
- Young male presented with painful fluctuant swelling between the gluteal folds. Per Rectal Examination is painless. The probable diagnosis is: Pilonidal Sinus. *(NEET PATTERN 2016)*

BLOOD VESSELS

- NOT true regarding amputation surgery in Thromboangiitis Obliterans patients: Sympathectomy is useful in all patients.
  (DNB PATTERN 2002)
- Raynaud's phenomenon is associated with Systemic Sclerosis. *(DNB PATTERN 2005)*
- Deep vein thrombosis is best diagnosed by Doppler.
  (DNB PATTERN 2001)
- Visceral aneurysms are most common in Splenic Artery.
  (DNB PATTERN 2007)
- Risk of thromboembolism is highest with—Femoral vein thrombus. *(DNB PATTERN JUNE 2008)*
- Trendelenburg's operation is seen in Varicose veins.
  (DNB PATTERN JUNE 2012)
- Best way to control external hemorrhage is Direct pressure.
  (DNB PATTERN JUNE 2012)
- Buerger's disease involves Artery, vein and nerve.
  (DNB PATTERN JUNE 2012)
- An adult patient with leg pain and gangrene of toe. His ankle to brachial pressure ratio would be less than 0.3.
  (DNB PATTERN JUNE 2011)

- Feature of acute limb ischemia: pain, pallor, paresthesia, pulselessness, paralysis. no cyanosis.
  (DNB PATTERN DEC 2010)
- Best method to treat large port wine Hemangioma: Pulsed dye laser (Selective autothermolysis).
  (DNB PATTERN DEC 2010)
- Raynaud's phenomenon sequence—Pallor, Cyanosis, Rubor.
  (DNB PATTERN JUNE 2008)
- Hemangioma is a compressible tumor.
  (DNB PATTERN JUNE 2009)
- Raynaud's phenomenon is NOT seen in JRA.
  (DNB PATTERN JUNE 2009)
- Capillaries fill fast in the following type of Shock: Septic Shock. *(FMGE PATTERN MAR 2013)*
- Artery cannulated most often for invasive blood pressure monitoring: Radial Artery. *(FMGE PATTERN MAR 2013)*
- Radial artery is cannulated to measure: Blood Pressure.
  (FMGE PATTERN MAR 2013)
- Most common complication of central venous line: Sepsis.
  (FMGE PATTERN MAR 2013)
- Seldinger needle is used for: Arteriography.
  (FMGE PATTERN MAR 2010)
- In Abdominal aortic aneurysm, the indication for surgery is when size of aneurysm is more than: 5.5 cm.
  (DNB PATTERN OCT 2013)
- Cut off for surgery in Abdominal Aortic Aneurysm in asymptomatic patients is: >5.5 cm. *(NEET PATTERN 2018)*
- NOT a sign of Thromboembolism: Virchow's sign.
  (NEET PATTERN 2013)
- Boyd's Perforator vein is most frequently located: In the proximal calf. *(NEET PATTERN 2014)*
- Femoral Artery is NOT a contributor to the Circle of Death.
  (NEET PATTERN 2014)
- Most common site of Acute Limb Ischemia from an Embolic Event: Femoral Bifurcation. *(NEET PATTERN 2014)*
- Ankle Brachial Pressure Index (ABPI) Suggesting Imminent Necrosis is: <0.3 *(NEET PATTERN 2016)*
- Commonest site of Peripheral Arterial Aneurysm: Popliteal.
  (NEET PATTERN 2015)
- Cirsoid Aneurysms of the Scalp are derived from: Superficial Temporal Artery. *(NEET PATTERN 2016)*
- Most common presentation of DVT is: Charley Horse Cramp. *(NEET PATTERN 2016)*

LYMPHATIC SYSTEM

- Milroy's disease is lymphoedema which is familial.
 (DNB PATTERN 2002)
- True about lymphangioma is lymphangioma progress slowly and may invade local tissue. *(DNB PATTERN JUNE 2011)*
- MC type primary lymphedema—lymphedema praecox (80%). *(DNB PATTERN DEC 2010)*
- MC bacterial infection with lymphedema—streptococcus.
 (DNB PATTERN DEC 2010)
- Carcinoma NOT spreading by lymphatics—Basal Cell Carcinoma. *(DNB PATTERN JUNE 2008)*
- Lymphangiosarcoma occurs in Lymphedema. It is a rare tumor that develops as a complication of long standing lymphedema (>10 yrs).
- Buerger's disease—does not involve lymphatics.
 (DNB PATTERN DEC 2009)

BRAIN

- N-Myc amplification is seen in Neuroblastoma.
 (DNB PATTERN 2004)
- Commonest site of meningomyelocele is Lumbosacral.
 (DNB PATTERN 2006)
- Pseudoclaudication is due to compression of Cauda Equina.
 (DNB PATTERN 2007)
- Diabetes Mellitus is NOT a complication of transection of the Pituitary. *(DNB PATTERN 2007)*
- Most common neurologic condition associated with head injury is: Altered consciousness. *(DNB PATTERN 2007)*
- Ganglion is collection of neurons outside CNS.
 (DNB PATTERN DEC 2011)
- Most common site of brain metastasis is cerebral cortex.
 (DNB PATTERN JUNE 2011)
- Management of epidural abscess is immediate surgical evacuation. *(DNB PATTERN JUNE 2011)*
- Lucid interval is seen in EDH. *(DNB PATTERN DEC 2010)*
- Common site for extradural hematoma is temporoparietal area. *(DNB PATTERN JUNE 2012)*
- Commonest functional tumor of pituitary: Prolactinoma.
 (DNB PATTERN JUNE 2009)
- Enlargement of pituitary tumor after adrenalectomy is called Nelson's syndrome. *(DNB PATTERN JUNE 2009)*
- MC cause of hypersecreting pituitary tumor: Pituitary Adenoma. *(DNB PATTERN DEC 2009)*

Surgery

- In Traumatic Brain Injury, the cerebral perfusion pressure should be maintained at: 70-90 mm Hg.
  (DNB PATTERN OCT 2013)

BURNS

- Blood transfusion is indicated in 50% superficial burns. *(DNB PATTERN 2005)*
- Splitting is the treatment of Burns of Hand. *(DNB PATTERN 2001)*
- Early cause of death due to burns is Shock. *(DNB PATTERN 2001)*
- Sunburns are first degree burns. *(DNB PATTERN 2007)*
- Myoglobinuria is seen in which burns electric burn. *(DNB PATTERN JUNE 2012)*
- A patient suffered from 3rd degree burn of right upper limb, 2nd degree burn of right lower limb, and 1st degree burn of whole of back. Total percentage of burn will be 45% (pix). *(DNB PATTERN JUNE 2011)*
- Curling ulcer is associated with—Burns. *(DNB PATTERN JUNE 2008)*
- Blisters are seen in superficial second degree burns. *(DNB PATTERN JUNE 2009)*
- Fluid of choice in resuscitation of burns patient: Ringer Lactate. *(FMGE PATTERN 2012, MAR 2013)*
- Rule of Nine in burns was proposed by: Alexander Wallace. *(FMGE PATTERN 2004)*
- Whole hand burns represent what percent of total body surface area?–1%. *(FMGE PATTERN MAR 2012)*
- According to Rule of Nine, burns involving perineum are: 1%. *(FMGE PATTERN MAR 2009)*
- Initial method to prevent infection in Burns patient: Handwashing. *(FMGE PATTERN MAR 2013)*
- Escharotomy is done in: Burns. *(FMGE PATTERN SEP 2012)*

BREAST

- Commonest secondaries of Carcinoma Breast is in Bone. *(DNB PATTERN 2000)*
- Most Common Site of breast metastasis: Bone (vertebra) lumbar > femur > thoracic > rib. *(DNB PATTERN DEC 2010)*
- Contralateral breast metastasis is most common in Lobular Carcinoma Breast. *(DNB PATTERN 2001)*
- Breast carcinoma with best prognosis: Colloid carcinoma, if tubular Ca is not in choice. *(DNB PATTERN 2002, 2005)*

- 30-year-old lady with inflammatory breast carcinoma, with negative axillary node and negative hepatic spread is best managed by Multimodal treatment. *(DNB PATTERN 2002)*
- Taxol is NOT used in Ca Breast. *(DNB PATTERN 2006, 2007)*
- Bleomycin is NOT used in Ca Breast. *(DNB PATTERN JUNE 2008)*
- Pain along medial aspect of arm in a postmastectomy patient is due to Intercostobrachial neuralgia. *(DNB PATTERN JUNE 2010)*
- Histological variety of breast carcinoma with best prognosis is Tubular Ca. *(DNB PATTERN JUNE 2011)*
- Peau d' orange appearance of breast is due to obstruction of dermal lymphatics. *(DNB PATTERN JUNE 2009, JUNE 2012)*
- Triple assessment includes: Clinical examination, Mammogram, FNAC. NOT Bone Scan. *(DNB PATTERN DEC 2010)*
- Conservative surgery NOT advisable in Ca breast, if there is subareolar lump. *(DNB PATTERN DEC 2010)*
- Breast cancer related with—Early menarche. *(DNB PATTERN JUNE 2008)*
- Investigation important in Breast conservation surgery: Sentinel Node Biopsy. *(DNB PATTERN 2002)*
- Lymphatic spread from upper outer quadrant of Breast does not occur to Parasternal Nodes. *(DNB PATTERN 2001)*
- Acute mastitis commonly occurs during Lactation. *(DNB PATTERN 2000)*
- Drug of choice for estrogen receptor positive breast cancer Tamoxifen. *(DNB PATTERN JUNE 2012)*
- Common presentation of duct papilloma of breast is bloody nipple discharge. *(DNB PATTERN JUNE 2011)*
- Paget's disease–97% ass with underlying invasive Carcinoma breast, underlying tumor lying within 2 cm of the nipple. *(DNB PATTERN DEC 2010)*
- Maximum risk of invasive breast Ca seen with atypical ductal hyperplasia (ADH). *(DNB PATTERN DEC 2010)*
- Preserved structure during breast reconstruction: P. major. *(DNB PATTERN JUNE 2009)*
- Sarcoma botyroides is also known as embryonal rhabdomyosarcoma. *(DNB PATTERN JUNE 2009)*
- Nerve which get damaged during breast surgery: Axillary nerves, Medial pectoral nerve, long thoracic nerve, Thoracodorsal nerve. *(DNB PATTERN JUNE 2009)*

- Young woman who received mantle radiation in childhood is likely to develop–Ca thyroid/Ca Breast.
(DNB PATTERN JUNE 2008)
- Treatment of Choice of Cystosarcoma Phyllodes: Wide Local Excision. *(NEET PATTERN 2016)*
- Tingling and Numbness over the posteromedial part of upper arm after Modified Radical Mastectomy is most likely to be due to injury to: Intercostobrachial Nerve.
(NEET PATTERN 2015)
- Treatment of Choice of Zuska's Disease is: Antibiotics, Incision and Drainage.
(NEET PATTERN 2015)
- Zuska's disease: recurrent nonlactational peridictal mastitis. New Mammography Screening Guidelines recommend Mammography to be routinely offered every 2 years after 50 years. *(NEET PATTERN 2015)*
- Van Nuys Prognostic Index is NOT based on: Estrogen Receptor status. *(NEET PATTERN 2018)*
- Van Nuys Prognostic Index for Ductal Carcinoma In Situ(DCIS) is based on: Size and Grade of DCIS, margins and age of the patient.

PROSTATE

- NOT used in treatment of Carcinoma Prostate: 5 fluorouracil. *(DNB PATTERN 2005)*
- Commonest mode of spread of Carcinoma prostate is: Blood vessel spread. *(DNB PATTERN 2000)*
- MC site of carcinoma prostate is Peripheral.
(DNB PATTERN JUNE 2012)
- Prostate cancer is best diagnosed by Transurethral USG.
(DNB PATTERN DEC 2011)
- Normal level of PSA in males is <4 ng/ml.
(DNB PATTERN JUNE 2011)
- True about PSA—Lipoprotein/Measured by immunoassay/ Sensitive and specific to differentiate between Ca and BPH.
(DNB PATTERN JUNE 2008)
- Gleason's scoring is done for prostate Ca.
(DNB PATTERN 2007)

SPLEEN

- Massive splenomegaly is seen in Hairy Cell Leukemia.
(DNB PATTERN 2003)
- Most common infection in post splenectomy patients is: Pneumococcal. *(DNB PATTERN 2003)*

- ❑ Disseminated Herpes Zoster is NOT common in post splenectomy cases. *(DNB PATTERN 2001)*
- ❑ In India, Splenectomy is most commonly done for indication of trauma. *(DNB PATTERN 2000)*

LUNG AND CHEST WALL

- ❑ Most common primary source for Brain secondaries: Lung. *(DNB PATTERN 2003)*
- ❑ Tietz syndrome usually develops at the second costal cartilage. *(DNB PATTERN 2000)*
- ❑ Adson's test—Cervical rib. *(DNB PATTERN 2006)*
- ❑ Poorest prognosis lung cancer: Small cell carcinoma. *(DNB PATTERN 2007)*
- ❑ Popcorn calcification is pathognomonic of Hamartoma. *(DNB PATTERN 2007)*
- ❑ MC tumor metastasizing to brain is Lung. *(DNB PATTERN JUNE 2012)*
- ❑ Marker of small cell cancer of lung is chromagnin. *(DNB PATTERN DEC 2011)*
- ❑ Mesothelioma-Decreasing incidence reflects ban on use of asbestos. *(DNB PATTERN JUNE 2008)*
- ❑ Family history is not associated with–Lung cancer. *(DNB PATTERN JUNE 2008)*
- ❑ Lung injury with good prognosis–Open pneumothorax. *(DNB PATTERN JUNE 2008)*
- ❑ Potato nodes are a feature of Sarcoidosis (Symmetric massive bilateral massive lymphadenopathy on chest X-ray). *(DNB PATTERN JUNE 2008)*
- ❑ Most common primary of metastatic bone tumor in male: Lung. *(DNB PATTERN JUNE 2009)*
- ❑ Lung injury with bad prognosis is tension pneumothorax. *(DNB PATTERN JUNE 2009)*
- ❑ Best sign indicating adequate functioning of the Intercostal drain: Movement of column in intercostal bottle. *(AIIMS PATTERN 2017)*

GENITAL SYSTEM

- ❑ Commonest type of Hypospadias: Glandular. *(DNB PATTERN 2000)*
- ❑ Most common tumor in undescended testis is: Seminoma. *(DNB PATTERN 2006)*
- ❑ Treatment of hydrocele in children is: Herniotomy. *(DNB PATTERN 2006)*

- Three glass test, shreds are present in first glass only. Most probable diagnosis is Urethritis.
(DNB PATTERN JUNE 2012)
- Testis is involved but epididymitis is spared in Syphilis.
(DNB PATTERN DEC 2011)
- Testicular teratoma has all markers except CEA.
(DNB PATTERN JUNE 2011)
- Testicular teratoma in adults is malignant.
(DNB PATTERN JUNE 2011)
- Perineal hematoma after trauma is due to rupture of bulbar urethra. *(DNB PATTERN JUNE 2011)*
- High inguinal orchiectomy for teratoma testes with involved epididymitis is what stage? Stage 1.
(DNB PATTERN JUNE 2011)
- Pain of external hemorrhoids is carried by pudendal nerve.
(DNB PATTERN JUNE 2011)
- Most common type of hypospadias is glandular.
(DNB PATTERN JUNE 2011)
- Painless Hematuria is NOT seen in cystitis.
(DNB PATTERN DEC 2009)
- Positive Prehn's sign is elevation of testes reduces pain of epididymitis. *(DNB PATTERN DEC 2010)*
- NOT a cause of painless hematuria—Acute Cystitis.
(DNB PATTERN JUNE 2008)
- Narrowest part of male urethra—External urethral meatus.
(DNB PATTERN JUNE 2008)
- Congenital hydrocele is treated by herniotomy.
(DNB PATTERN JUNE 2009)
- Hutch Diverticulum: Congenital Bladder Diverticulum seen in Boys. *(DNB PATTERN AUG 2013)*
- Hutch diverticulum is seen in: Bladder.
(DNB PATTERN JUNE 2014)

MISCELLANEOUS

- Van der Hoeve syndrome consists of blue sclera, fragile bones and conductive deafness. *(DNB PATTERN 2005)*
- Non irritant fluid to peritoneum is Blood.
(DNB PATTERN 2001)
- On 7th postoperative day, abdominal wound shows pink sanguineous discharge. It suggests impending wound dehiscence. *(DNB PATTERN 2001)*
- Intravenous antibiotics for prophylaxis should be given along with premedication. *(DNB PATTERN 2001)*

- Rectus cutting incision—Maryland incision.
  (DNB PATTERN JUNE 2008)
- Seen in tumor lysis syndrome—hypocalcemia.
  (DNB PATTERN DEC 2011)
- Not an immediate cause of death—Septicemia.
  (DNB PATTERN DEC 2011)
- Most common retroperitoneal sarcoma is Liposarcoma.
  (DNB PATTERN DEC 2011)
- Allen's test for integrity of palmar arch tests—patency of both ulnar and radial arteries. *(DNB PATTERN DEC 2011)*
- Content of epiplocele is Omentum.
  (DNB PATTERN DEC 2011)
- After trauma, hypovolemic shock can be due to all except head injury. *(DNB PATTERN JUNE 2011)*
- Most common site of rhabdomyosarcoma is orbit.
  (DNB PATTERN JUNE 2011)
- MC soft tissue tumor of adults: Malignant Fibrous Histiocytoma. *(DNB PATTERN DEC 2010)*
- Vertical banding gastroplasty (stomach stapling)—Morbid Obesity. *(DNB PATTERN DEC 2010)*
- Butcher's thigh is accidental injury to major vessels in thigh or groin (penetrating wound of femoral triangle due to knife slipping while boning meat). *(DNB PATTERN DEC 2010)*
- Patient with BAT presents wirth BP90/60, PR 124 INV to be done-FAST. *(DNB PATTERN DEC 2010)*
- Tripod fracture is seen in zygomatic bone. Costen's syndrome refers to neurological pain associated with temporomandibular jt. Most radio sensitive tissue is—Bone marrow.
  (DNB PATTERN JUNE 2008)
- Most common site of Actinomycetes—Jaw.
  (DNB PATTERN JUNE 2008)
- Clot of size of fist accounts for blood loss of—500 ml.
  (DNB PATTERN JUNE 2008)
- Skin grafts stored at 4 degree Celsius can survive up to 2 weeks. *(DNB PATTERN JUNE 2008)*
- Treatment of T4N0M0 stage of head and neck carcinoma: Surgery and Radiotherapy. *(DNB PATTERN JUNE 2008)*
- Management of Desmoid tumor: Wide excision.
  (DNB PATTERN JUNE 2008)
- Dr Christian Barnard–associated with world's first successful human to human heart transplant.
  (DNB PATTERN DEC 2009)
- Phantom limb is based upon law of projection.
  (DNB PATTERN DEC 2009)

- Most common type of Intussusception: Idiopathic.
  (DNB PATTERN DEC 2009)
- Pain from parietal pericardium is transmitted through Vagus nerve. *(DNB PATTERN DEC 2009)*
- Silver sulfadiazine is effective against Pseudomonas and is used in burns patients. *(DNB PATTERN DEC 2009)*
- Vitamin to be corrected in Obstructive jaundice—Vitamin K.
  (DNB PATTERN DEC 2009)
- Patient with hepatic insufficiency is being planned for surgery. Vitamin deficiency which has to be treated first is Vitamin K.
  (DNB PATTERN DEC 2009)
- Posterior perforation of peptic ulcer drains into Omental Bursa. *(DNB PATTERN DEC 2009)*
- Respiration is NOT a component of Glasgow Coma Scale.
  (DNB PATTERN DEC 2009)
- Lahshal Classification is for: Cleft Lip and Palate.
  (NEET PATTERN 2013)
- Trapezoid of disaster includes: triangle of doom laterally and triangle of pain medially. *(NEET PATTERN 2014)*
- Most common presentation of Desmoid Tumor: Abdominal Lump. *(AIIMS PATTERN 2017)*
- Common cause of Chronic Pancreatitis: Alcohol Use.
  (NEET PATTERN 2018)
- TRUE about Keloids: It contains Growth Factors.
  (NEET PATTERN 2018)
- Layers cut during Fasciotomy: Skin, subcutaneous tissue, superficial and deep fascia. *(NEET PATTERN 2018)*
- Calculate GCS of patient, 25 year old looking confused, opening eyes in response to pain, localises to pain: 11
  (NEET PATTERN 2018)
- A patient opens eye to painful stimulus, saying inappropriate sentences and able to spontaneously move all 4 limbs. GCS score will be: 11 *(AIIMS 2017 PATTERN)*

LEVEL II: HIGH YIELD FACTORS

Table 13.1: General surgery

Intra-abdominal pressure during Laparoscopic surgery	12-15 mm Hg
Amount of blood which can be removed from the body without change in Pulse rate/Blood Pressure	10-15%

Contd...

Contd...

Aspirin should be stopped	1 week prior to elective surgery
Ideal gas for laparoscopy	CO_2
Single most effective preventive measure in the hospital to prevent Nosocomial Infection	Hand washing
Most common opportunistic infection in organ transplant	Cytomegalovirus
Glasgow Coma scale score less than 7 is classified as	Coma

Table 13.2: Transplantation

1st heart transplant	Dr Christiaan Barnard, 1967
Transplantation of Human Organs Act by Govt of India	1994
Liver transplantation was first done by	Starzl
Most important HLA for organ transplantation	HLA D
Amputated digits are preserved in	Plastic bags in ice
Graft from sister to brother	Allograft
Graft from mother to son	Allograft
Commonest malignancy in renal transplant recipient	Skin cancer

Table 13.3: Cleft lip and palate

Cleft lip	Fusion of maxillary process with medial nasal process
Primary defect in Pierre Robin syndrome	Micrognathia
Unilateral cleft lip is associated with	Posterior displacement of Alar cartilage
Commonest type of cleft lip palate	Combined with cleft palate
Rhinoplasty is done at the age	16 years
Timing of repair of cleft lip	Between 3 and 6 months
Timing of repair of cleft	Between 6 and 18 months

Table 13.4: Burns

Most important aspect of management of Burns in first 24 hours	Fluid resuscitation
Most important cause of death in Burns in the early period	Hypovolemic shock

Contd...

Contd...

Ideal temperature of water to cool the Burns patient	15 degree
Minimum hourly urine output to be ensured to maintain adequate tissue perfusion in burns	30-50 ml/hour
Late death in burns is due to	Sepsis
Iced water should NOT be used on burns because	It can cause cutaneous vasoconstriction and can extend thermal damage
Most common infection in burns	Pseudomonas
Commonest ulcer in burns scar	Squamous cell carcinoma

Table 13.5: Skin and reconstructive surgery

Best dressing	Skin
Universal tumor	Lipoma
Abbe Estlander flap	Lip
First structure to be repaired in hand Injury	Skin
Skin grafting is absolutely contraindicated in	Streptococcus infection
Skin graft survives in the first 48 hours due to	Plasma imbibition
Wolfe's graft	Full thickness graft
Thiersch graft	Partial thickness graft

Table 13.6: Hernia

Viscera forms wall of	Sliding hernia
During hernia surgery, hernia sac should be opened at	Fundus
Most common content in hernia en Glissade	Sigmoid colon
Commonest hernia in female	Indirect inguinal hernia
Spigelian hernia is seen in	Subumbilical region
Most common hernia to strangulate	Femoral hernia
Hernia least likely to strangulate	Direct inguinal hernia
Mayo's operation is done for	Umbilical hernia

Table 13.7: Breast

Commonest site of carcinoma breast	Upper outer quadrant
Commonest site of secondaries of Carcinoma breast	Bone

Contd...

Contd...

Most malignant breast cancer	Mastitis carcinomatosa
Flap commonly used in breast reconstruction	TRAM flap
Most important prognostic factor for Carcinoma breast in females and males	Axillary lymph node status
Commonest type of carcinoma breast	Infiltrative ductal
Multicentric and bilateral	Lobular carcinoma
Best prognosis histological variant	Colloid (Mucinous)
Peau D orange appearance is due to	Lymphatic permeation

Table 13.8: Thyroid

Bone metastases common in	Hurthle cell tumor of thyroid
Most common histological variant of thyroid malignancy	Papillary
Medullary carcinoma thyroid arises from	Parafollicular C cells
FNAC is not useful in	Follicular carcinoma
Metastasis into thyroid gland most commonly occurs from	Carcinoma breast
Pulsatile vascular skeletal metastasis	Follicular carcinoma
Amyloid stroma is seen in	Medullary carcinoma
Most common solitary thyroid nodule	Follicular adenoma

Triangle of Doom	Medial Boundary Vas Deferens Lateral – Gonadal Vessels **Contents:** External Iliac Artery External Iliac Vein Inferior Epigastric Vessels.
Triangle of Pain	Superolateral border: Iliopubic tract Inferomedial border: Gonadal vessels. Lateral Border: Peritoneal reflection. **Contents:** Femoral Nerve. Femoral Branch of Genitofemoral Nerve. Lateral Femoral Cutaneous Nerve.
Trapezoid of Disaster	Anatomical Area formed by combining the Triangle of Death and the Triangle of Doom
Circle of Death (Corona Mortis)	Vascular Ring formed by anastomosis of Aberrant Obdurator Artery with the normal obdurator artery arising from a branch of the internal iliac artery. Aberrant Obdurator Artery can be damaged during Femoral Hernia repair

14. Obstetrics and Gynecology

"If you want to know how strong a country's health system is, look at the well being of its mothers."

—*Hilary Clinton*

REFERENCES

- *Novak's Gynecology, 15th ed.*
- *William's Obstetrics, 24th ed.*

LEVEL I: BASIC REPEATS

OBSTETRICS

- Hypertension in pregnancy causes Korotkoff's sound: phase 5. *(DNB PATTERN JUNE 2008)*
- The cardiac output returns to the pre-pregnancy state in 4 weeks. *(DNB PATTERN JUNE 2012)*
- Female with 37 wks pregnancy with grade 3 placenta preaevia, bleeding per vaginum with uterine contractions. Most appropriate management would be Emergency LSCS. *(DNB PATTERN JUNE 2012)*
- Commonest indication of classical caesarean section: Dense adhesion in lower uterine segment. *(DNB PATTERN JUNE 2012)*
- Purpose of Partogram to monitor progress of labor. *(DNB PATTERN JUNE 2012)*
- Cardinal movements during labor are in the following order: Engagement, descert, Flexion, Internal Rotation, Extensio, External Rotation and Expulsion. *(DNB PATTERN JUNE 2012)*
- A sure sign of labor: Breakage of Bag of Waters. *(DNB PATTERN JUNE 2012)*
- LH surge occurs how many hours before ovulation? 24-48 hrs. *(DNB PATTERN JUNE 2012)*
- Cervix dilatation suggestive of onset of labor is 3–5 cm. *(DNB PATTERN JUNE 2012)*
- Palmer sign seen in pregnancy is rhythmic contraction of uterus. *(DNB PATTERN JUNE 2012)*
- Peak HCG levels are seen by what intrauterine age? 8–10 weeks. *(DNB PATTERN JUNE 2012)*
- NOT true during Pregnancy: Decrease in Renal Plasma flow. *(DNB PATTERN JUNE 2012)*

- Least teratogenic potential is for HIV. *(DNB PATTERN JUNE 2012)*
- As per latest WHO guidelines, when a tubectomy operation cannot be done? 7–14 days. *(DNB PATTERN JUNE 2012)*
- Tubectomy done during 7–14 days would cause a sharp drop in milk output.
- The most common side effect of Progesterone only pills is irregular bleeding. *(DNB PATTERN JUNE 2012)*
- Legally MTP is defined up to 140 days. *(DNB PATTERN JUNE 2012)*
- Not required for the diagnosis of Bacterial vaginosis is plenty of lactobacilli. *(DNB PATTERN JUNE 2012)*
- Lower 1/3rd of vagina is formed by urogenital sinus. *(DNB PATTERN JUNE 2012)*
- Mifepristone is contraindicated in Ectopic pregnancy. *(DNB PATTERN JUNE 2012)*
- In recurrent abortions, all tests are to be done except TORCH infection screening. *(DNB PATTERN DEC 2011)*
- Neurological defect seen in fetus of diabetic mother is Caudal regression, situs inversus, spina bifida, hydrocephaly, anencephaly. *(DNB PATTERN DEC 2011)*
- Ratio of fetal weight and placental weight at term is 6:1. *(DNB PATTERN DEC 2011)*
- Placenta develops from deciduas basalis and chorion frondosum. *(DNB PATTERN DEC 2011)*
- Weight gain in normal pregnancy is 10–12 kgs. *(DNB PATTERN DEC 2011)*
- Total iron requirement during pregnancy is 1000 mg. *(DNB PATTERN DEC 2011)*
- Most common cause of perinatal mortality in twins is Prematurity. *(DNB PATTERN DEC 2011)*
- Percentage of breech presentation is 3%. *(DNB PATTERN DEC 2011)*
- Amniocentesis is done at what intrauterine age? 8–10 weeks. *(DNB PATTERN DEC 2011)*
- Peak levels of HCG are by what intrauterine age? 8–10 weeks. *(DNB PATTERN DEC 2011)*
- LCHAD deficiency is associated with fatty liver of pregnancy, HELLP syndrome, Liver failure. *(DNB PATTERN DEC 2011)*
- Late deceleration is due to uteroplacental insufficiency. *(DNB PATTERN DEC 2011)*
- Commonest cause of postpartum hemorrhage: Uterine atony. *(DNB PATTERN 2000)*

- Longest diameter of fetal skull: Mentovertical. *(DNB PATTERN 2000)*
- Commonest cause of Pyometra: Carcinoma cervix. *(DNB PATTERN 2000)*
- Most common fungal infection in 3rd trimester of pregnancy is Candida Albicans. *(DNB PATTERN 2001)*
- Most consistent sign in disturbed ectopic pregnancy: Pain. *(DNB PATTERN 2001)*
- Shortest diameter is obstetric conjugate. *(DNB PATTERN 2002)*
- Commonest type of ectopic pregnancy with rupture: Isthmic. *(DNB PATTERN 2002)*
- Alpha fetoprotein is decreased in Down's syndrome. *(DNB PATTERN 2002)*
- Sphingomyelin lecithin ratio is measured for assessing the maturity of Lung. *(DNB PATTERN 2003)*
- MTP act was passed in the year 1971. *(DNB PATTERN 2003)*
- Polycystic ovarian disease is associated with Adrenal hyperplasia. *(DNB PATTERN 2004)*
- Syphilis is transmitted in 28th week of pregnancy. *(DNB PATTERN 2005)*
- Litzmann's obliquity is Posterior asynclitism. *(DNB PATTERN 2007)*
- Naegele's Obliquity is Anterior Asynclitism.
- Burns Marshall technique is used to deliver the after coming head. *(DNB PATTERN 2007)*
- At term amniotic fluid volume is: 800 mL. *(DNB PATTERN JUNE 2008)*
- Amniotic fluid contain: Glucose, some Fructose No Galactose. *(DNB PATTERN JUNE 2008)*
- Oligohydramnios is associated with: Renal Agenesis. *(DNB PATTERN JUNE 2008)*
- Early amniocentesis is done at 12–14 wks. *(DNB PATTERN JUNE 2008)*
- Immune rejection of fetus prevented by: HCG. *(DNB PATTERN JUNE 2008)*
- Shortest diameter of Pelvic Cavity: Interspinous diameter. *(DNB PATTERN JUNE 2008)*
- Large Chorioangioma associated with: Polyhydramnios. *(DNB PATTERN JUNE 2008)*
- Frog eye appearane is seen in: Anencephaly.
- This is also called MICKEY MOUSE APPEARANCE: *(DNB PATTERN JUNE 2008)*

- Cervical change pregnancy: Increased Collagen/Increased Hyluronic Acid and Increased Glandular Structure.
  (DNB PATTERN JUNE 2008)
- Immediate complication 10U of Oxytcin bolus: Hypotension.
  (DNB PATTERN JUNE 2008)
- Oxytocin levels are NOT reduced by: Suckling.
  (DNB PATTERN JUNE 2008)
- Drug contraindicated in pregnancy: Enalapril.
  (DNB PATTERN JUNE 2008)
- Not a tocolytic: Misoprostol. *(DNB PATTERN JUNE 2008)*
- Not a steroid synthesis inhibitor: Mifepristone.
  (DNB PATTERN JUNE 2008)
- A 30-yr-old female with endometrial hyperplasia DOC: Medroxyprogesterone. *(DNB PATTERN JUNE 2008)*
- HELLP syndrome recurrence rate: 2%.
  (DNB PATTERN JUNE 2008)
- $MgSO_4$ to prevent seizure: 4 to 7 mg/mL.
  (DNB PATTERN JUNE 2008)
- Earliest fetal anomaly to be detected by USG: Anencephaly.
  (FMGE PATTERN MAR 2013)
- Glycosylated Hemoglobin in a pregnant lady should be less than: 6%. *(FMGE PATTERN MAR 2013)*
- Weight gain during pregnancy is: 12 kg.
  (FMGE PATTERN MAR 2012, MAR 2013)
- Weight of placenta at term: 550 gms.
  (FMGE PATTERN MAR 2013)
- Correct for urinary system changes in Pregnancy: GFR is increased. *(FMGE PATTERN MAR 2013)*
- Most sensitive test for detecting Iron depletion in pregnancy: Serum Ferritin. *(FMGE PATTERN MAR 2013)*
- In pregnancy, calculation of EDD considers the: First day of last menstruation. *(FMGE PATTERN MAR 2013)*
- Internal Podalic version is done for the: Second Twin.
  (DNB PATTERN AUG 2013)
- Amniotic fluid turnover occurs in: 1 day.
  (DNB PATTERN AUG 2013)
- **ZAVANELLI MANEUVER:** pushing back the delivered fetal head into the birth canal in case of Shoulder dystocia to perform a Caesarean section. *(DNB PATTERN AUG 2013)*
- MIRROR SYNDROME: Polyhydramnios + Hydrops Fetalis
  (DNB PATTERN AUG 2013)
- Also called Ballantyne Syndrome or Triple Oedema.
- Worst prognosis among valvular diseases in pregnancy is for: Aortic Stenosis. *(DNB PATTERN AUG 2013)*

- What is known as Pregnancy tumor? Pyogenic Granuloma. *(DNB PATTERN OCT 2013)*
- Earliest sign of Intrauterine death: Gas in Blood vessels. *(DNB PATTERN OCT 2013)*
- Most common cardiovascular condition causing Maternal death in Pregnancy: Pulmonary Hypertension. *(DNB PATTERN OCT 2013)*
- Maximum cardiac output is seen at: 30–34 weeks of Pregnancy. *(FMGE PATTERN SEP 2009)*
- pH of vagina in pregnancy: 4. *(FMGE PATTERN SEP 2009)*
- Increase in cardiac output seen in pregnancy is: 40%. *(FMGE PATTERN MAR 2010)*
- Increase in plasma volume seen in pregnancy is: 40–50%. *(FMGE PATTERN MAR 2010)*
- Plasma level of hCG in pregnancy doubles every: 2 days. *(FMGE PATTERN SEP 2010)*
- During pregnancy, maximum level of hCG is reached in: 70 days. *(FMGE PATTERN MAR 2007)*
- Change noticed in diastolic blood pressure in pregnancy: Decline of 5–10 mm Hg. *(FMGE PATTERN MAR 2010)*
- Fetal adrenals secrete which hormone predominantly: Cortisone. *(FMGE PATTERN MAR 2009, SEP 2010)*
- At what age does placenta take over Progesterone production? 12 weeks. *(DNB PATTERN JUNE 2014)*
- **McAfee Johnson Regime**: is used for Placenta Previa. *(FMGE PATTERN JUNE 2014)*
- Weight gain during second stage of pregnancy is: 5–7 kg. *(FMGE PATTERN JUNE 2014)*
- Lowest pregnancy rates for: ML Cu 375. *(NEET PATTERN 2014)*
- Dose of Progesterone released by MIRENA per day: 20 microgram. *(NEET PATTERN 2014)*
- Most common reason for discontinuation of IUCD use: Abnormal Uterine Bleeding. *(NEET PATTERN 2014)*
- NOT a risk factor for Ectopic Pregnancy: Condom. *(NEET PATTERN 2014)*
- Ideal contraceptive after Molar Pregnancy: Oral Contraceptive Pills. *(NEET PATTERN 2016)*
- IVF with Intracytoplasmic Sperm Injection is indicated when Total motile sperm count is less than: 1–5 million. *(NEET PATTERN 2016)*
- MTP is allowed till: 140 days as per MTP Act. *(NEET PATTERN 2016)*

- Metabolic Change which occurs during Hyperemesis Gravidarum: Hyperthyroidism. *(NEET PATTERN 2015)*
- Most common cause of BREECH presentation: Prematurity. *(NEET PATTERN 2016)*
- Most common Occipito Posterior position: Right Occipito Posterior. *(NEET PATTERN 2016)*
- Softening of Lower Uterine Examination on Bimanual examination is known as: HEGAR'S SIGN. *(NEET PATTERN 2015)*
- Incidence of Scar Rupture in previous LSCS is about: 1-2%. *(NEET PATTERN 2015)*
- During twin gestation, if division takes place on the 7th day, then the result would be: Diamniotic Monochorionic. *(NEET PATTERN 2015)*
- Drug used for enhancement of foetal lung maturity: Dexamethasone. (NEET PATTERN 2018)
- Best time to do the QUADRUPLE TEST: 15–20 weeks. *(NEET PATTERN 2018)*
- Quadruple Test includes:
    - Alpha Feto Protein. (AFP)
    - Human Chorionic Gonadotropin. (HCG)
    - Unconjugated Estriol.
    - Inhibin A.
- NOT a cause of secondary PPH: Placenta Praevia. *(NEET PATTERN 2018)*
- Recommended Daily Allowance of Iodine in pregnant women in micrograms: 250 micrograms/day. *(NEET PATTERN 2018)*

GYNECOLOGY

- pH of adult vagina is 4.5. *(DNB PATTERN 2006)*
- Mean pH of vagina during Pregnancy: 4 *(NEET PATTERN 2014)*
- pH of vagina is lowest during: Pregnancy. *(NEET PATTERN 2016)*
- pH of vagina after Ovariectomy: 7–7.5
- pH of vagina at Menopause: 7–7.5
- Weight of nulliparous uterus is 40–60 gm. *(DNB PATTERN DEC 2011)*
- Size of uterus in inches is: 3*2*1. *(DNB PATTERN 2003)*
- Provided that one secondary oocyte is produced in each menstrual cycle, how many secondary oocytes are on an average produced during the reproductive life of a human female? 420. *(DNB PATTERN JUNE 2012)*

- Cornification index or Eosinophilic index indicates Estrogenic effect. *(DNB PATTERN 2004)*
- Corpus Luteum of menstruation presents for: 14 days. *(DNB PATTERN 2005)*
- B lynch suture is applied on Uterus. *(DNB PATTERN 2007)*
- Latzko operation is done for: Vesicovaginal Fistula. *(DNB PATTERN JUNE 2008)*
- Partial Hydatidiform mole is associated with: Triploidy. *(DNB PATTERN JUNE 2008)*
- Commonest site of metastasis of Hydatidiform mole is Lung. *(DNB PATTERN 2007)*
- Karyotype of complete mole is 46XX. *(DNB PATTERN DEC 2011)*
- Which type of trophoblastic disease has worst prognosis? Postpartum. *(DNB PATTERN DEC 2011)*
- Chorionic Villi are absent in Choriocarcinoma. *(DNB PATTERN JUNE 2008)*
- Commonest presentation of Choriocarcinoma: Bleeding. *(DNB PATTERN JUNE 2008)*
- hCG is a tumor marker for Choriocarcinoma. *(DNB PATTERN 2006)*
- A risk factor for Choriocarcinoma: After full-term pregnancy. *(DNB PATTERN DEC 2011)*
- Definitive treatment of Adenomyosis is Hysterectomy. *(DNB PATTERN DEC 2011)*
- Most common site of Endometriosis: Ovary. *(DNB PATTERN DEC 2011)*
- Commonest degenerative changes seen in Uterine Myoma: Hyaline degeneration. *(DNB PATTERN 2003)*
- Pain in fibroid is NOT due to Hyaline degeneration. *(DNB PATTERN DEC 2011)*
- Retention of urine is seen in Anterior type of cervical fibroid. *(DNB PATTERN 2006)*
- Tuberculosis most commonly affects Fallopian tubes. *(DNB PATTERN 2004)*
- Best tubal function test is Laparoscopy. *(DNB PATTERN 2004)*
- Bonney's test is done for Stress Incontinence. *(DNB PATTERN 2006)*
- Bartholin's cyst adenitis is caused by Gonococcus. *(DNB PATTERN 2006)*

- Treatment of choice for Bartholin's abscess is Marsupialization. *(DNB PATTERN JUNE 2012)*
- Whiff test is done for Bacterial Vaginosis. *(DNB PATTERN DEC 2011)*
- Smear of vaginal discharge shows budding yeast cells.
- Causative agent is Candida. *(DNB PATTERN DEC 2011)*
- Female patient presents with reddish vagina and greenish discharge, the probable diagnosis is: Trichomonas vaginitis. *(DNB PATTERN 2002)*
- Polymenorrhea is NOT a feature of Polycystic Ovarian Disease. *(DNB PATTERN 2001)*
- Alpha fetoprotein is NOT increased in Down syndrome. *(DNB PATTERN DEC 2011)*
- Endometrial cancer is NOT associated with Dysgerminoma. *(DNB PATTERN DEC 2011)*
- Bodies found in Granulosa cell tumor: Call-Exner bodies. *(DNB PATTERN 2004)*
- Schiller Duval bodies are seen in Endodermal Sinus Tumor. *(DNB PATTERN 2005)*
- In a 25-yr-old female, cystitis is best treated by Nitrofurantoin. *(DNB PATTERN JUNE 2012)*
- Oral Contraceptive Pills are contraindicated in suspected breast cancer, heart disease and thromboembolism. *(DNB PATTERN DEC 2011)*
- Absolute contraindication of Hormone Replacement Therapy: Breast cancer. *(DNB PATTERN DEC 2011)*
- A female comes with normal breast development but scanty pubic hair is suffering from Testicular Feminization Syndrome *(DNB PATTERN DEC 2011)*
- Most commonly associated Human Papilloma virus associated with Cancer cervix is HPV 16. *(DNB PATTERN DEC 2011)*
- Agent implicated in Carcinoma cervix: Human Papilloma virus. *(DNB PATTERN 2002)*
- Most common symptom of Uterint Tuberculosis is: Infertility. *(DNB PATTERN OCT 2013)*
- Drug of choice for chemotherapy of Cervical Cancer: Cisplatin. *(DNB PATTERN OCT 2013)*
- Most common cause of Ruptured Uterus in India: Obstructed Labor. *(DNB PATTERN OCT 2013)*
- Treatment of Endometrial cyst > 5 cm: Laparoscopy. *(DNB PATTERN AUG 2013)*
- Marker of Endodermal Sinus Tumor: Alpha Fetoprotein. *(DNB PATTERN AUG 2013)*

- Kallmann syndrome: Hypogonadism with Anosmia and GnRH deficiency. *(DNB PATTERN AUG 2013)*
- Karyotype of Incomplete Mole: 69 XXY. *(DNB PATTERN AUG 2013)*
- Succenturiate Lobe of placenta: Smaller separate lobe of placenta with increased risk of Postpartum hemorrhage. *(DNB PATTERN AUG 2013)*
- Most common complication of Intrauterine Device: Bleeding. *(FMGE PATTERN MAR 2013)*
- Non-invasive method for locating an expelled IUD: USG. *(FMGE PATTERN MAR 2013)*
- Conventional contraception is: Condoms. *(FMGE PATTERN SEP 2006)*
- Other conventional contraceptives
    - Diaphragm
    - Vaginal Foam.
- Lifespan of CuT 380 A is: 10 years. *(FMGE PATTERN SEP 2011. MAR 2013, NEET PATTERN 2015)*
- Contraceptive supplied by Government of India free of cost: MALA-N. *(FMGE PATTERN SEP 2006)*
- Oral contraceptives predispose to: Cerebral Stroke. *(FMGE PATTERN MAR 2011)*
- Oral contraceptives prevent development of: Ovarian Malignancy. *(FMGE PATTERN MAR 2011)*
- Technique of CuT insertion: Pushing. *(FMGE PATTERN MAR 2010)*
- Which subtype of Papilloma virus has maximum chance of causing Carcinoma cervix? HPV 16,18. *(FMGE SEP 2012, MAR 2013)*
- Incidence of Vulval TB: <2%. *(DNB PATTERN JUNE 2014)*
- Whiff Test is used for: Gardnerella vaginalis. *(FMGE PATTERN JUNE 2014)*
- Feature of Physiological Vaginal Discharge: Cyclical. *(NEET PATTERN 2014)*
- Normal blood loss during Menstruation: 30–40 mL. *(NEET PATTERN 2014)*
- Physiologic Leukorrhea is least likely in Prepubertal Girls. *(NEET PATTERN 2014)*
- Most common cause of vulval discharge in an 8-yr-old prepubertal girl: Non-specific Vulvovaginitis. *(NEET PATTERN 2016)*

- Investigation of Primary Amenorrhea in a girl with full development of secondary sexual characteristics should be performed by: 16 yrs. *(NEET PATTERN 2014)*
- FSH LH levels in TURNER'S SYNDROME: High FSH, High LH. *(NEET PATTERN 2014)*
- Multiple Corpora Lutea cysts are NOT a feature of STEIN-LEVENTHAL SYNDROME. *(NEET PATTERN 2014)*
- Most common presenting symptom of Carcinoma Cervix is: Vaginal Bleeding. *(NEET PATTERN 2014)*
- MEIGS SYNDROME is associated with which ovarian tumor? FIBROMA. *(NEET PATTERN 2014)*
- A 60-yr-old with primary adenocarcinoma of the Uterus presents with large complex ovarian mass and ascites. Diagnosis is: KRUKENBERG TUMOR. *(NEET PATTERN 2014)*
- Next Investigation in a patient presenting with primary amenorrhea and normal secondary sexual characteristics: USG of Uterus. *(NEET PATTERN 2015)*
- SWISS CHEESE pattern Endometrium is seen in: Metropathia Hemorrhagica. *(NEET PATTERN 2016)*
- Anovulatory DUB is NOT a part of HALBAN'S DISEASE. *(NEET PATTERN 2016)*
- Pain in the Right Upper Quadrant due to adhesion inflammation between the liver and the diaphragm is known as: FITZ-HUGH-CURTIS SYNDROME. *(NEET PATTERN 2016)*
- Most common site of origin of Carcinoma Cervix is: Endocervical or Transitional Zone. *(NEET PATTERN 2015)*
- Sarcoma Botryoides arises most commonly from: Vagina. *(NEET PATTERN 2015)*
- Most common site of origin of Sarcoma Botryoides: Head and Neck >Vagina.
- Most common genital site of origin of Sarcoma Botryoides: Vagina
- Coffee Bean Nuclei are seen in: Brenner Tumor. *(NEET PATTERN 2015)*
- Most common indication of a Posterior Colpotomy: Drainage of Pelvic Abscess. *(NEET PATTERN 2015)*
- The term **COUVELAIRE UTERUS** is used in relation to: Uteroplacental Apoplexy. *(NEET PATTERN 2015)*
- Follicular Endometrium is NOT seen in **ARIAS-STELLA REACTION**. *(NEET PATTERN 2016)*

- Indication for Hormonal Therapy in Post menopausal women: Hot Flushes. *(NEET PATTERN 2018)*
- In Uterine Prolapse, whether the ring pessary is in place is known by: NOT getting expelled after an increase in intra abdominal pressure. *(NEET PATTERN 2018)*

LEVEL II: HIGH YIELD FACTOIDS

Table 14.1: Female reproductive system

Uterus measures	Normal position of uterus
	Fallopian tube measures
Internal diameter of Fallopian tube	9 cm * 6.5 cm * 3.5 cm
Widest and longest part of Fallopian tube	Anteverted anteflexed
Shortest and narrowest part of Fallopian tube	10 cm in length
Doderlein's bacillus	8 mm
	Ampulla
	Interstitial part
	Forms lactic acid which maintains the pH of vagina at 4.5

Table 14.2: Genital fistulae and stress incontinence

Chassar Moir technique	Treatment of vesicovaginal fistula
Martius graft or Gracilis muscle graft	Vesicovaginal fistula
Boari Flap operation	Ureteric fistulae
Youssef's syndrome	Cyclical hematuria caused by Bladder Endometriosis
Cyclical Hematuria	Common symptom of Vesicouterine fistula
Marshall's test	Stress Incontinence
Cotton Swab stick test/Stress Test	Other tests for Genuine Stress Urinary Incontinence

Table 14.3: Gestational trophoblastic diseases

Highest incidence of Hydatidiform Mole	South-East Asia
Recurrence rate of Hydatidiform Molar pregnancy	2%
Androgenesis	Feature of Complete Mole
Choriocarcinoma most commonly occurs	Following evacuation of hydatidiform mole
Most common site of metastasis of Choriocarcinoma	Lung

Contd...

Contd...

Patient should NOT conceive	For a year after receving chemotherapy for Choriocarcinoma
Most effective chemotherapeutic agent in choriocarcinoma	Methotrexate
Purple hemorrhagic projections into the vagina are pathognomonic of	Choriocarcinoma

Table 14.4: Endometriosis and adenomyosis

Endometriosis is most common in	Japan
Chocolate cysts of the ovary	Endometriosis
Powder burn spots are characteristic of	Endometriosis
Most common symptom of Endometriosis	Dysmenorrhea
Gold standard for the diagnosis of Endometriosis	Laparoscopy
Menorrhagia with accompanying dysmenorrhea is a sign of	Adenomyosis

Table 14.5: Ovarian tumors

Hobnail cells	Mesonephroid Tumor
Walthard cell rests	Brenner Tumor
Reinke Crystals	Hilus Cell Tumor
Schiller-Duval bodies	Endodermal Sinus Tumor

Table 14.6: Bartholin's gland/Gartner's cyst

Bartholin's gland location	Posterolaterally to the vaginal orifice
Bartholin's duct opening	On the inner side of Labium minus
Bartholin's gland	Compound racemose gland/lined by low columnar epithelium
Most common cause of Bartholinitis	Gonococci
Treatment of Bartholin's cyst	Antibiotics
Treatment of Bartholin's abscess	Drainage
Bartholin's gland tumor	Usually adenocarcinoma and treatment is Radical Vulvectomy
Treatment of asymptomatic Gartner's cyst	Leave alone
Treatment of symptomatic Gartner's cyst causing Dyspareunia	Marsupialization

Table 14.7: Genital tuberculosis

Least common site of Genital TB	Vagina/vulva
Most common type of spread of Genital TB	Hematogeneous spread
Hysterosalpingography is contraindicated in Pelvic TB	As it can lead to reactivation of TB
Pipe stem fallopian tubes	Genital TB
Tobacco pouch appearance of Fallopian tubes	Genital TB

Table 14.8: Carcinoma cervix

Most common genital cancer in India	Carcinoma Cervix
Viral etiology for Carcinoma cervix	Human Papilloma virus 16,18,31,33.HSV -2
Human papilloma viruses include	More than 70 types based on genetic homology
Papilloma viruses causing invasive cervical carcinoma	HPV 16,18,31,33,45 (high risk)
Papilloma viruses causing Condylomas or benign lesions	HPV 6,11,42,44 (low risk)
Papilloma viruses causing Verruca vulgaris or common warts	HPV 1,2,3,4
90% cervical intraepithelial neoplasia caused by 100% squamous cell cancers of the cervix	90% cervical intra epithelial neoplasia caused by: Human Papilloma Virus. 100% squamous cell cancers of the cervix contains: Human Papilloma Virus.
Commonest Human Papilloma virus causing invasive cervical cancer	HPV 16
Most specific HPV for invasive cervical cancer	HPV 18
Oncoproteins produced by HPV	E6/E7
A single Pap smear in a lifetime reduces the risk of cervical cancer by	50%
Yearly screening of all women between 21 and 64 reduces the risk of cervical cancer by	91%
New tumor marker for dysplastic Carcinoma cervix cells	AgNOR or Silver stained Nuclear Organizer Regions
Latest classification scheme for Pap smear	Bethesda system
Schauta's operation/Mitra's operation	Carcinoma cervix stages 1B and II A
Quadrivalent vaccine available for Carcinoma cervix	Gardasil
Bivalent vaccine available for Carcinoma cervix	Cervarix

Table 14.9: STD

Strawberry cervix	Trichomonas vaginalis
Diamond media	Culture of Trichomonas vaginalis
Feinberg-Whittington media	Culture of Trichomonas vaginalis
Clue cells	Bacterial vaginosis
Commonest sexually transmitted infection	Chlamydia Trachomatis
Groove sign	Lymphogranuloma inguinale
Donovan bodies	Granuloma inguinale

Table 14.10: Fibromyomas

Womb stones are	Calcareous degeneration of uterine fibroids
Most common cause of red degeneration of fibroid	Pregnancy
Inversion of uterus is caused by	Submucosal fundal myoma
Infertility and recurrent pregnancy loss is commonly seen with	Submucosal myoma
Hydroureter and hydronephrosis are complications of	Broad ligament fibroids
Retention of urine/urinary frequency more in	Anterior and Posterior fibroids lodged in the Pouch of Douglas
Adenomyosis is differentiated from Fibroids in that	Uterus is tender in case of Adenomyosis.
Uterus > 12 weeks size or irregularly enlarged uterus	favors a diagnosis of Fibromyoma over Adenomyosis

Table 14.11: Miscellaneous named questions

Ward-Mayo repair	Commonest surgery for Uterovaginal prolapse
Manchester operation/Fothergill operation	Uterine prolapse
Rotterdam II criteria	Polycystic Ovarian syndrome
Meig Syndrome	Ascites and pleural effusion accompanying benign ovarian fibroma
Pseudo-Meigs syndrome	Ascites and pleural effusion accompanying other tumors like cystic fibromyomas/Brenner tumor/thecoma/Granulosa cell tumor
Rokitansky's protuberance	Mature Cystic Teratoma
Lipschutz ulcer	Occurs on labia minora and introitus and etiology is Epstein-Barr virus

Contd...

Contd...

Bonney's hood incision	Used to remove a posterior fibroid
Halban/Moscowitz procedures	Enterocoele correction
Yuzpe regimen	Combined use of estrogen and progesterone for emergency contraception

CONTRACEPTION

Use and Forget Reversible Contraceptive devices	ParaGard T 380A and Mirena
Replacement Time period of CuT380A	10 years
Replacement Time period of Mirena	5 years
Treatment of choice of contraception after Molar Pregnancy	OCP
Effective Life of Nova CuT-200	5 years
Multiload CuT 250	3 years
Multiload CuT 375	3 years
CuT 380Ag	4 years
CuT 380S	2.5 years
Lippes Loop	Several years
Mechanism of Action of Copper T	Copper exerts toxic action on Sperms and inflammatory reaction in the Endometrium
Mechanism of Action of Hormonal Devices	Act by release of Progesterone which suppresses the estrogenic activity hindering the maturation of endometrium and preventing implantation of fertilized ova

15. Pediatrics

"Live neither in the past, nor in the future, but let each day's work absorb your entire energies, and satisfy your widest ambition."
—*William Osler*

REFERENCE
- *OP Ghai Essential Pediatrics, 9th ed.*

LEVEL I: BASIC REPEATS

GENERAL

- What is the dose of Isoniazid in children? 10–15 mg/kg. *(DNB PATTERN JUNE 2012)*
- At what age is a child's height expected to be 100 cm? 4 yrs. *(DNB PATTERN JUNE 2012)*
- Baby starts speaking sentence of few words at what age? 2 yrs. *(DNB PATTERN DEC 2009)*
- First sign of puberty in females is Thelarche. *(DNB PATTERN DEC 2009)*
- Earliest indication of sexual maturation in a girl is Thelarche. *(DNB PATTERN 2007)*
- In females, growth spurt is maximum in: Tanner stage III, Axillary stage III. *(DNB PATTERN DEC 2011)*
- First set of milk teeth appear at what age? 6 months. *(DNB PATTERN DEC 2009)*
- First permanent teeth to erupt are the first molars. *(DNB PATTERN 2007)*
- Brown fat NOT present in Cheek. *(DNB PATTERN JUNE 2008)*
- Fore milk does NOT contain Fat. *(DNB PATTERN JUNE 2008)*
- Blood specimen for thyroid screening in a neonate is obtained on cord blood. *(DNB PATTERN 2007)*
- Definition of childhood is under what age? 12 years. *(DNB PATTERN DEC 2009)*
- Percentage rise in length of infant in first year of life is: 50%. *(DNB PATTERN 2000)*
- Creeping upstairs is NOT a function of 3-year-old child. *(DNB PATTERN 2001)*

- Fetal movements are NOT a part of IUGR assessment.
  (DNB PATTERN 2001)
- Hypoglycemia in infants more than 24 hrs of age is defined as blood glucose levels less than 45 mg/dL.
  (DNB PATTERN JUNE 2011)
- Moro's reflex is abnormal after 12 weeks.
  (DNB PATTERN 2002)
- Newborn baby are prone to hypoglycemia because of low body glycogen reserve. *(DNB PATTERN JUNE 2009)*
- True about Gomez classification of malnutrition of children is: weight is the only parameter. *(DNB PATTERN DEC 2009)*
- Classification of Malnutrition which is independent of the weight of the child : McLaren Classification.
  (DNB PATTERN DEC 2010)
- Severe Hypothermia in a neonate is temperature <32 degree.
  (DNB PATTERN DEC 2010)
- This response is seen in newborns as a measure of thermogenesis? Shivering. *(DNB PATTERN JUNE 2011)*
- Low birth weight baby is the one whose birth weight is: less than 2500 g. Low Birth weight <2500 g.
  - Very Low Birth Weight <1500 g.
  - Extreme Low Birth Weight < 1000 g.

  (DNB PATTERN JUNE 2009)
- SGA baby is one whose body weight is: less than 10th percentile. *(DNB PATTERN JUNE 2009)*
- True hermaphroditism is when tissues of both ovaries and testes are present. *(DNB PATTERN JUNE 2009)*
- A child having IQ of 25 falls under which category? Dependent. *(DNB PATTERN JUNE 2010)*
- As per RCH II, Vitamin A dosage at 9 months of age is: 1 lakh units. *(DNB PATTERN JUNE 2011)*
- Most common Cause of Jaundice in newborn: ABO Incompatibility. *(DNB PATTERN AUG 2013)*
- Most common cause of Acute Laryngotracheobronchitis: Parainfluenza 1, 2. *(DNB PATTERN AUG 2013)*
- Definition of Neonatal period: from birth to 28 days.
  (DNB PATTERN AUG 2013)
- Meconium is seen in upper small intestine by: 3 months Intrauterine Life. *(DNB PATTERN AUG 2013)*
- Child crawls by: 7th–8th month.
  (DNB PATTERN AUG 2013)
- Very Low Birth Weight is less than: 1500 gm.
  (FMGE PATTERN MAR 2013)

- Anterior fontanelle ossifies by: 18 months.
  (FMGE PATTERN 2007)
- Moro Reflex disappears by: 3 months.
  (FMGE PATTERN MAR 2010)
- A 10-year-old child with mental age of 2 yrs will have an IQ level of: 20. *(FMGE PATTERN MAR 2013)*
- First sign of sexual maturity in boys: Testicular enlargement.
  (FMGE PATTERN SEP 2010)
- Child attains a height of 100 cm at: 4 yrs.
  (FMGE PATTERN MAR 2011, SEP 2012)
- Average gain of height in first year is: 25 cm.
  (DNB PATTERN NOV 2013)
- At what age do permanent first teeth appear? 6 yrs.
  (DNB PATTERN NOV 2013)
- NOT a correct sign of good attachment of a baby to the breast: Lower areola more visible.
  (FMGE PATTERN SEP 2012)
- Common cause of neonatal hypoglycemia is: Infant of Diabetic mother. *(FMGE PATTERN MAR 2013)*
- Physiological jaundice in a term baby lasts up to: 10 days.
  (FMGE PATTERN MAR 2005, SEP 2010)
- Most common cause of pathological jaundice on first day of life is: Rh incompatibility. *(FMGE PATTERN MAR 2008)*
- Most common cause of Neonatal mortality in India: Prematurity. *(FMGE PATTERN MAR 2013)*
- Most common birth defect in North India: Neural Tube Defects (Spina Bifida). *(DNB PATTERN NOV 2013)*
- Non-appearance of social smile even after: 8 weeks is considered abnormal. *(FMGE PATTERN SEP 2011)*
- Both chest and head is lifted at what time? 6 months.
  (FMGE PATTERN SEP 2012)
- In boys, 1st sign of sexual maturity: Testicular growth.
  (FMGE PATTERN SEP 2012)
- When does child know his gender? 2½ to 3 yrs.
  (FMGE PATTERN SEP 2012)
- Extremely Low Birth Weight is: Less than 1000 g.
  (FMGE PATTERN JUNE 2014)
- Percentiles depicted with color coded lines in WHOs new Growth Chart contains which percentiles? 3rd, 15th, 50th, 85th and 97th. *(NEET PATTERN 2014)*
- Recommended Target Preductal saturations of neonates to be ensured at 5 min after birth: 80-85%.
  (NEET PATTERN 2014)

- Ideal site for bone marrow aspirate in infants: Upper end of tibia. *(NEET PATTERN 2014)*
- Heart rate is not a part of the Pediatric Assessment Triangle. *(NEET PATTERN 2015)*
- Handedness is established by 3 years of age. *(NEET PATTERN 2015)*
- Last fontanelle to close: Anterior Fontanelle. *(NEET PATTERN 2018)*
- 1st fontanelle to close: Posterior fontanelle (2–3 months after birth).
  - Posterior 2–3 months
  - Sphenoidal 6 months
  - Mastoid 6–18 months
  - Anterior 1–3 years.

METABOLIC AND NUTRITIONAL DISEASES

- In Rickets, NOT seen is increased ACID phosphatase. *(DNB PATTERN DEC 2009)*
- True of Vitamin D resistant Rickets? Defect in Proximal Tubular Reabsorption. *(DNB PATTERN JUNE 2011)*
- In an 8-year-old girl with symptoms of Rickets, lab investigations show serumcalcium 7.2 mg/dL. Serum phosphate 2.3 mg/dL, alkaline phosphatase 2420 IU/L. The most probable diagnosis is: Nutritional Rickets. *(DNB PATTERN DEC 2010)*
- Craniotabes is NOT seen in Kernicterus. *(DNB PATTERN 2006)*
- Metabolic Acidosis is associated with Acetazolamide. *(DNB PATTERN 2003)*
- Child with diarrhea having deep and rapid respiration. The diagnosis is: Metabolic Acidosis. *(DNB PATTERN 2001)*
- Epiphyseal dysgenesis is a feature of Hypothyroidism. *(DNB PATTERN 2003)*
- In Hyperparathyroidism, serum Ca is increased, serum phosphorus is decreased. *(DNB PATTERN 2000)*
- Breast milk is deficient in Vitamin D. *(DNB PATTERN AUG 2013)*
- Specific sign of Kwashiorkor is: Pitting edema. *(FMGE PATTERN SEP 2007)*
- Breastfeeding should be initiated within: Half-an-hour. *(FMGE PATTERN SEP 2009)*
- Acute malnutrition in a child is clinically assessed by: Weight for Height (Wasting). *(FMGE PATTERN SEP 2010)*

- Best index of chronic malnutrition: Height for Age (Stunting). *(FMGE PATTERN SEP 2010)*
- Waterlow classification of Malnutrition takes into account: Weight for Height and Height for Age. *(DNB PATTERN NOV 2013)*
- Combined indicator to reflect both Acute and Chronic Malnutrition: Weight for Age.
- Black colored urine is seen in: Alkaptonuria. *(FMGE PATTERN JUNE 2014)*

> Alkaptonuria Fact File
> NITISINONE–New Drug under trial for Alkaptonuria which reduces urinary Homogenetisic Acid levels.
> Pigmentation of Heart valves occur in: Alkaptonuria
> Pigmentation of Tympanic Membranes, Heart valves, Larynx, Ear cartilages [concha, antihelix and finally helix] and skin occurs in Alkaptonuria.
> Small joints are usually SPARED in Ochronotic Arthritis.
> Intervertebral disc calcification occurs in alkaptonuria.
> Coronary artery calcification occurs in alkaptonuria.

- Stoss Therapy is used for: Vitamin D deficiency Rickets. *(NEET PATTERN 2014)*
- Enzyme deficiency which causes Lesch Nyhan Syndrome: Hypoxanthine Guanine PhosphoRibosyl transferase. (HGPRTase). *(NEET PATTERN 2018)*

CVS

- Wide splitting of the second heart sound is characteristic of ASD. *(DNB PATTERN 2004)*
- ASD is NOT a cause of pansystolic murmur. *(DNB PATTERN 2000, 2002)*
- Not seen in Fallot's tetrology: ASD. *(DNB PATTERN 2000, 2002)*
- Single S2 is a feature of Tetrology of Fallot. *(DNB PATTERN 2004)*
- Pentology of Fallot: TOF + ASD. *(DNB PATTERN 2009)*
- NOT a treatment for cyanotic spells in TOF: Isoprenaline administration. *(DNB PATTERN 2002)*
- NOT an association of TOF: Right-sided aortic arch. *(DNB PATTERN JUNE 2008)*
- ASD patient with murmur similar to MR and left axis deviation of 40 degrees is having floppy mitral valve. *(DNB PATTERN JUNE 2009, DEC 2009)*

- Most common cause of death in PDA is: Cardiac failure. *(DNB PATTERN DEC 2009)*
- Congestive heart failure in children is best diagnosed by: Tachycardia and tender hepatomegaly. *(DNB PATTERN 2000)*
- Sure sign of cardiac failure in an infant: Liver enlargement. *(DNB PATTERN 2000, 2004)*
- Commonest cause of heart failure in infancy: Congenital heart disease. *(DNB PATTERN 2007, 2009)*
- Cardiac defect common in Down's syndrome: Atrioventricular septal defect. *(DNB PATTERN 2000)*
- Congenital long QT syndrome is associated with Neonatal bradycardia. *(DNB PATTERN 2007)*
- Most common valve associated with Rheumatic Heart Disease: Mitral valve. *(DNB PATTERN JUNE 2008)*
- NADA's criteria is for Heart Disease. *(DNB PATTERN JUNE 2008)*
- Single umbilical artery is associated with: congenital anomalies in 10–20% cases. *(DNB PATTERN JUNE 2008)*
- CVS Anomaly commonly seen in Turner's syndrome: Coarctation of Aorta. *(DNB PATTERN AUG 2013)*
- Most common presentation of Double Aortic Arch in infants is: Tracheal compression symptoms. *(DNB PATTERN NOV 2013)*
- Children borne to mothers with SLE are likely to get: Complete heart block. *(DNB PATTERN 2008)*
- Most common Congenital Heart Disease associated with Down's Syndrome: Atrioventricular Septal Defect. *(NEET PATTERN 2015)*
- Complete Heart Block in Neonatal Lupus is related to: Anti-RO Antibodies. *(NEET PATTERN 2016)*
- Tetrology of Fallot, Vaginal Atresia and Polydactyly is seen together in: Mccusick Kaufman Syndrome. *(JIPMER PATTERN 2017)*
- Pott's Shunt: Shunt from Left Pulmonary Artery to Descending Aorta. *(JIPMER PATTERN 2017)*
- Pott's Shunt is mainly used for decompression of Pulmonary Hypertension.

RENAL SYSTEM

- NOT true about Wilm's tumor: presents at 5 yrs of age. *(DNB PATTERN DEC 2011, JUNE 2012)*
- In minimal change disease, 90% cases respond to short course of steroid therapy. *(DNB PATTERN 2004)*

- Steroids are useful in Minimal Change Disease. *(DNB PATTERN 2003)*
- Commonest nephrotic syndrome in child: Minimal change disease. *(DNB PATTERN 2005)*
- Second most common cause of Nephrotic Syndrome in Child: Focal Segmental Glomerulosclerosis (FSGS). *(NEET PATTERN 2014)*
- Berger nephropathy is due to deposition of IgA and C3. *(DNB PATTERN 2007)*
- Decreased serum cholesterol is NOT a feature of Nephrotic syndrome. *(DNB PATTERN 2007)*
- Most common cause of Hypertension in a child: Chronic glomerulonephritis. *(DNB PATTERN 2008)*
- Most common cause of renal artery stenosis in India in children: Takayasu aortoarteritis. *(DNB PATTERN 2009)*
- Kidney attains Adult level GFR by what age? 1–2 years. *(NEET PATTERN 2015)*
- A 10-year-old boy presented with cola coloured urine, oliguria for 3 days, facial puffiness and edema. Urine albumin is positive and C3 levels are reduced. BP is 130/80 mm Hg. There is history of skin infection 2 weeks back. The next line of management is: Conservative management. *(JIPMER 2017 PATTERN)*
- Urine Osmolality in Pre Term is: 600 mOsm/kg. *(JIPMER 2017 PATTERN)*

CNS

- A newborn has been brought with seizures refractory to treatment and a continuous bruit through the anterior fontanelle. CT shows midline lesion with hypoechogenicity and dilated lateral ventricles. Most probable diagnosis is: Vein of Galen Malformation. *(DNB PATTERN JUNE 2010)*
- Most common cause of seizure in newborn on day 1 is Hypoxia. *(DNB PATTERN DEC 2010)*
- Generalized 3–4 Hz spike and slow wave complexes on EEG are seen in Juvenile Myoclonic Epilepsy. *(DNB PATTERN DEC 2009)*
- Hypsarrhythmia seen in: West syndrome (infantile spasm). *(DNB PATTERN JUNE 2008)*
- NOT a common cause of meningitis under age of 8 years: Staph aureus. *(DNB PATTERN DEC 2010)*
- Commonest cause of Meningitis in postneonatal period is: Streptococcus Pneumoniae. *(DNB PATTERN 2006)*

- Most common form of intracranial hemorrhage in preterm neonate is: Subependymal hemorrhage.
  (DNB PATTERN 2002)
- SSPE is a complication of Measles. *(DNB PATTERN 2002)*
- NOT true about Guillain-Barre syndrome: Autonomic disturbances are rare. *(DNB PATTERN 2002)*
- Treatment of febrile convulsions is based on control of fever. *(DNB PATTERN JUNE 2009)*
- NOT a cause of infantile tremor syndrome—Vitamin B1 deficiency. *(DNB PATTERN JUNE 2009)*
- Most common cause of acquired Aqueductal Stenosis: Mumps. *(DNB PATTERN NOV 2013)*
- In a small child diagnosed with Hemophilus Influenza Meningitis, the investigation to be done before discharging him form the hospital: BERA. *(DNB PATTERN NOV 2013)*
- Drug of choice for Benign Rolandic Epilepsy: Gabapentin. *(NEET PATTERN 2014)*
- NOT useful for diagnosing SSPE: Antibody in Blood. *(NEET PATTERN 2014)*

RESPIRATORY SYSTEM

- What is true about Alpha 1 antitrypsin deficiency? Severe pulmonary disease. *(DNB PATTERN JUNE 2011)*
- True about Alpha 1 antitrypsin deficiency is: deficiency of protease inhibitor, autosomal recessive and may cause cholestatic jaundice. *(DNB PATTERN JUNE 2009)*
- Viral disease which does NOT cause pneumonia? Mumps. *(DNB PATTERN JUNE 2011)*
- A child is said to have nocturnal asthmatic attacks 2 times in a week, day time attack is 3 times or more, can be categorized as Moderate persistent Asthma.
  (DNB PATTERN JUNE 2010)
- Best treatment of Bronchial Asthma: Avoidance of antigen. *(DNB PATTERN 2008)*
- NOT a component of APGAR scoring: Respiratory rate. *(DNB PATTERN DEC 2010)*
- Pathogenetic organism in Bronchiolitis: Respiratory Syncytial virus. *(DNB PATTERN 2003)*
- Gastric Aspirate Shake Test is used for the bedside test for: Respiratory Distress Syndrome. *(NEET PATTERN 2014)*
- Least common opportunistic fungus causing pulmonary infection in children: Sporothrix. *(NEET PATTERN 2014)*
- Most common cause of Croup in children: Parainfluenza. *(NEET PATTERN 2016)*

- Hecht's Pneumonia is typically seen in: Measles.
  (NEET PATTERN 2016)
- Round Pneumonia is typically seen with: Streptococcal Pneumonia. *(NEET PATTERN 2016)*
- Most important cause of under 5 mortality is: Respiratory Infections. *(DNB PATTERN 2005)*
- Hyaline membrane is NOT a feature of Staphylococcus Pneumoniae. *(DNB PATTERN 2002)*
- Treatment of breath holding spells is: Iron.
  (DNB PATTERN NOV 2013)
- Congenital Lobar Emphysema is COMMONEST in Left Upper Lobe. *(JIPMER 2017 PATTERN)*

GIT

- Management of 1-week-old baby with imperfortate anus and meconuria is: Diversion colostomy with sleeve resection followed by pull through. *(DNB PATTERN JUNE 2011)*
- Most common gastrointestinal malignancy of childhood is: Lymphoma. (DNB PATTERN DEC 2009)
- Vomiting on first day of birth is NOT seen in Pyloric Stenosis. *(DNB PATTERN JUNE 2009)*
- Least common site of volvulus in children is: Colon.
  (DNB PATTERN JUNE 2009)
- Gas reaches colonic end in a newborn by 8–10 hrs.
  (DNB PATTERN JUNE 2011)
- Neonate after 12 hrs of birth passes black colored meconium. True is: Normal finding. *(DNB PATTERN 2000)*
- Malena ia NOT a feature of Celiac Disease.
  (DNB PATTERN 2001)
- A 10-month-infant developed a watery diarrhea 2 days after routine visit to pediatrician. Probable diagnosis is: Rotavirus Diarrhea. *(DNB PATTERN 2002)*
- Most common cause of acute infantile gastroenteritis is: Rota virus. *(DNB PATTERN DEC 2011)*
- Rotor's syndrome is NOT a cause of Unconjugated Hyperbilirubinemia. *(DNB PATTERN 2004)*
- Enzyme deficiency after an attack of severe infectious enteritis: Lactase. *(DNB PATTERN 2007)*
- Percentage of dose given as basal insulin in bolus basal regimen in children is: 25–50%.
  (DNB PATTERN NOV 2013)
- Conjugated Bilirubin is increased in: Rotor syndrome.
  (DNB PATTERN NOV 2013)

- Vaccine withdrawn because of increased risk of Intussusception: Japanese Encephalitis (JE). *(NEET PATTERN 2015)*

PEDIATRIC HEMATOLOGY

- Commonest hematological malignancy in children: ALL. *(DNB PATTERN 2001, 2004)*
- Vitamin associated with Hemolytic Anemia in Preterm Babies: Vitamin K. *(DNB PATTERN 2005)*
- Large doses of Vitamin K in a newborn causes Hemolytic Anemia. *(DNB PATTERN JUNE 2011)*
- Treatment of choice in Thalassemia Major: Blood transfusion and Desferrioxamine. *(DNB PATTERN 2007)*
- Non-Immune Hydrops is seen in: Alpha thalassemia major. *(DNB PATTERN DEC 2010)*
- Pawn Ball Megakaryocytes are a feature of Myelodysplastic Syndrome. *(DNB PATTERN 2007)*
- Iron and folic acid supplementation of 6 months to 10-year-old children is 20 mg elemental iron and 100 mg folic acid. *(DNB PATTERN JUNE 2011)*
- According to WHO, cut off level for hemoglobin in child for Anemia is: 11 gm. *(DNB PATTERN JUNE 2012)*
- RBC Lifespan in Preterm babies: 35–50 days. *(JIPMER PATTERN 2017)*

SYNDROMES

- True about Turner's syndrome: Normal intelligence. *(DNB PATTERN JUNE 2009, DEC 2011)*
- McCune-Albright syndrome is characterized by: Cafe au lait macules. *(DNB PATTERN JUNE 2011)*
- Most common cause of death in Klinefelter syndrome is: Infections. *(DNB PATTERN DEC 2011)*
- In Hutchinson's triad in a new born child, what is not seen? Cataracts. *(DNB PATTERN JUNE 2009)*
- Follicular Conjunctivitis is NOT a part of Hutchinson's triad. *(NEET PATTERN 2016)*

> HUTCHINSON'S TRIAD includes Malformed Incisors, Vestibular Deafness and Interstitial Keratitis ... in Congenital Syphilis.
>
> HUTCHINSON'S PUPIL–in raised ICT
>
> HUTCHINSON'S TEETH–Peg-shaped Upper Central Incisors
>
> HUTCHINSON'S RULE/SIGN–Herpes Zoster Ophthalmicus.

- Down's syndrome is Trisomy 21. *(DNB PATTERN 2008)*
- Precocious puberty is seen in McCune-Albright syndrome. *(DNB PATTERN 2000)*
- Most common cardiac anomaly in Turner's syndrome: Bicuspid Aortic Valve. *(DNB PATTERN NOV 2013)*
- Karyotype in Testicular Feminising syndrome is: 46XY. *(DNB PATTERN NOV 2013)*
- NOT true about Fragile X syndrome: Pigmented nevi. *(DNB PATTERN NOV 2013)*
- Sandifer syndrome due to GERD is confused with: Seizures. *(DNB PATTERN NOV 2013)*
- Polyarticular JIA involves more than how many joints? 4 *(NEET PATTERN 2014)*
- Single most common defect in Congenital Rubella Syndrome is: Deafness. *(NEET PATTERN 2014)*
- Congenital Rubella Syndrome Classical Triad DOES NOT include MENTAL RETARDATION. *(NEET PATTERN 2015)*
- GOLDENHAR SYNDROME is associated with the abnormal development of: 1st and 2nd branchial arches. *(NEET PATTERN 2015)*
- Osteogenesis Imperfecta with normal dentition and sclera is: OI Type IA. *(JIPMER PATTERN 2017)*
- NOT a feature of DiGeorge's Syndrome: Impaired B cell immunity. *(JIPMER PATTERN 2017)*
- Impaired T cell immunity is seen in DiGeorge's Syndrome. *(JIPMER PATTERN 2017)*
- NOT seen in Foetal Alcohol Syndrome: Macrocephaly. *(JIPMER PATTERN 2017)*

MISCELLANEOUS

- NOT a common feature of Duchenne Muscular Dystrophy is: Distal muscle involvement. *(DNB PATTERN JUNE 2011)*
- NOT a feature of Myotonic dystrophy: Proximal muscle weakness. *(DNB PATTERN JUNE 2010)*
- A 5-year-old child presents with enlarged liver, uncontrolled hypoglycemia and ketosis. Most probable diagnosis is: Glycogen storage diseases. *(DNB PATTERN JUNE 2011)*
- A female child presents with hypertension, hyperpigmentation and virilization, she is most likely to be suffering from deficiency of 11-beta-hydroxylase deficiency. *(DNB PATTERN JUNE 2011)*

- As per immunization schedule, Hepatitis A vaccine is recommended at 2 yrs. *(DNB PATTERN DEC 2010)*
- Most common cause of Acute epiglottitis in children is: Haemophilus influenzae type B. *(DNB PATTERN DEC 2010)*
- Most common cause of congenital adrenal hyperplasia is deficiency of: 21 alpha hydroxylase. *(DNB PATTERN DEC 2010)*
- NOT true about Kernicterus: not associated with increased morbidity. *(DNB PATTERN DEC 2010)*
- A 3-yr-old presents with recurrent stridor, what is the most probable Diagnosis? Laryngotracheobronchitis. *(DNB PATTERN DEC 2009)*
- BCG is a live attenuated bacterial vaccine. *(DNB PATTERN JUNE 2009)*
- Hirsutism is NOT seen in Testicular feminization. *(DNB PATTERN JUNE 2010)*
- Most common thyroid tumor in children is: Papillary carcinoma. *(DNB PATTERN DEC 2011)*
- Hydrocephalus is NOT a feature of Congenital Rubella. *(DNB PATTERN DEC 2011)*
- Most common childhood malignancy: ALL. *(DNB PATTERN AUG 2013)*
- Congenital Toxoplasmosis is detected by: IgM. *(DNB PATTERN AUG 2013)*
- In Henoch-Schonlein Purpura, renal involvement is NOT seen generally if no involvement till–1 month after onset. *(DNB PATTERN NOV 2013)*
- Most common cause of death in Rett syndrome: Uncontrolled Seizures. *(Ref: Rett Syndrome Association Website.)* *(NEET PATTERN 2013)*
- A 7-year-girl from Bihar presented with 3 episodes of massive hematemesis and malena. No history of Jaundice.
- On examination, large spleen with non-palpable liver and mild ascites.
- Portal vein not seen on USG.
- LFT is normal and endoscopy shows esophageal varices. What is the diagnosis?
- Extrahepatic Portal vein obstruction. *(FMGE PATTERN JUNE 2014)*
- In Visceral Leishmaniasis, yield is highest from: Spleen. *(NEET PATTERN 2015)*
- Maximum Score in the New Ballard Score is: 50. *(NEET PATTERN 2016)*
- As per the LUND-BROWDER chart, the body surface area for which region does not change with age? Arm. *(NEET PATTERN 2016)*

- Seen in Tourette's syndrome :
  - Echolalia
  - Coprolalia
  - Symptoms unmasked by Methyl Phenidate.

  (JIPMER PATTERN 2017)

  Ans: All are correct.

- Most common cause of Neonatal Blindness: Neisseria gonorrhoea. *(NEET PATTERN 2018)*
- Lorenzo's Oil is used as a treatment for: Adrenoleukodystrophy. *(JIPMER PATTERN 2017)*
- Vaccine not included in Indradhanush Mission: Japanese Encephalitis. *(NEET PATTERN 2018)*
- Identify the congenital malformation in the image given below: *(NEET PATTERN 2018)*

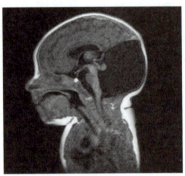

Ans: Dandy Walker Syndrome.

MORE FAQ ON CONGENITAL ANOMALIES....

Complete or partial absence of brain sulcation	Lissencephaly
Parallel Non-converging Cerebral Ventricles and Dilated occipital horns in CT is diagnostic of:	Corpus Callosal Agenesis
Chiari Type I malformation	Herniation of Peg-like cerebellar tonsils through foramen magnum
Chiari II	Caudal displacement of the brainstem and inferior part of the cerebellum into upper cervical spinal canal. Also Lumbar Meningomyelocele.
Chiari III	Chiari II features + a low occipital or high cervical encephalocoele
Chiari IV	Severe Cerebellar Hypoplasia or Absent Cerebellum

Cond...

Cond...

Dandy-Walker Malformation	Absence or hypoplasia of the Cerebellar vermis + associated hypoplasia of the cerebellar hemispheres (WINGED APPEARANCE of the cerebellar hemispheres) + Enlarged Fourth ventricle + Posterior Fossa cysts
VACTERL Syndrome	Vertebral and Vascular Abnormalities (Right-sided Aortic Arch) Anal AND Auricular Malformations Cardiac abnormalities like VSD Tracheoesophageal Fistula (TE) Renal Abnormalities Limb Malformations
Congenital Hypertrophic Pyloric Stenosis (CHPS)	Bull's Eye Lesion Doughnut Appearance—Ultrasonological Features which indicate CHPS Lack of NO synthase Olive shaped mass on palpation Hypertrophy of Pyloric circular muscle

LEVEL II: HIGH YIELD FACTORS

Table 15.1: Breast milk

Bifidus factor	Promotes growth of lactobacillus
Bile salt stimulated lipase (BSSL)	Is cidal toward Amoeba and Giardia
PABA	Protects against Malaria
Lactoferrin	Inhibits E. coli
Preterm Milk	High fat/High protein/High sodium/Low carbs
Fore Milk	Rich in proteins
Hind Milk	Rich in fat
Transitional Milk	Milk secreted during 3 days to 2 weeks
Mature Milk	Follows Transitional Milk
Human Milk lacks Vitamins	D and K
Amino acid absent in Breast Milk	Glycine
Exclusive Breastfed babies are prone to	Iron deficiency Anemia/Scurvy/Hemorrhagic Disease of Newborn

Table 15.2: Syndromes

Lutembacher's syndrome	Ostium secondum ASD + MS
Laurence-Moon-Biedl syndrome	Retinitis Pigmentosa/Obesity/Mental Retardation/Polydactyly
Pierre Robin syndrome	Mandibular Hypoplasia + Cleft Palate + Glossoptosis
Lowe's syndrome	Hypophosphatemic Rickets + Amino Aciduria

Cond...

Cond...

Alport's syndrome	Hematuria + Sensorineural deafness + Ocular Anomaly
Vogt-Koyanagi-Harada syndrome	Face/Scalp Hypopigmentation + Bilateral Anterior Uveitis
Osler-Weber-Rendu syndrome	Hereditary Hemorrhagic Telangiectasia + AV malformation

Table 15.3: Congenital heart disease

Pink Fallot	VSD + Mild PS
Fallot's Triology	ASD + RVH + PS
Fallot's Tetrology	Perimembranous VSD + RVH + Infundibular PS + Overriding of Aorta
Fallot's Pentology	Fallot's tetralogy + ASD
Machinery murmur	PDA
Differential Cyanosis	PDA
Blalock-Taussig shunt	In TOF between SCA and Pulmonary Artery
Waterson's shunt	In TOF between Ascending Aorta and Right Pulmonary Artery
Pott's shunt	In TOF between Descending Aorta and Left Pulmonary Artery
Most common defect in ASD	Ostium secondum defect
Most commonly associated with Down's syndrome	Ostium primum ASD

Table 15.4: Respiratory system

Monospot test	Infectious Mononucleosis
Cyanotic spells commonly occur between	6 months and 5 yrs
Treatment of Cyanotic spells	No specific treatment required
Recommended drug for Acute Respiratory Illness in ARI program	Cotrimoxazole
Atypical lymphocytes in IMN should be	10%

Table 15.5: CNS

Scarf Sign	Floppy Infant
Most common type of JRA in boys	Pauciarticular type 2
Most common type of JRA	Pauciarticular type 1
Gower's sign	Duchenne Muscular Dystrophy

Cond...

Cond...

In Acute Flaccid Paralysis	Two stool samples should be collected 24 to 48 hrs apart within 14 days of onset of paralysis for virus isolation
Mitochondrial Myopathies	Kearns-Sayre syndrome/ Leber's Hereditary Optic Neuropathy/ MELAS/MERRF
Definitive diagnosis of Duchenne Muscular Dystrophy	Muscle Biopsy

Table 15.6: Teratogenicity

Accutane Embryopathy	Isotretinoin
Fractured Chromosomes	LSD
Minamata Disease	Mercury
Gray Baby syndrome	Chloramphenicol
Pyloric Stenosis	Erythromycin
Hypoplasia of Nasal bones	Warfarin
Neural Tube defects	Valproate
Clear cell Adenocarcinoma vagina	Diethylstilbesterol

MALNUTRITION

Country with Highest burden of Childhood Under nutrition in the world: India

National Family Health Survey (NFHS) 3 conducted in 2005-2006.

According to NFHS 3, the percentage of childhood Under nutrition in India: 40%

Maximum level of underweight children in India: Chhattisgarh, Bihar, Jharkhand and Madhya Pradesh.

Minimum level of underweight children in India: Punjab, Kerala, Jammu and Kashmir and Tamil Nadu.

WELCOME CLASSIFICATION

Based on Weight For Age and Presence/Absence of Oedema

60–80% weight for age	Underweight
60–80% with oedema	Kwashiorkor
<60%	Marasmus
<60% with oedema	Marasmic Kwashiorkor.

GOMEZ CLASSIFICATION

Based on Weight For Age

>90%	Normal
76–90%	Mild (1st degree) Malnutrition
61–75%	Moderate (2nd degree) Malnutrition
<60%	Severe (3rd degree) Malnutrution

MCLAREN CLASSIFICATION

Based on Weight for Height at a particular age.

>110%	Obesity
90–110%	Normal
85–90%	Underweight (Mild PEM)
75–85%	Moderate PEM
<75%	Severe PEM

WATERLOW CLASSIFICATION

Based on degree of WASTING (Weight for Height) and Stunting (Height for Age)

Stunting	Wasting	Degree of Pem
87.5–95%	80–90%	Mild/Grade 1
80–87.5%	70–80%	Moderate/Grade 2
<80%	<70%	Severe/Grade 3

IAP CLASSIFICATION

Based on Weight for Age of the standard

>80%	Normal
71–80%	Grade 1 (Mild Malnutrition)
61–70%	Grade II (Moderate Malnutrition)
51–60%	Grade III (Severe Malnutrition)
<50%	Grade IV (Very Severe Malnutrition)

WHO CLASSIFICATION

Based on Weight for Height/Height for Age/presence of Edema

WHO recommends the use of Z scores or Standard Deviation Scores (SDS)

SD Score = Observed Value – Median Reference Value/ Standard Deviation of Reference Population

SD Score	
– 2 to – 3	Moderate Malnutrition
Less than – 3	Severe Malnutrition
+2 to +3	Overweight
More than +3	Obesity
Edema present	Edematous Malnutrition

16 Dermatology

"Start where you are. Use what you have. Do what you can."
—*Arthur Ashe*

REFERENCES
- *Harrison's Principles of Internal Medicine, 19th ed.*
- *Indian Journal of Dermatology Venereology and Leprology.*

LEVEL I: BASIC REPEATS

PSORIASIS

- Not a premalignant condition of skin: Psoriasis.
  (DNB PATTERN JUNE 2012)
- Pseudoismorphic phenomenon is seen in Warts.
  (DNB PATTERN JUNE 2010)
- Koebner's phenomenon is seen in Lichen planus/Psoriasis/Molluscum Contagiosum. *(DNB PATTERN JUNE 2009)*
- Also in Kaposi Sarcoma, Warts, Vitiligo, DLE.
- Most common site affected by psoriasis is: Extensor surface.
  (DNB PATTERN DEC 2009)
- Nikolsky's test is NOT positive in: Psoriasis.
  (DNB PATTERN 2000)
- This is treated with PUVA therapy: Psoriasis.
  (DNB PATTERN 2003)
- Berkeley Membrane is seen in: Psoriasis.
  (DNB PATTERN 2003)
- Koebner's phenomenon is seen in: Psoriasis.
  (DNB PATTERN 2003)
- Bleeding spots are seen in removal of plaques with Psoriasis.
  (DNB PATTERN JUNE 2009)
- True regarding Munro Microabscesses is: Debris consists of Neutrophils. Pautrier's Microabscesses contain Malignant Lymphocytes. They are seen in Mycosis Fungoides and Sezary syndrome. *(DNB PATTERN JUNE 2009)*
- Photochemotherapy is useful in: Psoriasis.
  (DNB PATTERN 2000)
- Koebner's phenomenon is associated with: Psoriasis.
  (DNB PATTERN AUG 2013)

- Nail lesion in Psoriasis is due to lesion in: Proximal Nail Matrix. *(DNB PATTERN AUG 2013)*
- Tiny bleeding spots after removal of deep scales in Plaque Psoriasis is: Auspitz Sign. *(NEET PATTERN 2016)*
- Von Zombusch Disease is a type of Acute Generalised Pustular Psoriasis. It is the most severe form of Psoriasis. *(NEET PATTERN 2015)*

FAQ PSORIASIS

- Auspitz Sign
- Koebner's Phenomenon
- Grattage Test
- Candle Grease Sign
- Oil Drop Sign
- Burkeley's membrane
- Woronoff Ring
- Munro Micro abscesses
- Silvery Scales
- Onycholysis
- Proximal Nail Matrix Lesion
- Nail Pitting

- **KOEBNER PHENOMENON** *(Ref: Thappa DM*
The isomorphic phenomenon of Koebner. Indian J Dermatol Venereol Leprol 2004;70:187-9)

True Isomorphic phenomenon	Psoriasis, Lichen Planus and Vitiligo
Pseudoisomorphic phenomenon	Koebner's phenomenon seen in infectious diseases Warts Molluscum contagiosum Behcet's disease Pyoderma gangrenosum
Occasionally occurring Isomorphic phenomenon	Hailey Hailey Disease Darier's disease Kaposi's sarcoma Erythema multiforme
Reverse Koebner response	Area of psoriasis clears following injury - This is called Reverse Koebner's response. Also in Vitiligo – spontaneous repigmentation of vitiligo patches distant from the autologous skin graft sites. **('Remote Reverse Koebner Response')**

LICHEN PLANUS

- Koebner's phenomenon is seen in Lichen planus/Psoriasis/ Molluscum Contagiosum. *(DNB PATTERN JUNE 2009)*

BULLOUS DISEASES

- Dapsone used in the treatment and therapeutic diagnosis of Dermatitis Herpetiformis. *(DNB PATTERN DEC 2010)*
- Not true about Dermatitis Herpetiformis—Lesions have epidermal bullae. *(DNB PATTERN DEC 2010)*
- Which of the following is a subepidermal blistering disorder? Bullous pemphigoid. *(DNB PATTERN JUNE 2009)*
- A person presents with haemorrhagic fluid in tense blister at dermoepidermal junction. Most probable diagnosis is Pemphigoid. *(DNB PATTERN DEC 2009)*
- Epidermal bullae are seen in Pemphigus vulgaris. *(DNB PATTERN DEC 2009)*
- Tzanck test is positive in the Pemphigus foliaceus and Pemphigus vegetans. Also in Pemphigus Vulgaris and Pemphigus Erythematosus. *(DNB PATTERN 2000, 2001)*
- Bulla spread sign is seen in: Pemphigus vulgaris. *(DNB PATTERN 2000)*
- Drug effective in Dermatitis Herpetiformis is: Dapsone. *(DNB PATTERN 2002)*
- Most common type of Pemphigus in India: Pemphigus vulgaris. *(FMGE PATTERN 2008)*
- Histological feature of Pemphigus: Acantholysis. *(FMGE PATTERN 2010)*
- Flaccid bullae with mucosal involvement and intraepidermal acantholysis are typical of: Pemphigus Vulgaris. *(NEET PATTERN 2016)*

TUBEROUS SCLEROSIS

- Earliest feature of Tuberous Sclerosis is Ash leaf spot. *(DNB PATTERN DEC 2011, JUNE 2009)*
- Skin lesions in Tuberous Sclerosis does NOT include: Acanthosis nigricans. *(DNB PATTERN 2007)*

LEPROSY AND LEPRA REACTIONS

- Most infective stage of Leprosy is: Lepromatous. *(DNB PATTERN JUNE 2009)*
- Young boy, single hypoanaesthetic patch over hand and thickened ulnar nerve, diagnosis is: Tuberculoid Leprosy. *(DNB PATTERN 2002)*
- A 7-year-old child from Bihar is having hypopigmented anaesthetic patch on his face. What is the most probable diagnosis? Indeterminate leprosy. *(DNB PATTERN DEC 2009)*

- Which of the following is NOT used in Lepra reaction? Rifampicin. *(DNB PATTERN DEC 2011)*
- Type 2 Lepra reaction is found in: Lepromatous Leprosy. *(DNB PATTERN 2001)*
- Drug used in Lepra reaction is: Thalidomide/Clofazimine/Chloroquine *(DNB PATTERN 2002)*
- All can be used.
- Lepromin Test is strongly positive in: Tuberculoid Leprosy (TT). *(FMGE PATTERN MAR 2013)*

ACNE VULGARIS

- Oral retinoid is used in the treatment of Acne vulgaris. *(DNB PATTERN 2000, 2001)*
- Acid that is increased in acne comedones is Palmitic Acid. *(DNB PATTERN JUNE 2011)*
- Linoleic Acid is decreased and Palmitic Acid is increased in Acne Vulgaris.

ACRODERMATITIS ENTEROPATHICA

- True about Acrodermatitis Enteropathica is Lifelong treatment required. *(DNB PATTERN JUNE 2011)*
- Dose of Zinc used in Acrodermatitis enteropathica is 2 mg/kg. 1-3 mg/kg/day is the range of Zinc dosage in Acrodermatitis Enteropathica. *(DNB PATTERN JUNE 2009)*

PITYRIASIS VERSICOLOR AND PITYRIASIS ROSEA

- Pityriasis versicolor is caused by Malassezia furfur. *(DNB PATTERN 2000, JUNE 2011)*
- Selenium sulphide is indicated in: Tinea Versicolor. *(DNB PATTERN 2007)*
- Lesions of Pityriasis Rosea are distributed mostly on the: Trunk. *(DNB PATTERN 2003)*
- Hanging curtains sign is seen in Pityriais rosea. *(DNB PATTERN JUNE 2010)*
- Hanging curtains/Falling curtains Sign: Pityriasis Rosea. *(DNB PATTERN AUG 2013, NEET PATTERN 2016)*
- Christmas Tree Arrangement of skin lesions is seen in: Pityriasis Rosea. *(DNB PATTERN NOV 2013)*
- Other named descriptions frequently asked in Pityriasis Rosea:

  ➤ Herald Patch
  ➤ Herald Plaque

- Inverted Fir Tree Arrangement of lesions on trunk
- Cigarette Paper scales
- Cigarette Paper Scars : in Tertiary Syphilis.
- Mother Patch

MISCELLANEOUS

- Palpable purpura is caused by all except Giant cell arteritis. *(DNB PATTERN DEC 2011)*
- Vit D is synthesised by Keratinocytes. *(DNB PATTERN DEC 2011)*
- NOT true about Solar urticaria: Common in females between 20-40. *(DNB PATTERN JUNE 2011)*
- Most common site of Necrobiosis Lipoidica Diabeticorum: Front of leg. *(DNB PATTERN JUNE 2011)*
- Parakeratosis is defined as retained nuclei in stratum corneum cells. *(DNB PATTERN JUNE 2011)*
- Rapid, diffuse, excessive hair loss after three months of pregnancy is due to Telogen effluvium. *(DNB PATTERN JUNE 2011)*
- Fox Fordyce disease is a disorder of Apocrine glands. *(DNB PATTERN JUNE 2011)*
- Follicular hyperkeratosis is due to the deficiency of Vitamin A. *(DNB PATTERN DEC 2010)*
- Groton's sign is seen in Dermatomyositis. *(DNB PATTERN JUNE 2011)*
- Chancroid is caused by Haemophilus ducreyi. *(DNB PATTERN DEC 2010)*
- Heliotrope rash is seen in Dermatomyositis. *(DNB PATTERN JUNE 2010)*
- Dermatomyositis
  - Holster's Sign
  - Shawl Sign
  - Mechanic Hand Lesion
- Which of the following causes allergic contact dermatitis through air? Parthenium. *(DNB PATTERN JUNE 2010)*
- Urticaria pigmentosa is a feature of Mast cells. *(DNB PATTERN JUNE 2009)*
- Tumor not caused by PUVA is Cutaneous T cell lymphoma. *(DNB PATTERN JUNE 2009)*
- Echtyma gangrenosum is caused by Pseudomonas aeruginosa. *(DNB PATTERN DEC 2009)*
- Pathergy test is positive in Behcet's disease. *(DNB PATTERN DEC 2009)*

- A 5-year old boy presents with itchy excoriated papules and elevated IgE levels. Most probable diagnosis is: Atopic Dermatitis. *(DNB PATTERN DEC 2009)*
- Commonest cutaneous eruption in SLE: Erythema of light exposed area. *(DNB PATTERN 2000, 2001)*
- Commonest venereal disease in India: Gonorrhoea. *(DNB PATTERN 2000)*
- Drug which produce fixed drug eruptions: Phenolphthalein/Aspirin/Dapsone/Furosemide. *(DNB PATTERN 2001)*
- Onycholysis is NOT seen in Nephrotic Syndrome. *(DNB PATTERN 2002)*
- Hemophilus Ducreyi causes: Soft chancre. *(DNB PATTERN 2002)*
- Increased level of Ig E is seen in: Atopy. *(DNB PATTERN 2003)*
- Mycosis Fungoides is a: T cell lymphoma. *(DNB PATTERN 2003)*
- Photosensitive rash is common in: Erythropoeitic Protoporphyria. *(DNB PATTERN 2003)*
- Frei's test is diagnostic of: Lymphogranuloma venereum. *(DNB PATTERN 2006, 2007)*
- Leukonychia is known as Gift Spots. *(DNB PATTERN 2007)*
- Commonest site of Atopic Dermatitis: Anti cubital fossa. *(DNB PATTERN 2007)*
- Definitive diagnosis of Sporotrichosis—generally depends on Culture. *(DNB PATTERN 2007)*
- Young female complains of genital wart. Agent implicated is: Human Papilloma virus. *(DNB PATTERN 2001, 2007)*
- Acanthosis nigricans is due to carcinoma of: Colon. *(DNB PATTERN 2007)*
- Pitting of nails can be seen in: Alopecia Areata. *(DNB PATTERN 2007)*
- Furuncle is caused by: Staphylococcus. *(DNB PATTERN 2008)*
- Causative agent of scabies is: Mite. (Sarcoptes Scabei). *(DNB PATTERN 2008)*
- Hepar Lobatum is seen in: Congenital Syphilis. *(FMGE PATTERN MAR 2013)*

> - Buttonhole Sign: Neurofibromatosis Type 1.
> - Barnett's Sign: Scleroderma
> - Nikolsky's Sign: Acantholysis.

- Buschke Ollendorf Sign is seen in: Secondary Syphilis. *(DNB PATTERN NOV 2013)*

- Bullous Impetigo is caused by: Staphylococcus Aureus. *(FMGE PATTERN MAR 2013)*
- Dennie Morgan Fold is characteristic of: Atopic Dermatitis. *(FMGE PATTERN MAR 2013)*
- Chronic paronychia is of: Fungal etiology. *(FMGE PATTERN MAR 2013)*
- Mineral causing skin Allergy: Nickel. Nickel Cobalt can cause skin allergy.
- Antibiotics with risk of Contact Dermatitis: Neomycin, Bacitracin. *(FMGE PATTERN MAR 2013)*
- Target lesions are associated with: Erythema Multiforme. *(DNB PATTERN AUG 2013)*
- Extra layer of skin present in the epidermis of palms and soles: Stratum Lucidum. Stratum Lucidum contains Transitional Cells. *(NEET PATTERN 2016)*
- Bromhidrosis affects Sebaceous glands. *(NEET PATTERN 2016)*
- Contact dermatitis known as Scourge of India is caused by: Parthenium. *(NEET PATTERN 2016)*
- Mucocutaneous Pemphigus Vulgaris is characterised by antibodies against: Desmoglein 1 and Desmoglein 3. *(NEET PATTERN 2016)*
- Carpet Tack Sign is seen in: DLE. *(NEET PATTERN 2016)*
- Asboe Hansen Sign is used to demonstrate: Acantholysis. *(NEET PATTERN 2016)*
- Dew Drop on rose petal lesions are typical of: Chicken Pox *(NEET PATTERN 2015)*
- Coral Red fluorescence on Wood's lamp in Erythasma results from: Coproporphyrin 111. *(NEET PATTERN 2015)*
- ANTENNA sign is seen in: KERATOSIS PILARIS. *(NEET PATTERN 2016)*
- Shingles is caused by: Herpes Zoster. *(NEET PATTERN 2018)*
- Sulfur Granules occur in infections caused by: Actinomyces israelii. *(NEET PATTERN 2018)*
- Identify the following lesion. *(NEET PG 2018)*

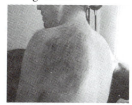

Ans: Becker Nevus.

- Cutis Marmorata occurs due to exposure to: Cold Temperature. *(NEET PATTERN 2018)*

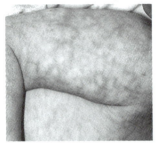

- A child has a rash like seen in the picture. His family history is positive for Asthma. What is the possible diagnosis? *(NEET PATTERN 2018)*

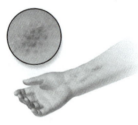

Ans: Allergic Contact Dermatitis.

ERYTHEMA MULTIFORME

- Target Lesions
- Iris Lesions
- Bull's Eye Lesions

- Vagabond's disease: Pediculosis Corporis. *(DNB PATTERN AUG 2013)*
- Salt and Pepper skin is seen in: Scleroderma. *(DNB PATTERN NOV 2013)*
- Asboe Hansen Sign is negative in: Staphylococcal Skin Scalded Syndrome. *(DNB PATTERN NOV 2013)*
- Asboe Hansen sign is positive in: Pemphigus vulgaris Nikolsky's sign is positive in SSSS/TEN also!!
- Hanifin Rajka criteria is used in: Atopic Eczema. *(NEET PATTERN 2013)*
- Hunan Hand is seen in: Contact Dermatitis associated with Capsaicin. (Chili Burn). *(NEET PATTERN 2013)*
- Tapir Nose is seen in: Rhinoscleroma. *(DNB PATTERN AUG 2013)*
  - Also called Hebra Nose/Hippopotamus Nose.

- Herpes Gladiatorum, common in wrestlers is caused by: HSV 1. *(DNB PATTERN AUG 2013)*
- Koenen tumor is seen in: Tuberous Sclerosis. *(DNB PATTERN JUNE 2014)*
- Spindle cells are seen in which tumor–Synovial Sarcoma. *(DNB PATTERN JUNE 2014)*

LEVEL II: HIGH YIELD FACTORS

Table 16.1: Psoriasis

Sausage Digits/**Arthritis Mutilans**: Psoriatic Arthritis Psoriasis of intertriginous areas is called **Inverse Psoriasis** Lithium/Beta blockers/antimalarial medications can **exacerbate**

Psoriasis

Pustules of Kogoj

Salmon coloured plaque covered by silvery scale

Loss of **stratum granulosum**

Auspitz sign

Munro Microabscesses

Topical Vit D analogue used in Psoriasis: **Calcipotriene**

Drug of choice for **Psoriatic Arthropathy. Oral Methotrexate**

Drug of choice for **Psoriatic Erythroderma** and **Pustular Psoriasis**: **Oral Retinoid**

Grattage test is done for Psoriasis

Thimble pitting of nail plate is seen in Psoriasis

Test tubes in a Rack appearance

Table 16.2: Lichen planus

Wickham Striae

Saw toothing of rete ridges

Civatte Bodies or Colloid Bodies—necrotic basal cells in Lichen Planus

Interface dermatitis

"Pruritic, purple, polygonal, planar papules, and plaques"

Table 16.3: Bullous diseases

Subcorneal blistering	Pemphigus foliaceus
Suprabasal blistering	Pemphigus vulgaris
Subepidermal blistering	Bullous pemphigoid and Dermatitis Herpetiformis
Most common histologic denominator in all forms of Pemphigus	Acantholysis

Contd...

Contd...

Table 16.3: Bullous diseases

FISH NET Appearance: Pemphigus Vulgaris. Dermatitis Herpetiformis: Associated with Gluten Sensitivity	Pemphigus Vulgaris associated with Gluten sensitivity
IgA deposition Nikolsky's sign (Manual pressure leading to epidermal separation)	Dermatitis Herpetiformis classically seen in Pemphigus
Nikolsky's sign	NOT specific and is also seen in Toxic epidermal Necrolysis/ Steven Johnson syndrome
Pemphigus is associated with	Thymoma/Myasthenia gravis

Table 16.4: Mycosis fungoides

Histological characteristic feature is: Sezary Lutzner cells

CD4 positivity

Pautrier Microabscesses characteristic

Epidermotropism

Indolent T cell lymphoma

Total skin electron beam radiation is the treatment for Mycosis Fungoides in the early stage

Table 16.5: Sexually transmitted diseases

Chancre Redux	Early Syphilis
School of fish and Rail Road appearance	Chancroid
Pseudoelephantiasis of labia	Calymmatobacterium granulomatosis
Rhagades	Congenital Syphilis
Higaumenakis sign	Congenital Syphilis
Hutchinson's teeth/Saddle nose/ Sabre Tibia/Mulberry Molars	Congenital Syphilis
Condyloma lata	In secondary syphilis
Diagnosis of Syphilis	Dark Field Microscopy
Esthiomene or elephentiasis of vulva	Lymphogranuloma venereum
Most common venereal disease in India	Gonorrhoea
Testis is spared and epididimis is involved in	Gonorrhoea
Pseudobubo	Donovanosis
Painless indurated ulcers	Syphilis
Soft tender ulcers	Chancroid

Contd...

Contd...

Table 16.5: Sexually transmitted diseases	
Groove's sign	Lymphogranuloma venereum
Lymphadenopathy is NOT seen in	Donovanosis

FAQ - NAIL CHANGES

Leukonychia	Tuberculosis/Hodgkin's/Leprosy
Koilonychia	Iron deficiency Anemia, Plummer Vinson Syndrome.
Pterygium of Nail[Q]	Lichen planus
Middle nail matrix involvement[Q] Distal Nail matrix involvement[Q] Terry's Nail	Lichen planus Characteristically seen in Cirrhosis of Liver. Also in DM/ Rheumatoid Arthritis.
Shoreline Nails	Severe Drug reactions – Type 2 Lepra Reaction
Nail Patella Syndrome (Fong Disease)[Q]	Hypoplasia of Patella and nails with cataract/heterochromia of iris.
Yellow Nail Syndrome	Chronic Ankle Oedema/Hypoalbuminemia
Half Half Nails	Chronic Renal Failure
Shell Nail Syndrome	Bronchiectasis
Mees lines[Q]	Arsenic poisoning/Dissecting aneurysm/Chronic renal failure
Muehrcke's Lines[Q]	Chronic Hypoalbuminemia
Beau's Lines[Q]	Mitotic Arrest – Child Birth, Measles
Koenen's periungual fibroma[Q]	Tuberous Sclerosis
Oil Drop Sign[Q] Subungual hyperkeratosis Onycholysis	Sclerosis Psoriasis Oil Drop Sign: Psoriasis Subungual Hyperkeratoses: Psoriasis Onycholysis: Psoriasis
Proximal nail matrix involvement[Q]	Psoriasis
Azure Lunulae[Q]	Bluish colouration in proximal lunular portion of nail in Wilson's Disease.
Spotted Lunulae	Alopecia Areata
Onychophagia	Nail Biting
Onychotillomania	Compulsive nail picking
Hapalonychia	Thinning and softening of nails in Malnutrition, Myxedema, Leprosy, Raynaud's
Melanonychia	Blackish discolouration of nail plate due to nevocellular nevus in nail matrix

Contd...

Contd...

Hippocratic Nails	Clubbing
Triangular nicking of the free edge of the Nail plate	Darier's disease
Sausage shaped dilated capillary loops on nail folds	Dermatomyositis
Unguis incarnatum	Ingrowing nails

SCABIES

Rate of burrowing in scabies	2 mm/day
No of scabies eggs laid daily	2-3
Average number of mites found on the body of a person suffering from Scabies is	10-15
Predominant symptom of Scabies	Pruritus, worse at night
Characteristic lesion of Scabies	Burrow
Length of scabies burrow	<1 cm long
Shape of Scabies Burrow like channels	S shaped/tortuous/zig zag thread
Incubation period of Scabies	1 month
Face and neck are characteristically spared in	Scabies in ADULTS
Imaginary circle connecting main sites of scabies infestation	Circle of HEBRA
Scabies is an example of Scybala	Water related Dis
Primary syphilitic chancre developing on the scabetic lesion on the external genitals particularly penis	Scabies Galeusus
Scabies in patients who are on topical or systemic corticosteroids	Scabies Incognito
Intensely pruritic reddish brown nodular lesions on axillae, scrotum, chest, groin, penile skin	Nodular Scabies
Woods light examination in Scabies	Grey white in distinctive linear configuration

ATOPIC DERMATITIS

Pallor of skin of face and periorbital pallor	Head Light Sign
Thinning of lateral eyebrows in Atopic Dermatitis	Hertoghe's Sign
Linear transverse fold just below the lower eyelids	Dennie Morgan Fold

Contd...

Ophthalmologic association of Atopy	Posterior Capsular Opacity/ Keratoconus
Blanching of skin at the site of stroking with blunt object	White dermographism

BULLOUS DISEASES

Familial Benign Chronic Pemphigus is known as:	Hailey Hailey Disease
Row of Tombstones appearance of basal cells of the epidermis	Pemphigus vulgaris
On lateral pressure with finger tip, on normal skin surrounding a blister, epidermal separation occurs	Nikolsky Sign
Nikolsky's sign is also present in:	Toxic Epidermal Necrolysis/ Steven Johnson Syndrome.
Pressure on blister causes peripheral extension of the bulla due to passage of fluid between loosely adherent cells of epidermis	Asboe Hansen sign
Characteristic histological feature of Pemphigus vulgaris	Intraepidermal clefts that result from Acantholysis.
Most common histological denominator in all types of Pemphigus	Acantholysis
Subcorneal Blistering	Pemphigus foliaceus
Suprabasal Blistering	Pemphigus vulgaris
FISH NET appearance on Immunofluorescence studies	Pemphigus vulgaris
Drugs causing Pemphigus vulgaris	Rifampicin/Pencillamine/ Penicillin/Captopril
Endemic form of Pemphigus foliaceus in Brasil	Fogo Selvagem
Pemphigus which has both the clinical features of Lupus Erythematosus and Pemphigus	Pemphigus erythematosus (Senear Usher syndrome)
Worst prognosis Pemphigus	Pemphigus vulgaris
Acantholysis is ABSENT in	Bullous Pemphigoid
Age group of Bullous Pemphigoid	Elderly
Anti Basement membrane antibodies are seen in	Bullous Pemphigoid
Drugs causing Bullous Pemphigoid	Furosemide/Phenacetin
Bullous Pemphigoid may be associated with:	Myasthenia Gravis, Thymoma, Ulcerative colitis, Rheumatoid Arthritis

Contd...

Contd...

Dermatitis Herpetiformis is also known as	Duhring's disease
Anti endomysial IgA antibodies are seen in	Dermatitis Herpetiformis
Characteristic feature of Dermatitis Herpetiformis	Papillary tip neutrophilic abscess
Drug of choice of Dermatitis Herpetiformis	Dapsone
Dermatitis Herpetiformis patients should strictly avoid:	Gluten
Gluten is present in:	Wheat, Barley, Oats and Triticale
Gluten consists of proteins :	Gliadin and Glutenin
Bullous disease which develops in second trimester of pregnancy	Pemphigoid gestationis or Herpes gestationis (old name)
Pemphigoid gestationis remits by:	Spontaneous remission 3 months after delivery
Treatment of choice for all types of Pemphigus including Herpes gestationis	Steroids.

WOOD'S LAMP

Wood's Lamp produces:	Long wave ultraviolet light
Wavelength of Wood's Lamp light	365 nm.
Mechanism of Wood's Lamp	Filtering an ultraviolet light source with Barium Silicate Glass containing Nickel Oxide.
Coral Red fluorescence	Erythrasma – Corynebacterium minuttismum
Pink	Porphyria
Greenish yellow	Pseudomonas infection
Golden yellow	Tinea versicolor
Yellow green	Tinea capitis
Yellow	Tetracycline induced discolouration

IMPORTANT PSEUDO SIGNS IN DERMATOLOGY

Pseudo Koebner's phenomenon	Molluscum Contagiosum, Verrucae
Koebner's isomorphic phenomenon	Psoriasis, Lichen planus
Pseudo Darier's Sign	Congenital smooth muscle Hamartoma, Becker's nevus

Contd...

Darier's Sign	Urticaria pigmentosa
Pseudo Nikolsky's Sign	TEN/SSSS
Nikolsky's Sign	Pemphigus
Pseudo Porphyria cutanea tarda	Furosemide and Erythropoeitin therapy
Pseudo Bowen's Disease	Bowenoid Papulosis
Pseudo Leser Trelat Sign	Seborrheic Keratoses after Cytarabine treatment for AML
Leser Trelat Sign	Abrupt appearance of multiple seborrheic keratoses most commonly associated with 1. Nasopharyngeal Carcinoma 2. Acute Myeloid Leukemia
Pseudo Hutchinson's Sign	Non melanoma skin cancers producing peri ungual hyperpigmentation
Hutchinson's Sign	Peri ungula hyperpigmentation seen in sub ungual melanoma
Pseudo Kaposi's Sarcoma	Stewart Bluefarb syndrome
Pseudo Dermatomyositis	Chronic Hydroxyurea therapy
Pseudo Rheumatoid nodule	Granuloma Annulare
Pseudo Scleroderma	Scleredema
Pseudo Lupus vulgaris	Blastomyces dermatidis
Lupus Vulgaris	TB
Pseudo Botryomycosis	Pyogenic Granuloma
Botryomycosis	Staphylococcus aureus
Pseudo Sporotrichosis	Mycobacterium marinum (Fish Tank Granuloma)
Pseudo Furuncle	Dermal Myiasis
Pseudo Mycetoma	Dermatophytosis
Pseudo Bubo: Donovanosis Pseudo Groove's Sign: Granuloma Inguinale (Donovanosis)	Donovanosis (Granuloma inguinale)
Pseudo Elephantiasis: Donovanosis Bubo: Chancroid/LGV	Chancroid/LGV
Groove's Sign of Greenblatt: Lymphogranuloma Venereum (LGV)	LGV

Ref: Kudur MH, Himani M. "Pseudo" conditions in Dermatology: Need to know both real and unreal. Indian J Dermatol Venereol Leprol. 2012;78:763-73.

SIGNS IN DERMATOLOGY

Antenna Sign	Keratosis Pilaris
Barnett's Sign (Scleroderma Neck Sign)	Scleroderma
Breakfast, Lunch and Dinner Sign	Bed Bug (Cimex lectularis)
Buschkke Ollendorff Sign	Secondary Syphilis
Butterfly Sign	Prurigo nodularis + Neurodermatitis
Romana's Sign	Trypanosoma cruzi
Coral Bead Sign	Multicentric Reticulohistiocytosis.
Coudability Sign	Alopecia areata
Friar Tuck Sign	Trichotillomania
Gorlin's Sign	Ehler Danlos Syndrome
Groove Sign of Goldblatt	Lymphogranuloma venereum
Hang Glider Sign	Scabies
Hamburger Sign	Trichotillomania
Holster Sign	Dermatomyositis
Queen Anne's Sign	Same as Hertoghe's Sign
INGRAM'S Sign	Progressive Systemic Sclerosis
Love's Sign	Glomus Tumor
Matchbox Sign	Delusional Parasitosis
Meffert's Sign	Fordyce's Disease
Mizutani Sign	Seen in Raynaud's phenomenon
Nazzaro's Sign	Follicular Hairy Hyperkeratosis
PAVITHRAN'S Nose sign	Exfoliative Dermatitis

17. Anesthesia

*"My dear Sir,
Everybody wants to have a hand in the great discovery. All I will do is to give a hint or two as to names.......
The state should, I think, be called Anaesthesia...."*

—Letter from Oliver Wendell Holmes to William Morton, 1846.

REFERENCE
- Miller's Anaesthesia, 8th ed.

LEVEL I: BASIC REPEATS

KETAMINE

- Increased intracranial tension is seen in Ketamine. *(DNB PATTERN DEC 2010)*
- Not a bradycardia-producing anesthetic: Ketamine. *(DNB PATTERN DEC 2009)*
- Anesthesia of choice in child with cyanotic heart disease: Ketamine. *(DNB PATTERN DEC 2009)*
- Anesthetic of choice in Status asthmaticus: Ketamine. *(DNB PATTERN JUNE 2011)*
- Anesthetic agent associated with Hallucination is: Ketamine. *(DNB PATTERN 2001)*
- Dissociative anesthesia is associated with ketamine. *(DNB PATTERN 2003, 2006, 2007)*
- Ketamine raises intraocular pressure. *(DNB PATTERN 2000, 2005)*
- General anesthetic agent causing sympathetic stimulation: Ketamine. *(FMGE PATTERN SEP 2011)*
- Ketamine is the preferred anesthetic agent in: Bronchial asthma. *(NEET PATTERN 2016)*
- Ketamine acts primarily at: NMDA receptor. *(NEET PATTERN 2015)*
- Inducing Agent of choice in Tetrlogy of Fallot: Ketamine. *(DNB 2015 PATTERN)*

PROPOFOL

- Which of the following intravenous induction agents is the most suitable for day care surgery? Propofol. *(DNB PATTERN DEC 2010, 2011)*

- Safe-inducing agent in Malignant Hyperpyrexia: Propofol
 (DNB PATTERN 2007)
- Propofol Infusion Syndrome is NOT associated with: Hypokalemia. *(NEET PATTERN 2015)*

PROPOFOL-RELATED INFUSION SYNDROME (PRIS)
- Typical features: NEW ONSET METABOLIC ACIDOSIS and cardiac dysfunction.
- Related to dose (4 mg/kg/hr) and duration (>48 hrs) of Propofol Therapy.
- Other features: R–Renal failure and Rhabdomyolysis.
  H–Hyperkalemia, Hyperlipidemia and Hepatomegaly.

SUCCINYL CHOLINE

- Malignant hyperthermia is most commonly precipitated by Succinyl Choline. *(DNB PATTERN 2000, 2004, JUNE 2010)*
- Muscle relaxant which increases intracranial pressure: Suxamethonium. *(DNB PATTERN 2007)*
- Succinyl choline is the muscle relaxant associated with Masseter spasm. *(DNB PATTERN 2002, 2006)*
- Succinyl choline is not contraindicated in Hepatic Failure. *(DNB PATTERN 2007)*

BUPIVACAINE

- Most cardiotoxic local anesthetic is: Bupivacaine. *(DNB PATTERN JUNE 2010)*
- Local anesthetic that is not used topically is: Bupivacaine. *(DNB PATTERN JUNE 2011)*
- Anesthetic agent of choice as epidural anesthesia in labor is: Bupivacaine. *(DNB PATTERN DEC 2009)*

ATRACURIUM

- Hoffman degradation is seen in which muscle relaxant? Atracurium. *(DNB PATTERN JUNE 2011)*
- Skeletal muscle relaxant of choice in liver and renal disease is Atracurium. *(DNB PATTERN DEC 2011)*

COCAINE

- Local anesthetic associated with vasoconstriction and mydriasis is: Cocaine. *(DNB PATTERN 2003)*
- Effect of cocaine on blood vessels: Vasoconstriction. *(DNB PATTERN JUNE 2011)*

- Local anesthetic with a vasoconstrictor action: Cocaine.
  (DNB PATTERN 2005)

SEVOFLURANE, DESFLURANE, METHOXYFLURANE

- Anesthesia of choice in induction in day care surgery in children is: Sevoflurane. *(DNB PATTERN JUNE 2010)*
- The anesthetic agent which has rapid onset and rapid recovery and is most desirable for day care surgical procedures is: Desflurane. *(DNB PATTERN 2002, 2004)*
- High output renal failure is caused by Methoxyflurane.
  (DNB PATTERN 2000, 2005)

GALLAMINE

- Gallamine is excreted mainly through Kidney.
  (DNB PATTERN JUNE 2011)
- Contraindicated in renal failure: Gallamine.
  (DNB PATTERN 2000)

TRICHLOROETHYLENE

- Soda lime circuit is NOT seen in anesthesia with Trichloroethylene. *(DNB PATTERN 2001, 2005)*
- Tachypnea is seen with Trilene.
  (DNB PATTERN 2001, 2003, 2004, 2006)

NITROUS OXIDE

- Gas formed in liquid form is: N_2O.
  (DNB PATTERN DEC 2009)
- Bone marrow depression is caused by: N_2O.
  (DNB PATTERN JUNE 2011)
- True regarding Nitrous Oxide: Blunts Ventilatory/Pulmonary response to Hypoxia. *(FMGE PATTERN MAR 2013)*
- Pin Index of Nitrous Oxide is: 3,5.
  (FMGE PATTERN MAR 2013)
- Inhalational anesthetic with second gas effect: Nitrous Oxide.
  (DNB PATTERN AUG 2013)

ANESTHESIA DEVICES AND PROCEDURES

- Ventilator pressure release valve stuck in closed position can result in Barotrauma. *(DNB PATTERN 2008)*
- Color of Oxygen cylinder is Black with white shoulders.
  (DNB PATTERN DEC 2010)

- Colour of Ethylene cylinder is: Red. *(DNB PATTERN 2004)*
- Fixed oxygen delivery device is: Venturi mask. *(DNB PATTERN JUNE 2010)*
- Maximum O_2 concentration attained in Venturi mask is: 60%. *(DNB PATTERN DEC 2009)*
- Foley's catheter of size 16 F means 16 mm circumference. *(DNB PATTERN JUNE 2010)*
- Armoured endotracheal tube is used in: Neurosurgery. *(DNB PATTERN DEC 2009)*
- Mapleson circuit used in children: Ayres T Tube. (Mapleson E). *(DNB PATTERN JUNE 2010)*
- Blind nasal intubation is contraindicated in: Base of skull fracture. *(DNB PATTERN DEC 2009)*
- Advantages of laryngeal mask are all except: Prevents aspiration. *(DNB PATTERN DEC 2009)*
- NOT related to difficult intubation: Increased Thyromental distance. Decreased Thyromental distance is related to difficult intubation. *(DNB PATTERN DEC 2011)*
- Mallampatti classification is for: Inspection of oral cavity before intubation.
- *Mnemonic for Mallampatti scores*: PUSH
  - Mallampatti 1 - **P**illars
  - Mallampatti 2 - **U**vula
  - Mallampatti 3 - **S**oft Palate
  - Mallampatti 4 - **H**ard Palate.
    (DNB PATTERN DEC 2009)
- The most important and decisive factor in CPR is Defibrillation. *(DNB PATTERN JUNE 2012)*
- The ratio of chest compression to manual ventilation for a single rescuer in CPR is: 30: 2 (ACLS 2010 guidelines) *(DNB PATTERN 2002, 2003)*
- For foreign body causing sudden choking, most appropriate first line of management is: Heimlich Manouevre. *(DNB PATTERN JUNE 2011)*
- Early and reliable indication of air embolism during anesthesia can be obtained by continued monitoring of End Tidal CO_2. *(DNB PATTERN 2008)*
- During rapid sequence intubation in a child after taking brief history and clinical examination, next step is: Administer oxygen. *(DNB PATTERN DEC 2010)*
- Pudendal nerve block involves: S2/S3/S4. *(DNB PATTERN DEC 2009)*
- Pulse oximetry gives an estimate of systemic arterial oxygen saturation. *(DNB PATTERN 2002, 2004)*

- First Endotracheal Intubation in history was done by: McEwen. *(DNB PATTERN AUG 2013)*
- Proper technique of Endotracheal intubation involves: Flexion of Neck and extension of Atlanto-occipital Joint. *(FMGE PATTERN MAR 2012)*
- Contraindicated during Endotracheal Intubation: Neck Flexion at Atlanto-occipital Joint. *(FMGE PATTERN MAR 2011)*
- When no cervical injury is suspected, a small pad is placed under the Occiput.
- This is the SNIFFING POSITION for Endotracheal Intubation.
- When cervical spine injury is suspected, these steps are omitted and neck is stabilised with the help of an assistant.
- Pressure on Thyroid cartilage during Intubation is given as: BURP (Backward, Upward and Rightward Pressure)
- Most common postoperative complication related to Intubation: Sore Throat. *(FMGE PATTERN MAR 2011)*
- Most common nerve used for monitoring during Anesthesia: Ulnar Nerve. *(FMGE PATTERN MAR 2013)*
- Most common muscle used for Neuromuscular monitoring in Anesthesia: Adductor Pollicis.
- Most common modality used for Neuromuscular monitoring in Anesthesia: Train of Four.
- Method to establish a safer airway in a patient with neck trauma, cricoid fracture with possibility of a difficult airway: Emergency Tracheostomy. *(FMGE PATTERN MAR 2011)*
- Site for External Cardiac Massage in Adults: Lower third of Sternum. *(FMGE PATTERN MAR 2009)*
- Depth of chest compression during CPR: 2 inches. *(FMGE PATTERN MAR 2013)*
- During CPR in adult, chest compressions are given at a rate of: 100 compressions/min. *(FMGE PATTERN SEP 2011)*
- Ratio of chest compression to breathing during CPR of newborn patient admitted to ICU is: 3:1. *(FMGE PATTERN MAR 2012, MAR 2013)*
- ASA classification is done for: Fitness, Status of patient. *(FMGE PATTERN MAR 2013)*
- Endotracheal concentration of Adrenaline in CPR for pediatric population is: 1:1000. *(FMGE PATTERN SEP 2012)*
- 1:10,000 in Adults. (0.01 mg/kg is the Endotracheal dose of Adrenaline).

- Curved Laryngoscope was invented by: McIntosh.
(DNB PATTERN AUG 2013)
- Pin Index of Oxygen is: 2,5. *(FMGE PATTERN MAR 2013)*
- Muscle Rigidity is a side effect of: Fentanyl.
(DNB PATTERN NOV 2013)
- Maximum Histamine release among Non-Depolarising skeletal muscle relaxants is: D Tubocurarine.
(DNB PATTERN AUG 2013)
- World Anesthesia Day: October 16.
(DNB PATTERN NOV 2013)
- William TG Morton is known as: Father of Anesthesia.
(DNB PATTERN NOV 2013)
- PEEP level at which alveolar cell recruitment occurs is: 10-12. *(DNB PATTERN NOV 2013)*
- Neuroleptanalgesia consists of: Droperidol and Fentanyl.
(DNB PATTERN NOV 2013)
- DISS (Diameter Index Safety System) is a low pressure safety system. *(NEET PATTERN 2015)*
- True about Gregg Effect: Increased Coronary flow improves LV systolic performance. *(NEET PATTERN 2015)*
- Rapid onset of action of an inhalational agent depends on: Low blood gas partition coefficient.
(NEET PATTERN 2016)
- Colour of Nirous Oxide cylinder in India is: Blue.
(NEET PATTERN 2016)
- Recommended sequence of premedication during elective intubation in a neonate is: Atropine >Fentanyl>Vecuronium.
(NEET PATTERN 2016)
- Murphy's Eye is seen in: Endotracheal Tube.
(NEET PATTERN 2018)
- Nerve commonly tested for adequacy of Anaesthesia: Median Nerve. *(NEET PATTERN 2018)*
- Mechanism of action of Curare type drugs as muscle relaxant: Act competitively on Acetyl Choline receptors blocking post synaptically. *(NEET PATTERN 2018)*
- Most effective circuit in spontaneous anaesthesia: Magill's circuit (Mapleson A). *(NEET PATTERN 2018)*

SPINAL AND EPIDURAL ANESTHESIA

- Dose of lignocaine for spinal anesthesia is: 5%.
(DNB PATTERN JUNE 2011)
- Not a complication of Epidural Anesthesia: DIC.
(DNB PATTERN DEC 2011)

- Not a complication of Epidural Anesthesia: Hypertension.
  (DNB PATTERN 2001, 2005)
- In spinal anesthesia, drug is deposited between Pia and Arachnoid. *(DNB PATTERN DEC 2011)*
- In spinal anesthesia, which fibres are affected earliest? Sympathetic preganglionic. *(DNB PATTERN DEC 2011)*
- Adverse effect of using Ephedrine over Phenyl Ephrine-induced hypotension in LSCS under Spinal Anesthesia: Acidosis. *(DNB PATTERN NOV 2013)*

MISCELLANEOUS

- Receptor responsible for malignant hyperthermia is Ryanodine receptor. *(DNB PATTERN DEC 2011)*
- The skeletal muscle relaxant Rocuronium is NOT excreted largely unchanged in urine. Rocuronium excretion is mostly through liver. Only 10% through kidney.
  (DNB PATTERN JUNE 2011)
- Which muscle is most resistant to neuromuscular blockage? Diaphragm. *(DNB PATTERN JUNE 2011)*
- Concentration of adrenaline used with lidocaine is: 1 in 2,00,000. *(DNB PATTERN DEC 2011)*
- All are amides except: Procaine. *(DNB PATTERN DEC 2011)*
- Mendelson's syndrome is due to pulmonary aspiration of gastric contents. *(DNB PATTERN DEC 2010)*
- Ether was first used as an anesthetic by: Morton. *(DNB PATTERN DEC 2009)*
- Dose of thiopentone is: 2.5%. *(DNB PATTERN DEC 2009)*
- Which inhalational agent is best uterine relaxant? Halothane. *(DNB PATTERN DEC 2009)*
- Composition of soda lime is: 4% NaOH, 95% $Ca(OH)_2$, 1% KOH. *(DNB PATTERN 2000)*
- Methemoglobinemia is caused by Prilocaine. *(DNB PATTERN 2001)*
- Drug used to reverse the effect of D tubocurarine – Neostigmine. *(DNB PATTERN 2001, 2005)*
- To counter central anticholinergic effect, the drug used is: Physostigmine. *(DNB PATTERN 2001)*
- Mechanism of local anesthetic action is stabilisation of membrane. *(DNB PATTERN 2001)*
- Best anesthetic agent for Acute Paronychia is: 1% Xylocaine. *(DNB PATTERN 2002)*
- Maximum safe dose of Lignocaine with Adrenaline is: 7 mg/kg weight. *(DNB PATTERN 2004)*

- Glycopyrollate does NOT cross the blood brain barrier.
  (DNB PATTERN 2002, 2003)
- Safest Local Anaesthetic: Prilocaine.
- Methemoglobinemia is caused by: Prilocaine.
  (DNB PATTERN 2004, 2007)
- Drug commonly causing anaphylaxis: Alcuronium.
  (DNB PATTERN 2007)
- Fastest route of absorption of local anesthetic is: Intercostal.
  (DNB PATTERN 2008)
- Local anesthetics act by inhibiting: Sodium channels.
  (FMGE PATTERN MAR 2012)
- Longest acting local anesthetic is: Dibucaine.
  (FMGE PATTERN MAR 2013)
- Most potent Local Anaesthetic: Dibucaine.
- Most stable Local Anaesthetic: Dibucaine.
- Fifth vital sign elicited by Anesthesiologists is: Pain.
  (NEET PATTERN 2016)
- Sixth vital sign during opiod administration: Sedation.
- Sedation with which drug is likely to resemble normal sleep? Dexmedetomidine. *(NEET PATTERN 2015)*
- Primary determinant of Local Anaesthetic Potency is: Lipid Solubility. *(NEET PATTERN 2015)*
- Amount of pressure exerted by a gas in a mixture is proportional to the percentage of gas in the mixture. This law is known as: Dalton's Law. *(NEET PATTERN 2016)*

LEVEL II: HIGH YIELD FACTORS

Table 17.1: Ketamine

Increases Muscle Tone/Pulse Rate/BP/IOP/ICP Causes Profound Analgesia

Anesthesia of choice in hypovolemic shock and hypotension

Associated with emergence psychotomimetic side effects like illusion, hallucination

Emergence delirium is a side effect

Pretreatment with Lorazepam decreases the chances of emergence side effects

Table 17.2: Propofol

Made up of soyabean oil, glycerol and egg lecithin, Milky white in colour and is a lipid emulsion. Injection of propofol is very painful

Dose-dependent myocardial suppression – hypotension with bradycardia reduces nausea and vomiting

Propofol can be given for child with Porphyria

Table 17.3: Succinyl choline

Shortest acting Muscle relaxant

Commonly used for Rapid sequence induction

Onset of action of Succinyl Choline: 10-30 seconds Duration of action of Succinyl choline: 3-5 minutes

Table 17.4: Local anesthetics

Bupivacaine NOT to be used in Bier's Block

Xylocaine 2% used in dose of 3-5 mg/kg

Xylocaine 2% with Adrenaline used in a dose of 5-7 mg/kg

Cocaine is used in Topical Anesthesia of eye

Table 17.5: Halothane

Bronchodilator and can be safely used in Asthma

NOT used in pregnancy because of increased postpartum hemorrhage

Drager Narko Test

Stored in amber-colored bottles

Thymol is added to halothane for stability

Table 17.6: Anesthesia devices and procedures

High-pressure cylinders	Are made of molybdenum steel
Boyle's machine operates on pin index safety system	Continuous flow principle to discourage incorrect cylinder attachment
Cyclopropane cylinder	Orange
N_2O	Blue
Entonox	Blue body with blue and white shoulder
Rebreathing prevention valve	Should be as near as possible from the patient
Rebreathing prevention valve	Should be installed at expiratory end
Venturi mask	Is a fixed performance or high flow oxygen delivery device
Maximum oxygen delivered by Venturi mask	60%
Maximum oxygen delivered by Nasal cannula	44%
Laryngeal Mask	Is used for difficult airway management during CPR
Laryngeal Mask Airway	Oropharyngeal abscess or mass is a contraindication

Table 17.7: Mapleson systems

Mapleson systems	Are basically for Anesthesia gas delivery
Efficiency of Mapleson systems for spontaneous respiration:	Mapleson A > D & E > C > B
Efficiency of Mapleson systems for assisted and controlled ventilation: Mapleson A	Mapleson D & E > B > C > A Magill's system
Mapleson A	System of choice for Spontaneous Breathing
Mapleson A	Flow rate = Minute
Mapleson A	Volume flow rate is 5 lit/min Water's system
Mapleson C	
Mapleson D	Bain's coaxial system
Mapleson D	Most effective in Controlled or Assisted ventilation
Mapleson E	Ayre's T tube
Mapleson E	Is for infants and young children
Mapleson E	Flow rate is 2-3 X Minute volume
Mapleson F	Jackson Rees modification of Ayre's T tube

HISTORY OF ANESTHESIA

Term Anesthesia was coined by	Oliver Wendell Holmes[Q]
World Anesthesia Day	16th October[Q]
Father of Anesthesia	William TG Morton, 1846[Q]
First physician to intubate the trachea orally	Sir William Macewen[Q]
Curved Laryngoscope was introduced by	Robert Mcintosh[Q]
Laryngeal Mask Airway was invented by	AJ Brian
Indirect Laryngoscopy	Manuel Garcia
Direct Laryngoscopy	Chevalier Jackson
Rapid Sequence Induction for preventing GERD	Brian A Sellick
Nitrous Oxide was first synthesized by:	Priestly
First spinal anesthesia in human beings	August Bier
First Anesthesia machine by	Edmund Gaskin Boyle

Contd...

CPR

	Infants (0–1 yr)	Children (1–14)	Adults
Rate	100/mt	100/mt	100/mt
Depth	1 inch	1-1/2 inches	2 inches
How to compress	2-3 fingers	Heel of one hand	Both hands (one over the other)
Compression area	Mid-Sternum	Mid-Sternum	Lower third of Sternum
Ratio	15:2 (two assistants)	15:2 (two assistants)	30:2
	30:2 (one rescuer)	30:2 (one rescuer)	

KETAMINE

Ketamine was synthesised by	Calvin Stevens
Ketamine is also known as (Street Names)	Kit Kat/Vitamin K(!)/Super K.
Ketamine anaesthesia was first administered in	Vietnam War
Urinary Bladder lesion caused by recreational use of Ketamine	Ulcerative Cystitis (Ketamine Vesicopathy)
Psychiatric Symptoms produced by Ketamine	Dissociative States – Derealization Depersonalisation **K HOLE** – Extreme Dissociation with Auditary and Visual Hallucinations.
Ketamine Metabolism	Liver (CYP)
Ketamine Excretion	Kidney (90%)
Biological Half Life	2.5-3 hrs.
Onset of Action	<5 min.
Duration of Action	Less than 1 hour
Other uses of Ketamine other than Anaesthesia	Post-operative Pain management Management of intractable pain Bronchodilator in the treatment of Severe Asthma. Tested as Rapid Acting Antidepressant in cases of Treatment Resistant Depression.

18 Psychiatry

"One day, in retrospect, the years of struggle will strike you as the most beautiful."
—*Sigmund Freud*

REFERENCE

- *Kaplan and Sadock's Comprehensive Textbook of Psychiatry, 10th ed.*

LEVEL I: BASIC REPEATS

SCHIZOPHRENIA

- Incidence of schizophrenia is 1%. (This is easy to remember schizophrenia is still number one in psychiatry).
  (DNB PATTERN DEC 2011)
- Drug of choice for schizophrenia in a patient with poor oral absorption is Olanzapine. (This is a tough one since only Olanzapine and Fluphenazine are injectables but still Olanzapine being second generation is considered better).
  (DNB PATTERN JUNE 2011)
- Schizophrenia is considered as a thought disorder.
  (DNB PATTERN DEC 2009)
- Schizophrenia is said to be caused by the overactivity of which dopaminergic system? Mesocortical dopaminergic system.
  (DNB PATTERN 2007)
- Poor prognostic factor in Schizophrenia: Gradual onset.
  (DNB PATTERN 2007, 2006)
- Neurotransmitter found in increased amounts in Schizophrenia: Dopamine. *(DNB PATTERN 2007)*
- Not a Schneider's first rank symptom: Delusion of self reference. *(DNB PATTERN 2000)*
- Antipsychotic induced akathisia is characterised by Motoric restlessness. *(DNB PATTERN 2008)*
- Haloperidol toxicity can cause Akathisia and QT prolongation. *(DNB PATTERN DEC 2011)*
- Delusions and Hallucinations are known as Psychotic symptoms. *(DNB PATTERN 2002)*
- Othello syndrome is delusion of infidelity.
  (DNB PATTERN DEC 2011)

- Othello – acronym for "OTHER FELLO." (Mnemonic Aid!!)
- Antipsychotic which increases mortality in Dementia: Haloperidol (Conventional antipsychotics > Atypical Antipsychotics > Non use) *(DNB PATTERN AUG 2013)*
- Fregoli syndrome: Delusion of hyper identification. (The patient believes that everybody he meets is the same person in disguise) *(DNB PATTERN AUG 2013).*
  - Also called Positive Misidentification.

Capgras syndrome	Person believes that his family member is replaced by a double
Fregoli syndrome	Positive misidentification
Couvade syndrome	Person complains of obstetric symptoms during partner's pregnancy
Diogenes syndrome	Gross self neglect among elderly persons.

- Most common hallucination in Schizophrenia: Auditory. *(FMGE PATTERN MAR 2013)*
- Young patient with schizophrenia is intolerant to antipsychotic medications. Treatment to be given is: Clozapine. *(FMGE PATTERN MAR 2013)*
- Delusion is NOT a disorder of perception. *(NEET PATTERN 2016)*
- Delusional misidentification syndrome is: Capgras syndrome. *(2016)*
  - Capgras is a disorder of hypoidentification and Fregoli syndrome is a disorder of Hyperidentification. Both come under the category of Delusional Misidentification.
- Schizoid personality comes under which cluster? Cluster A. *(2016)*
  - Cluster A - Odd eccentric cluster – Schizoid, schizotypal and paranoid
  - Cluster B - Dramatic erratic cluster – Borderline, histrionic and antisocial
  - Cluster C - Anxious cluster – Anxious avoidant, dependent and obsessive compulsive
- Bleuler's criteria for Schizophrenia does NOT include Automatism. *(2016)*
  - Instead it includes autism.
- The skew theory of abnormal family pattern in Schizophrenia is more relevant in case of male children. *(NEET PATTERN 2016)*
- Extra pyramidal side effects are least for: Clozapine. *(NEET PATTERN 2018)*

MOOD DISORDERS

- Maximum burden psychiatric disease in society is DEPRESSION. *(DNB PATTERN JUNE 2009)*
- Unipolar depression > Self inflicted injuries > Alcohol use disorders Burden of Disease (WHO World Report 2001)
- Patient depressed for 3 years with less social interaction but normal sleep and appetite is suffering from: Dysthymia. *(DNB PATTERN DEC 2011)*
- NOT a risk factor for suicide in depression: Female sex. *(DNB PATTERN JUNE 2011)*
- Cognitive model of depression was given by Aaron Beck. *(DNB PATTERN 2008)*
- Aaron Beck's cognitive theory of depression deals mainly with negative thoughts or cognitions about self, future and the environment. NOT with negative thoughts about the past. *(DNB PATTERN DEC 2010)*
- Bipolar disorder type 2 is characterised by hypomania and Major Depressive Episodes. *(DNB PATTERN DEC 2009)*
- Most common psychiatric disorder in India: Depression. *(DNB PATTERN 2008)*
- Drug of choice in Manic depressive psychoses: Lithium. *(DNB PATTERN 2007)*
- True about Manic depressive psychoses: Symptoms remit completely between attacks. *(DNB PATTERN 2000)*
- Time criteria for manic syndrome is 1 week. *(DNB PATTERN JUNE 2010) (ICD 10 criteria).*
- Fluoxetine is used in which childhood condition: Depression. *(DNB PATTERN 2002)*
- Long term lithium use is associated with Hypothyroidism. *(DNB PATTERN 2008)*
- Not an antidepressant: Risperidone. *(DNB PATTERN 2002)*
- ECT is first line treatment in depression with suicidal risk. *(DNB PATTERN 2002)*
- Learned helplessness is typically seen in depression. *(DNB PATTERN 2004)*
- Major depressive disorder criteria as per ICD 10 duration should be more than: 2 weeks. *(DNB PATTERN AUG 2013)*
- Vitamin deficiency associated with depression: Vitamin D. *(NEET PATTERN DEC 2013)*
- Personality type associated with depression: Type D personality
- An old lady is getting very irritable. She shows unusual anger at the noise made by her children in the house and sometimes

beats the two children harmfully. What disorder does the lady have? – Depression. *(FMGE PATTERN MAR 2013)*

- A 30-year-old lady develops acute onset talkativeness to strangers, remains agitated and moves quickly from one task to another. Her diagnosis is: Mania. *(FMGE PATTERN MAR 2013)*

- Most important indication of Bright light treatment is: Seasonal affective disorder. *(NEET PATTERN 2016)*

- Repetitive transcranial magnetic stimulation (RTMS) is used in: Depression. *(NEET PATTERN 2016)*

- Mood stabilizer drug with Anti Suicide properties : Lithium. *(AIIMS MAY 2017 PATTERN)*

GENERAL PSYCHIATRY

- **Behavioural Sciences** includes social psychology, social anthropology and sociology but NOT political science. *(DNB PATTERN JUNE 2012)*

- Sociology is the science of human social behaviour.

- Sociobiology is a subset of evolutionary theory, analysing behaviour of organisms through an evolutionary view point.

- Psychosexual development theory was given by Sigmund freud. *(DNB PATTERN DEC 2010)*

- Medical student with normal weight, parotid abscess and dental caries has bulimia. (Anorexia is typically underweight and obviously oral lesions indicate overeating). *(DNB PATTERN DEC 2011)*

- True about Anorexia all except female male ratio is 2:1. *(DNB PATTERN JUNE 2011)*

- Female Male ratio in Anorexia is 10:1.

- Not a symptom of Anorexia nervosa: Menorrhagia. Amenorrhoea is commonly seen. *(DNB PATTERN 2000)*

- Not seen in Anorexia nervosa: repeated vomiting. *(DNB PATTERN 2004)*

- Young person with self mutilation and impulsivity has a borderline personality disorder. This is easy if you remember borderline is the same as emotionally unstable. *(DNB PATTERN DEC 2011)*

- Conversion disorder –Not true—is occurrence in late age. *(DNB PATTERN JUNE 2011)*

- Obnoxious smell and hallucinations seen in Temporal lobe lesions. *(DNB PATTERN JUNE 2011)*

- Gustatory hallucinations are commonly seen in temporal lobe epilepsy. *(DNB PATTERN 2008)*

- Vivid dreams are NOT a part of PTSD.
  (DNB PATTERN DEC 2010)
- Hallucinations can happen in PTSD even though PTSD is considered to be a neurotic disorder.
  (DNB PATTERN DEC 2010)
- Aggression is NOT part of Kubler-Ross stages of Grief.
  (DNB PATTERN DEC 2010)
- Number of stages in Elizabeth Kubler-Ross' stages of Grief? 5. *(2016)*
  > Denial/Anger/Bargaining/Depression/Acceptance. (DABDA)
- Delirium and dementia can be differentiated by altered sensorium. *(DNB PATTERN JUNE 2010)*
- Sensorium is usually clear in dementia except Lewy body dementia which can present with sudden fluctuations in orientation/sensorium.
- True about dual sex therapy is patient alone is not treated. (Dual sex therapy was started by two people, husband and wife – Masters and Johnson and is essentially for the couple. *(DNB PATTERN JUNE 2011)*
- A person laughs to a joke and then suddenly loses muscle tone. This is called Cataplexy. *(DNB PATTERN DEC 2009)*
- Conversion disorder component is Hysteric fits.
  (DNB PATTERN JUNE 2009)
- All are seen in generalised anxiety except fear of impending doom. This is generally seen in a panic attack.
  (DNB PATTERN JUNE 2009)
- Organicity is manifested usually by mood lability and perseveration.
- Neurosis: insight is preserved, no reality testing impairment.
- Psychosis: insight is lost, reality testing is impaired.
- Disease included in disability act: Mental retardation.
  (DNB PATTERN 2008)
- Oniomania is compulsive buying. *(DNB PATTERN 2008)*
- Perseveration is persistent and inappropriate repetition of the same thoughts. *(DNB PATTERN 2007)*
- In phobic neurosis, main defense mechanism used by the patient is avoidance. *(DNB PATTERN 2007)*
- Drug most useful in the treatment of OCD: SSRI.
  (DNB PATTERN 2006,2007, JUNE 2009)
- Differentiation of hysterical fit from epileptic fit: Hysterical fit occurs when people are watching. *(DNB PATTERN 2007)*
- Only absolute contraindication to ECT: Raised intracranial tension/Brain tumour. (This may raise the ICT indirectly).
  (DNB PATTERN 2000)

- Olfactory and gustatory hallucinations are seen in temporal lobe epilepsy. *(DNB PATTERN 2002)*
- Commonest type of phobia seen in clinical practice: Social phobia. *(DNB PATTERN 2004)*
- Pseudologia fantastica is typically seen in Munchausen's syndrome. *(DNB PATTERN 2004)*
- Capacity to make a will is called Testamentary capacity. *(DNB PATTERN 2004)*
- Classification in Psychiatry is for: Communication, control, comprehension *(DNB PATTERN AUG 2013)* *(Ref: Kaplan Sadock CTP, 9th ed. chap. 9.1)*
- Medical psychology: Use of psychological principles in the evaluation and treatment of diseases is known as Medical Psychology. *(NEET PATTERN DEC 2013)*
- Psychiatrist can give case file to: Patient. *(DNB PATTERN AUG 2013)*
- Sundowning is seen in: Dementia. *(DNB PATTERN AUG 2013)*
- Koro is associated with feeling of shrinking penis. *(DNB PATTERN AUG2013)*
- Which type of personality is related to cardiovascular consequences? Type A. *(NEET PATTERN DEC 2013)*
- The definition of obsession is: Recurrent and intrusive thought, feeling, idea or sensation. *(DNB PATTERN NOV 2013)*
- Area of brain involved in OCD: Basal ganglia. *(FMGE PATTERN 2004)*
- Expression and consequent release of previously repressed emotion is called: Abreaction *(NEET PATTERN 2018)*
- Total Score in MMSE: 30. *(NEET PATTERN 2018)*
- Squeeze Technique is a treatment for: Premature Ejaculation. *(NEET PATTERN 2018)*
- Freud's theory of dreams include all except: Correlation. *(NEET PATTERN 2018)*
- Freud's theory of dreams involve the processes of condensation, displacement and secondary elaboration.

CHILD PSYCHIATRY

- Tics, hair pulling and nail biting does not need any intervention in little children, as they are benign and self limiting. *(DNB PATTERN DEC 2011)*
- NOT a habit disorder: Temper Tantrums. *(NEET PATTERN 2018)*

- Rett's syndrome is the neuropsychiatric syndrome seen ONLY in females. *(DNB PATTERN DEC 2011)*
- A child finding difficulty to spell and read with normal IQ, normal social repertoire and normal vision has Dyslexia. *(DNB PATTERN JUNE 2011)*
- ADHD is comorbid with anxiety, sleep and language disorders but not with elimination disorders. *(DNB PATTERN DEC 2010)*
- M-CHAT (Modified Checklist for Autism in Toddlers) checklist is used for: Autism. *(DNB PATTERN AUG 2013)*
- Cause of death in Rett's syndrome: Respiratory failure. *(DNB PATTERN AUG 2013)*
- Child fights with other children frequently. He has disciplinary problem at school and steals things. Most likely diagnosis: Conduct disorder. *(FMGE PATTERN MARCH 2013)*
- La belle indifference is seen in: Conversion Disorder. (2016)
- Mental Retardation has been renamed as: Intellectual and Developmental Disability. *(NEET PATTERN 2018)*
- According to DSM 5 ADHD criteria, the symptoms of ADHD must have been manifest before the age of 12 yrs. *(JIPMER PATTERN)*

ALCOHOL AND OTHER SUBSTANCE USE DISORDERS

- Irresistible urge to drink alcohol is called DIPSOMANIA. *(DNB PATTERN JUNE 2011)*
- All are seen in alcohol withdrawal except hypersomnolence. *(DNB PATTERN DEC 2009)*
- Alcohol withdrawal is characterised by insomnia, for which the benzodiazepines will surely help. Delirium tremens is caused by alcohol withdrawal. *(DNB PATTERN JUNE 2010)*
- All are present in Delirium tremens except severe depression. *(DNB PATTERN JUNE 2010)*
- Delusions, anxiety and hallucinations are present.
- Main symptom of Korsakoff psychosis is confabulation. *(DNB PATTERN JUNE 2010)*
- Delirium tremens is characteristically seen in Chronic alcoholism. *(DNB PATTERN 2007)*
- Not a feature of delirium tremens: Orientation clear. *(DNB PATTERN 2001)*
- NOT a feature of morphine withdrawal: Constipation. *(DNB PATTERN 2002)*
- Opioid withdrawal state has sweating, diarrhea and vomiting but no polyuria. *(DNB PATTERN JUNE 2010)*

- Caffeine withdrawal does NOT cause hallucinations. *(DNB PATTERN DEC 2011)*
- Nicotine withdrawal does NOT cause Tachycardia. *(DNB PATTERN DEC 2011)*
- Physical withdrawal signs are absent in cannabis withdrawal. *(DNB PATTERN 2000)*
- Cannabis is associated with: Hypnagogic hallucinations. *(DNB PATTERN AUG 2013)*
- Delirium tremens is seen in: Alcohol withdrawal. *(DNB PATTERN AUG 2013/FMGE PATTERN MARCH 2013)*
- Drug used in long term maintenance of opioid dependence: Methadone. *(FMGE PATTERN MARCH 2013)*
- In a chronic alcoholic, Wernicke's encephalopathy can be prevented by: Thiamine supplementation. *(FMGE PATTERN MAR 2013)*
- Ophthalmoplegia is NOT a sign of Delirium tremens. *(NEET PATTERN DEC 2013)*
- Best representation of the Stages of Change in Transtheoretical model: Precontemplation – Contemplation – Preparation – Action – Maintenance. *(NEET PATTERN 2016)*
  - Stages of Change were proposed by Prochaska and Diclemente.
- Paranoid psychosis due to cocaine is seen in intoxication stage of cocaine use. *(NEET PATTERN 2016)*
- Synaesthesia or cross over of sensory perceptions is seen with: LSD. *(NEET PATTERN 2016)*
- Use of Illegal substances is NOT a criterion for drug dependence. *(NEET PATTERN 2016)*

PTSD AND ANXIETY DISORDERS

- Differentiating feature of PTSD in ICD 10: Should start within 6 months. *(DNB PATTERN OCT 2013)*
- Not feature of PTSD: Amnesia. *(DNB PATTERN OCT 2013)*
- Newer therapy for PTSD: Eye Movement desensitisation and reprocessing. *(DNB PATTERN OCT 2013)*
- A patient with history of Road Traffic Accident 2 months back complaints of dreams of accidents. He is able to visualise the same scene whenever he visits the place. Diagnosis is: Post Traumatic Stress Disorder. *(NEET PATTERN 2018)*
- 30 year old lady with sudden onset breathlessness, anxiety, palpitation and feeling of impending doom. Diagnosis is: Panic attack. *(FMGE PATTERN SEP 2012)*
- In Bulimia nervosa vs. Binge Eating, which is in favour of Binge Eating? *(DNB PATTERN JUNE 2014)* – Absence of compensatory behaviours like purging or laxative abuse.

- NOT true about Anorexia nervosa: Normal menstruation. *(DNB PATTERN JUNE 2014)*
- General Adaptation Syndrome (GAS) is seen in: Stressful situations. *(NEET 2016 PATTERN)*
- A lady washes her hand up to 40 times a day. Cognitive behavioural therapy for her should include: Response prevention. *(NEET 2016 PATTERN)*
- Use of Buspirone is: Anxiolytic. *(NEET PATTERN 2018)*

NARCOLEPSY AND SLEEP DISORDERS

- Hypocretin is associated with Narcolepsy. *(DNB PATTERN NOV 2013)*
- NOT true about narcolepsy: seen in NREM sleep. *(DNB PATTERN NOV 2013)*
- True about good sleep hygiene: same time for sleep and waking up daily. *(DNB PATTERN NOV 2013)*
- Delta waves on EEG are seen in: fully relaxed deep sleep. *(FMGE PATTERN MAR 2013)*
- 25 yr old woman with sudden collapse on hearing a bad news. Possible diagnosis is: Cataplexy. *(NEET 2016 PATTERN)*
- Anorexia is NOT a part of Klein-Levin syndrome. (Sleeping beauty syndrome). Hyperphagia is seen in this condition. *(NEET 2016 PATTERN)*
- Delay of return to sleep due to fear is NOT a feature of Pavor nocturnus. *(NEET 2016 PATTERN)*
- NREM Sleep is associated with: Night Terrors.. *(FMGE MAR 2013 PATTERN)*

LEVEL II: HIGH YIELD FACTORS

SCHIZOPHRENIA KEY POINTS

- Risk of Schizophrenia increases with increased paternal age/winter births/obstetric complications at the time of delivery.
- Cannabis can precipitate the symptoms of schizophrenia in people who are genetically vulnerable to get schizophrenia.
- Schizophrenia was referred to as Dementia precox by Kraepelin.
- Term schizophrenia was coined by Eugen bleuler.
- Bleuler's 4As – autistic thinking/abnormal associations/ambivalence/abnormal affect
- First rank symptoms were proposed by Schneider.

Contd...

Contd...

- FIRST RANK SYMPTOMS
  - Made act/affect/volition
  - Thought broadcast/insertion/withdrawal
  - Thought echo
  - Delusional perception
  - Somatic passivity
  - 2nd/3rd person auditory hallucinations.
- Most common type of hallucination in schizophrenia: Auditory
- Most common subtype of schizophrenia: Paranoid.

ANOREXIA/BULIMIA

- Only for Bulimia nervosa
  - Normal body weight
  - Normal menstruation
  - Callus on hand
  - Dental erosions
- Only for Anorexia nervosa
  - Low body weight
  - Amenorrhoea
  - Lanugo
  - Bradycardia/hypotension
  - Normochromic normocytic anemia
  - Elevated liver enzymes
  - Constipation
- Common to both eating disorders
  - Binge eating (may be seen in 25% anorexics also)
  - Female predominance (10:1 ratio)
  - Salivary gland enlargement

KORSAKOFF'S SYNDROME

- Classically present with confabulation.
- Immediate recall and implicit learning (learning procedures) preserved.
- Overall intact intelligence
- Striking anterograde amnesia (inabililty to form new memories)
- Retrograde amnesia less severe.

DELIRIUM

- Alcohol, opioid, benzodiazepines all produce withdrawal delirium.
- Delirium tremens – delirium, autonomic hyperactivity (tachycardia and hypertension) and frequent visual and tactile hallucinations in alcohol withdrawal.

Contd...

Contd...

- RUM FITS – Grand mal seizures in delirium tremens
- Peak incidence of seizures is on 2nd day of alcohol withdrawal.
- Antipsychotic frequently used in delirium tremens: Haloperidol.
- Most frequent type of hallucinations in delirium: Visual
- Most frequent type of delusions in delirium: Paranoid/Persecutory
- Hypoactive delirium is more common in elderly patients.
- EEG in delirium: diffuse slow wave or low voltage activity.
- **Opioid withdrawal:** Orificeal signs – Yawning, lacrimation, rhinorrhoea, vomiting, diarrhoea, cold turkey (gooseflesh) but NO POLYURIA.
- **Nicotine withdrawal:** Bradycardia, weight gain, constipation, insomnia, cough, mouth ulcers
- **Caffeine withdrawal:** Headache, fatigue, sleepiness, Flu like symptoms, concentration difficulties. Anxiety is NOT a valid symptom of Caffeine withdrawal. *(Comprehensive Textbook of Psychiatry 8th ed ch.11.4)* Cannabis withdrawal: anxiety, insomnia, appetite disturbance, and depression.
- **Alcohol withdrawal:** Tachycardia, hypertension, tremor (coarse), seizures, anxiety, visual/tactile hallucinations
- **Cocaine withdrawal:** Agitation, anxiety, alternating anorexia and hyperphagia, fatigue, and anhedonia.
- **Benzodiazepine withdrawal:** Illusions, hallucinations, depersonalisation, grand mal seizures.
- Epigenetic theory or Psychosocial theory – Erik erikson. Stages of cognitive development – Piaget

SIGMUND FREUD

- Oedipus complex/Electra complex
- Interpretation of Dreams
- Psychoanalysis

MAJOR RATING SCALES IN PSYCHIATRY

PANSS (Positive and Negative Symptoms of Schizophrenia)	Schizophrenia
HAM-D (Hamilton's Scale for Depression)	Depression
CARS (Childhood Autism Rating Scale)	Autism
YMRS (Young's Mania Rating Scale)	Mania
Connor's Scale	ADHD
M CHAT (Modified Checklist for Autism in Toddlers)[Q]	Autism
MADRS	Depression
CAGE Questionnaire[Q]	Alcoholism
Impact of Event Scale	PTSD
Los Angeles symptom checklist	PTSD

Contd...

Psychiatry

PSYCHOSURGERY

Started by:	Burckhardt
Word Psychosurgery coined by:	Egas Moniz
Nobel Prize for Psychosurgery:	Egas Moniz
Procedures:	Anterior cingulotomy/Limbic leucotomy/Subcaudate tractotomy/Anterior capsulotomy
Indications:	Depression/OCD
Currently NOT a treatment for	Antisocial personality disorder

❑ Reading up on the controversial **Ice Pick Lobotomist Walter Freeman** from Wikipedia (not in the last minute, of course) will definitely help you to remember this topic forever!

ELECTROCONVULSIVE THERAPY

Invented by:	Cerletti and Bini, 1938.
Primary indication:	Severe depression with suicidal ideation
Mechanism of action:	Not known
Other indications:	Mania/Catatonia > Schizophrenia
Other medical indications:	Neuroleptic malignant syndrome/Parkinsonism/Status epilepticus
Absolute contraindication:	Raised ICT/Papilloedema
Most important cognitive adverse effect:	Retrograde Amnesia
Pregnancy is only a Relative Contraindication for ECT.	
ECT is NOT the treatment of choice in Catatonia. (TOC is Benzodiazepine Trial.)	
Other adverse effects:	Anterograde amnesia and transient confusion

REPETITIVE TRANSCRANIAL MAGNETIC STIMULATION (RTMS)

Primary indication:	Major depressive disorder
Other indications:	OCD/Refractory auditory hallucinations
Major adverse effect:	Provokes GTCS in susceptible individuals.
Advantage over ECT:	Minimal risk for amnestic syndromes
Mechanism of action:	Neuronal depolarization (definitive MOA not clear)

DEEP BRAIN STIMULATION

Used primarily in Parkinson's disease
Middle thalamus or subthalamic nucleus is stimulated in PD
Psychiatric indications: OCD/Treatment resistant depression
Disadvantages: Invasive procedure, requires neurosurgery
Also known as Virtual limbic leucotomy

Contd...

PTSD

PTSD was initially described as	Post Vietnam syndrome
Other names for PTSD	Soldier's heart,
	Shell shock,
	Battle fatigue,
	Traumatic war neurosis,
	RAILWAY SPINE (some cases)
Genes involved in PTSD	RORA gene, STMN 1 gene coding for STATHMIN protein
STATHMIN in PTSD is related to	Re-experiencing symptoms
MRI finding in PTSD	Smaller hippocampal volume
Important rating scales for PTSD	Impact of event scale
	Los Angeles symptom checklist
	Trauma symptom checklist
Difference between DSM IV and ICD 10 criteria for PTSD	Symptom duration of > 1 month in DSM IV and onset of symptoms within 6 months in ICD 10
Reliving of traumatic event in PTSD	Flashback
Vivid memories or Recurring dreams are a feature of	PTSD
New treatment for PTSD	Eye Movement Desensitisation and Reprocessing (EMDR)

PSYCHIATRIC SYNDROMES

OTHELLO syndrome	Pathological jealousy
DE CLERAMBAULT syndrome	Delusion of love
CAPGRAS syndrome	Delusion of doubles; known person replaced by impostor (Hypoidentification)
FREGOLI syndrome	Hyperidentification or delusion that different people are in fact the same person who changes appearance or is in disguise.
DORIAN GRAY syndrome	Dysmorphophobia, Narcissistic personality traits and Paraphilia with excessive preoccupation with youth preservation efforts.
ADONIS complex	Type of Body dysmorphophobic disorder in which person becomes obsessed with body building but believes himself to be an insufficient weakling. Also called BIGAREXIA/MUSCLE DYSMORPHIA/REVERSE ANOREXIA.

Contd...

Contd...

OEDIPUS complex	Fixation/Sexual Involvement of Boy to his mother and rivalry towards father.
ELECTRA complex	Fixation/Sexual Involvement of Girl to her father and rivalry towards mother.
COTARD syndrome	Delusion that one is already dead, do not exist, putrefying or have lost one's own blood or internal organs. Also called WALKING CORPSE SYNDROME.
COUVADE syndrome	Also called Sympathetic Pregnancy in which a partner experiences some of the symptoms of an expectant mother.
DIOGENES syndrome	Extreme self neglect/Social withdrawal/Compulsive hoarding mostly in elderly individuals.
ALICE IN WONDERLAND syndrome	Micropsia—patient sees objects as much smaller than original.

19 Radiology

"I didn't think. I experimented."
Wilhelm Roentgen

REFERENCES

- *Diagnostic Radiology AIIMS – PGI – MAMC series.*

LEVEL I: BASIC REPEATS

CONVENTIONAL PROCEDURES (X-RAY AND CONTRAST PROCEDURES)

WILHELM ROENTGEN

- Father of Diagnostic Radiology
- Discovered X RAYS in 1895.
- Nobel Prize in Physics in 1901.
- Element 111 - Roentgenium is named after him.
- First Medical X-ray: of Anna Bertha Ludwig, wife of Roentgen.
- Used the CROOKE'S TUBE to discover X Rays.

- Plain X-ray abdomen ERECT view—Best X-ray view for Pneumoperitoneum. *(DNB PATTERN DEC 2011)*
- Most sensitive investigation for Pneumoperitoneum: CT scan.
- Other X-ray signs in Pneumoperitoneum: Rigler's sign/Football sign/Inverted V sign/Cupola sign
- X-ray abdomen SUPINE view—Best X-ray for Intestinal obstruction. *(DNB PATTERN DEC 2011)*
- X-ray for minimal right sided pleural effusion done in: Right lateral decubitus position. *(DNB PATTERN JUNE 2009)*
- Ipsilateral decubitus views also for minimal pneumothorax lesions.
- For visualization of Tracheal bifurcation, best radiographic view: Left posteroanterior oblique. *(DNB PATTERN 2000)*
- Lordotic view: Best view for Lung Apices and Lingular abnormalities.
- Dead bone in X-ray is MORE radio-opaque. *(DNB PATTERN JUNE 2009)*

- Radio-opaque appearance in Avascular Necrotic Bone.
- Disseminated small nodules with calcification in chest suggest Histoplasmosis. *(DNB PATTERN 2000)*
- **Apple Core** sign in Barium enema is seen in Carcinoma colon. *(DNB PATTERN JUNE 2010)*

> Apple Core lesion is a general description and so don't jump to the colon always since Apple Core lesions in barium MEAL is indicative of advanced esophageal carcinoma!

- Salt and Pepper appearance in skull in Hyperparathyroidism. *(Pepper for Parathyroid)* *(DNB PATTERN JUNE 2011)*
- **Hyperparathyroidism Bone within Bone** appearance in lateral view of skull X-rays. Hypoparathyroidism: **Basal Ganglia Calcification**.

OTHER FEATURES OF HYPERPARATHYROIDISM

- **Brown Tumor**
- **Tufting of Terminal phalanx**
- **Subperiosteal resorption of cortical bone.**

- **Bone within Bone** appearance is seen in Osteopetrosis. *(DNB PATTERN 2007)*
- Thickness of skull is increased in Thalassemia. *(DNB PATTERN 2005)*
- **Floating teeth** on X-ray seen in Histiocytosis X. *(DNB PATTERN 2003)*
- **Tram line calcification** seen in Sturge-Weber syndrome. *(DNB PATTERN 2007)*
- Hilar Dance in Fluoroscopy is seen in: Atrial Septal Defect *(DNB PATTERN 2004, 2005)*
- Left Atrial enlargement on chest radiograph appears as: Straightening of left heart border. It is an early feature of Mitral Stenosis. *(DNB PATTERN 2001)*
- Nipple sign in Chest X-ray has a sharp Lateral margin. *(DNB PATTERN 2008)*
  - Nipple Sign in Chest X-ray includes:
  - A sharp Lateral Margin
  - Poorly defined Medial Margin
  - This is to be differentiated from a Solitary Pulmonary Nodule.
- At the end of 1 year, no. of carpal bones seen in X-ray is 2. *(DNB PATTERN 2008)*
- At the end of 2 yrs, no of carpal bones seen is 3.
- Target element seen in Mammography is Molybdenum. *(DNB PATTERN JUNE 2010)*

- Positive Predictive Value in Mammography is: Around 20%
- False about Mammography: High positive predictive value.
  (DNB PATTERN JUNE 2010)
- Investigation of choice for Posterior Urethral Valve/Vesico-ureteral reflux is Micturating Cystourethrogram.
  (DNB PATTERN DEC 2010 JUNE 2012)
- Earliest signs of increased ICT is Erosion of dorsum sellae in adults and suture diastasis in children.
  (DNB PATTERN DEC 2011)
- Signs of raised ICT in child: separation of sutures/tense anterior fontanelle/silver beaten appearance of the bones.
  (DNB PATTERN 2007)
- Copper Beaten Skull is also a feature of Raised ICT in child.
- **Cork screw appearance**—Diffuse Esophageal spasm.
  (NEET PATTERN 2012, DNB PATTERN JUNE 2009)
- Corkscrew Collaterals in Thromboangitis Obliterans (TAO) OR Buerger's Disease.
  Rat tail appearance – *Carcinoma Esophagus*.
  (DNB PATTERN JUNE 2011)
- **Beak shaped distal esophagus** in Achalasia Cardia. **Snowman sign** in TAPVC. *(DNB PATTERN DEC 2009)*
- **Snowstorm appearance** in USG for Hydatidiform mole.
  (DNB PATTERN DEC 2011).
- Snowstorm sign in abdominal USG has been described for Hydatid cyst also. **Snowstorm appearance** in chest X-ray is seen in Miliary Tuberculosis.
- **Double Bubble sign** is seen in Duodenal Atresia.
- Single Bubble sign: Pyloric Stenosis
- Triple Bubble sign: Jejunal Atresia.
  (DNB PATTERN 2001, JUNE 2011)
- **Mercedes Benz sign** is seen in Gallstone.
  (DNB PATTERN DEC 2010)
- **Drooping Water Lilly sign** in IVU is seen in Upper pole renal mass. *(DNB PATTERN DEC 2010)*.
- **Water Lilly appearance** is with: Hydatid cyst.
  (DNB PATTERN 2004)
- **Water Lilly Sign/Rising Sun sign** in chest X-ray is suggestive of Ruptured Pulmonary Hydatid cysts.
  (DNB PATTERN 2007)
- Bead Cystogram is used for Stress Incontinence.
  (DNB PATTERN 2004)
- "Bird of Prey" sign in Barium study in Sigmoid Volvulus
  (DNB PATTERN 2008)

Radiology

- Air Bronchogram sign is seen in Consolidation. *(DNB PATTERN JUNE 2011)*
- **Egg shell calcification in chest X-ray** is seen in Silicosis, Sarcoidosis and Lymphoma. *(DNB PATTERN JUNE 2009)*
- Egg shell calcification in Silicosis. *(DNB PATTERN 2007)*
- Angiographic finding in Buerger's disease is **Corkscrew arteries.** *(DNB PATTERN JUNE 2009)*
- **String of Beads appearance** of renal artery is seen in Fibromuscular Dysplasia. *(DNB PATTERN 2005)*
- **Chain of Lakes appearance** is seen in Chronic pancreatitis. *(DNB PATTERN JUNE 2010)*
- Not a feature of Mitral stenosis: Lower lobe prominence of veins. *(DNB PATTERN JUNE 2009)*
- Snowman appearance on X-ray: Supracardiac TAPVC. *(NEET PATTERN 2012)*
- Figure of Eight Appearance on X-ray: Supracardiac TAPVC *(DNB PATTERN AUG 2013)*
- Scimitar sign on X-ray: Infracardiac TAPVC
- Infracardiac TAPVC is associated with Hypoplasia or Sequesteration of Right Lung.
- NOT seen on chest X-ray in Pulmonary Artery Hypertension: Narrowing of central arteries. *(NEET PATTERN 2012)*
- View taken for aortic window: LAO view. *(NEET PATTERN 2012)*
- Rat Tail appearance on Barium Swallow examination is seen in: Carcinoma esophagus. *(NEET PATTERN 2012)*
- Radio-opaque stone: Cysteine. *(NEET PATTERN 2012)*
- Right heart border is NOT formed by Left Atrium. *(NEET PATTERN 2012)*
- Superior most structure in normal X-ray: Coracoid process. *(NEET PATTERN 2012)*
- Colon is identified on X-ray by: Haustra. *(NEET PATTERN 2012)*
- Double Bubble sign is seen in: Duodenal Atresia. *(NEET PATTERN 2012)*
- Onion peel appearance is seen in: Ewing's sarcoma. *(NEET PATTERN 2012)*
- Perihilar fluffy opacities on chest X-ray is seen in: Sarcoidosis. *(NEET PATTERN 2012)*
- Sunray appearance on X-ray: Osteogenic Sarcoma. *(NEET PATTERN 2012)*
- Bone within Bone appearance is seen in: Osteopetrosis. *(NEET PATTERN 2012)*

- Calcification of intervertebral disc is seen in: Gout. *(NEET PATTERN 2012)*
- Rim sign in IVP: Polycystic Kidney. *(NEET PATTERN 2012)*
- Gray equals 100 rad. *(NEET PATTERN 2012)*
- Fraenkel's line is seen in: Scurvy. *(NEET PATTERN 2012)*
- Pseudofracture or Looser's zone is seen in: Osteomalacia. *(NEET PATTERN 2012)*
- Hypertranslucent Chest X-ray is NOT seen in Pneumonectomy. *(NEET PATTERN 2012)*
- Von Rosen's view is for CDH. *(NEET PATTERN 2012)*
- Trident Hand is seen in Achondroplasia. *(NEET PATTERN 2012)*
- Half life of Iodine 131 is: 8 days. *(NEET PATTERN 2012)*
- Most common radionuclide used for Bone Scan: Technetium 99. *(DNB PATTERN NOV 2013)*
- Most commonly used radioisotope for the treatment of Bone cancer: Strontium 89. *(DNB PATTERN NOV 2013)*
- Radioisotope used in PET scan: Fluoride 18. *(DNB PATTERN NOV 2013)*
- Carman Meniscus sign in Barium meal is pathognomonic of: Malignant gastric ulcer. *(FMGE PATTERN SEP 2003)*
- String sign of Kantor is seen in Crohn's disease. *(FMGE PATTERN MARCH 2013)*
- Thumb Print sign is seen in: Ischemic colitis. *(FMGE PATTERN MARCH 2011)*
- Radial Club Hand is associated with: Holt Oram Syndrome. *(DNB PATTERN AUG 2013)*
- Other associated syndromes: VATER syndrome/Fanconi's Anemia, TAR syndrome
- Madelung Deformity: dorsal and radial bowing of the radius resulting in cosmetic and functional deformity.
- A/W Turner's syndrome/Nail patella syndrome/Leri-Weill syndrome.
- Investigation of choice in Posterior Urethral Valve: Micturition Cystourethrogram. *(DNB PATTERN NOV 2013)*
- Gold Standard investigation for the diagnosis of swallowing disorders: Videofluoroscopy. *(DNB PATTERN NOV 2013)*
- First Indication of Left Atrial Enlargement in Mitral Stenosis is: Left Atrial Appendage Enlargement. *(NEET PATTERN 2013)*
- Arrow Headed Fingers on X-ray is suggestive of: Acromegaly. *(NEET PATTERN 2014)*
- Finger in Glove appearance in Chest X-ray is seen in: Bronchocele. *(FMGE PATTERN JUNE 2014)*

> It is also called Mickey Mouse Appearance or Rabbit Ear Appearance. It is usually caused by: Asthma/ABPA/Cystic fibrosis.

- Earliest Sign on Barium Enema in patients with Ulcerative Colitis: Mucosal Granularity. *(NEET PATTERN 2015)*
- Double Bubble on Abdominal X-ray: Duodenal Atresia. *(NEET PATTERN 2016)*
- Stippled Ribs are NOT seen in Hypothyroidism. *(NEET PATTERN 2015)*
- Luckenschadel skull is typically seen in Arnold Chiari Malformation. *(NEET PATTERN 2016)*
  Also associated with Meningocele, Meningomyelocele, Spina Bifida, Cleft Palate.
- Luckenschadel is also called Craniolacunia or Lacunar Skull.
- Luftsichel Sign: Chest X-ray PA view showing hyperlucent para-aortic crescent in Left Upper Lobe Collapse.
- Money Bag Appearance of skull is seen in: Pericardial Effusion. *(NEET PATTERN 2015)*
- Flask-shaped Heart is seen in: Pericardial Effusion. *(NEET PATTERN 2012)*

Pericardial Effusion:
- Pear-shaped Heart
- Purse-shaped Heart
- Flask-shaped Heart

- Most commonly used X-ray film for Mammography: Single film Single Emulsion. *(NEET PATTERN 2016)*
- KvP DOES NOT control Density of X-rays. *(NEET PATTERN 2016)*
- KvP is equal to: Peak voltage applied to the X-ray tube *(NEET PATTERN 2018)*
- KvP is Kilo voltage Peak: It determines the highest energy of X-ray photon.
- Increase in KvP shifts the X-ray spectrum to the right.
- The X-ray image shown below is indicative of: *(NEET PATTERN 2018)*

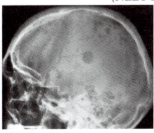

Ans: Multiple Myeloma (Punched out skull appearance).

- The following diagnostic test is called:

(NEET PATTERN 2018)

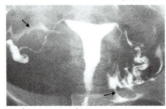

Ans: Hysterosalpingography

ULTRASONOGRAPHY (USG)

- Diagnostic Ultrasound in Medicine was pioneered by: Ian Donald.
- Cart wheel appearance/Wheel spoke appearance in USG is seen in Hydatid cyst. *(DNB PATTERN DEC 2010)*
- Solitary hypoechoic lesion of liver with septa and debri are seen in Hydatid cyst. *(DNB PATTERN DEC 2009)*
- INV of choice for minimal ascites is USG. *(DNB PATTERN JUNE 2009)*
- Min amount of fluid for diagnosing ascites through USG: 100 ml.
- Best investigation for a 4 mm nodule in pancreas is Endoscopic USG. *(DNB PATTERN JUNE 2010)*
- Asymmetric growth on ultrasound imaging is seen in: Anencephaly. *(DNB PATTERN 2002)*
- Best method of investigation in a case of Acute cholecystitis is: HIDA scan. *(DNB PATTERN 2002)*
- Neonate triangular cord sign on USG is seen in: Biliary atresia. *(NEET PATTERN 2012)*
- Congenital hypertrophic pyloric stenosis is diagnosed by: USG. *(NEET PATTERN 2012)*
- Beaded pattern with fimbrial fluid is seen in – TB of fallopian tube. *(NEET PATTERN 2012)*
- Ground glass ventricular septum is seen in: HOCM. *(NEET PATTERN 2012)*
- Technique using piezoelectric crystals: USG. *(NEET PATTERN 2012)*
- Initial investigation of choice for Intussusception: USG. *(FMGE PATTERN 2003)*
- Gold standard investigation for the diagnosis of cystic echinococcus: USG. *(FMGE PATTERN 2009)*
- Initial investigation of Amoebic Liver Abscess: USG. *(FMGE PATTERN 2009)*

- FAST Ultrasound is used to evaluate fluid in all regions Except: Pleura. *(NEET PATTERN 2014)*
- Most specific sign of Portal Hypertension on USG is: Recanalized Umbilical Vein. *(NEET PATTERN 2014)*
- Blue color on Color Doppler represents: Deoxygenated blood flow. *(NEET PATTERN 2015)*
- Sign of Hepatobiliary Ascariasis on Transverse Ultrasound: Bull's Eye Sign. *(NEET PATTERN 2016)*

COMPUTED TOMOGRAPHY (CT)

- Hounsfield units are used in CT scan. *(DNB PATTERN JUNE 2011)*
- Tesla in MRI, Voxel in functional MRI.
- Investigation of choice for Acute SAH: Noncontrast CT scan, not DSA/MRI. *(DNB PATTERN DEC 2011)*
- Most sensitive test for ureteric stones is Noncontrast CT scan. *(DNB PATTERN JUNE 2010)*
- Investigation of choice for Advanced renal tuberculosis: CT scan. *(DNB PATTERN JUNE 2011)*
- Investigation of choice for Neuroangiofibroma is Contrast enhanced CT. *(DNB PATTERN DEC 2009)*
- MRI was invented by: Raymond Damadian (controversial !)
- Nobel Prize in Medicine for pioneering MR imaging: Lauterbur and Mansfield.
- CT scan was invented by Geoffrey Hounsfield. *(DNB PATTERN 2003)*
- Central stellate scars on CT scan seen in Renal Oncocytoma. *(DNB PATTERN 2008)*

    Central Scar in CT
    - Renal Cell Carcinoma
    - Fibrolamellar Hepatocellular Carcinoma.
- Central dot sign in CT scan is seen in: Caroli's disease. *(DNB PATTERN 2008)*
- Best investigation for Bronchiectasis is HRCT. *(DNB PATTERN DEC 2010)*
- HRCT is the investigation of choice for Sarcoidosis, Pulmonary Fibrosis and Miliary Tuberculosis but NOT Aneurysm. *(DNB PATTERN DEC 2011)*
- Best imaging modality in Bronchogenic carcinoma: CT. *(NEET PATTERN 2012)*
- HU is a measure of: CT. *(NEET PATTERN 2012)*

- The most sensitive imaging modality for diagnosis of ureteric stones in a patient with acute colic is – Noncontrast CT of the abdomen. *(NEET PATTERN 2012)*
- How much area is covered by Spiral CT in 30 seconds? – Whole body. *(DNB PATTERN NOV 2013)*
- Best investigation for diagnosing abdominal aortic aneurysm is: CT Angiography. *(DNB PATTERN NOV 2013)*
- Sylvian Point is related to: Lateral cerebral sulcus. *(NEET PATTERN 2014)*
- Air and Water have Hounsfield units of: -1000 Air and 0 Water. *(NEET PATTERN 2014)*
- CT Angiography shown below is indicative of: *(NEET PATTERN 2018)*

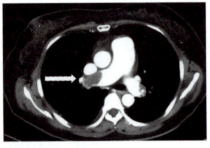

Ans: Pulmonary Embolism.

MAGNETIC RESONANCE IMAGING (MRI)

- Investigation of choice for Entrapment neuropathy is MRI. *(DNB PATTERN DEC 2010)*
- Investigation of choice for Vestibular Schwannoma: Gadolinium enhanced MRI. *(NEET PATTERN 2012)*
- Ice Cream Cone Appearance on MRI: Vestibular Schwannoma.
- Investigation of choice in Intramedullary space occupying lesion: MRI *(NEET PATTERN 2012)*
- Investigation of choice for Multiple Sclerosis: MRI. *(NEET PATTERN 2012)*
- Dawson's fingers are typically seen in: Multiple Sclerosis. *(DNB PATTERN NOVEMBER 2013)*
- Tiger eye sign on MRI: Hallervorden Spatz Disease. *(NEET PATTERN 2012)*
- Fat appears Bright in T1/Intermediate Bright in T2 sequences.
- Which looks same on T1 and T2 in MRI? Fat. *(NEET PATTERN 2012)*
- Earliest diagnosis of cerebral infarct is done by: Diffusion Weighted MRI. *(DNB PATTERN NOV 2013)*

- NOT TRUE about T1 weighted image in MRI: Fluid appears Bright. *(NEET PATTERN 2016)*

RADIOTHERAPY

- Oxygenation is effective during radiotherapy just before starting. *(DNB PATTERN DEC 2011)*
- In small cell lung carcinoma, prophylactic cranial irradiation is given. *(DNB PATTERN DEC 2011)*
- Prophylactic Cranial Irradiation is also given in ALL but currently has an ambiguous role.
- Most radiosensitive tumor is a dysgerminoma. *(DNB PATTERN JUNE 2011)*
- PET uses the tracer material FDG (Fluorodeoxyglucose *(DNB PATTERN JUNE 2010)*
- Another tracer isotope for PET scan: RUBIDIUM 82
- Gamma Knife is used in Stereotactic Surgery which is a form of Radiotherapy. *(DNB PATTERN JUNE 2010)*
- Linear Accelerator - two points to be put in reverse order.
- Linear Accelerator can also produce High Energy electrons.
- Linear Accelerator produces X-rays. *(DNB PATTERN DEC 2009, 2011)*
- Pure beta particle(electron) emitter is Phosphorus 32. *(DNB PATTERN DEC 2011)*
- Cyclotron produces gamma rays. Betatron produces X-rays. *(DNB PATTERN DEC 2011)*
- Radium on disintegration leads to Radon in gaseous form. *(DNB PATTERN JUNE 2010)*
- Half life of Radium 226 is 1600 years.
- Largest half life is for Radium: *(DNB PATTERN DEC 2009)*
- Not used in Brachytherapy—Iodine 131. *(DNB PATTERN DEC 2009)*
- Iodine 131 is not used because of carcinogenic potential. Iodine 125 is used for Brachytherapy.
- Cell most sensitive to radiation is: Lymphocyte. *(DNB PATTERN 2000, 2005)*
- Xeroradiography is used in the detection of Breast lesions. *(DNB PATTERN 2000)*
- Xeroradiography uses a charged Selenium plate.
- Device used for Xeroradiography: Scorotron. *(DNB PATTERN 2003)*
- Dye used for myelography is Myodil. *(DNB PATTERN 2000, 2003, 2005)*

- Meckel's diverticulum is best diagnosed by Tc 99 Pertechnetium scan. *(DNB PATTERN 2000)*
- Most radiosensitive tissue is Bone Marrow. *(DNB PATTERN 2003)*
- M in 99 Tc^m stands for Metastable. (Superscript m stands for Metastable. *(DNB PATTERN DEC 2010)*
- Shield used in Radiology is made up of Lead. *(DNB PATTERN JUNE 2009)*
- Fetus is MOST radiosensitive at 3–6 weeks. *(DNB PATTERN JUNE 2009)*
- Ideal Therapeutic Radio Isotope is: Strong Beta Low Gamma Emitter. *(NEET PATTERN 2016)*
- Example of Strong Beta Low Gamma emitter: Lutetium 177
- Infrared Rays do not belong to the category of Ionizing Radiation. *(NEET PATTERN 2016)*
- Nuclides with Identical Atomic Mass numbers but different Atomic numbers are called: Isobars. *(NEET PATTERN 2014)*

MISCELLANEOUS

- In Corrosive poisoning leading to stricture, the investigation of choice is Endoscopy. *(DNB PATTERN DEC 2011)*
- Thimble bladder is seen in Chronic Tubercular Cystitis. *(DNB PATTERN 2007)*
- Best investigation of choice for Dissecting Aortic Aneurysm is: MRI, CT, and Trans Esophageal Echo have the same sensitivity and specificity. *(Ref: Diagnostic Radiology AIIMS PGI MAMC)* *(DNB PATTERN NOV 2013)*
- Vertical Acetabular Roof is NOT seen in Achondroplasia. *(NEET PATTERN 2016)*
- Best investigation for the delineation of Parathyroid abnormalities: Sestamibi scan. *(AIIMS PATTERN 2017)*
- Negative Test on FDG PET SCAN is classically described for: Typical Pulmonary Carcinoid. *(AIIMS PATTERN 2017)*
- Small Cell Lung Carcinoma, Large Cell Neuroendocrine Carcinoma, and Atypical Carcinoid show increased uptake on FDG PET scan.
- Incidentally detected complex renal cyst is more likely to be- Angiomyolipoma.

(AIIMS PATTERN 2017)

- DSA scan shown below is indicative of:

(NEET PATTERN 2018)

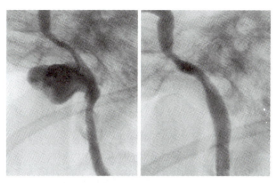

Ans: Internal Carotid Artery Pseudoaneurysm.

- **Yin Yang Sign** is seen in both true and false arterial aneurysms.
- The Thyroid Scan image shown below is indicative of:

(NEET PATTERN 2018)

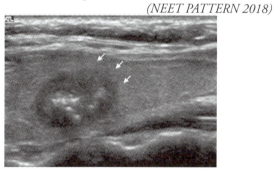

Ans: Medullary Carcinoma Thyroid (coarse clump of calcification.)

- The procedure shown below is called:

(NEET PATTERN 2018)

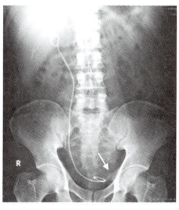

Ans: DJ stenting.

- The procedure shown below is: *(NEET PATTERN 2018)*

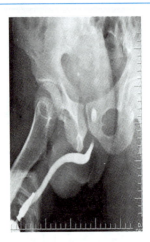

Ans: Retrograde Urethrogram (RGU)

ACHONDROPLASIA

- Funnel shaped foramen magnum
- Bullet shaped vertebra
- Posterior vertebral scalloping
- Trident pelvis
- Tombstone iliac wings
- Champagne glass pelvic inlet
- Trident hand
- Trumpet bone
- Chevron deformity of growth plate
- Rhizomelic shortening of femori and humeri.

LEVEL 2: HIGH YIELD FACTORS

TB AND RADIOLOGY

- Snowstorm appearance on CXR: Miliary Tuberculosis.
- Putty Kidney/Moth eaten calyx/Phantom calyx/Hydrocalyx: Renal Tuberculosis.
- Autonephrectomy in Renal TB.
- Thimble Bladder/interstitial cystitis: Tuberculous Bladder.
- Watermelon Sign: Tuberculous Prostatitis.
- Saw tooth Ureter/Pipe stem ureter: TB Ureter.
- Best investigation for early renal TB: IVU.
- Earliest urographic sign in Renal TB: loss of definition of minor calyx/feathery outline.
- Investigation of choice in advanced Renal TB: CT scan (to get more info on functional status/calcification).

- Coal Worker's Pneumoconiosis.

HRCT

- Thin collimation is used in HRCT.
- Thickness of individual sections are 1-2 mm (Usual CT 7-10 mm).
- Characteristic diagnostic patterns in HRCT seen in Sarcoidosis/Idiopathic Pulmonary Fibrosis/Lymphangitic Carcinoma/Eosinophilic Granuloma/Bronchiectasis.
- HRCT findings are not specific and has to be interpreted in the clinical context.
- Most common cause of Tree in Bud pattern: Bronchiolitis.
- Crazy pavement pattern: Pulmonary alveolar proteinosis/Pneumocystis carinii pneumonia.
- Ground glass opacities are nonspecific and can occur in many conditions including ARDS.

NAMED SIGNS IN THE GIT

- Rat tail sign: Carcinoma esophagus.
- Bird Beak sign: Achalasia Cardia.
- Corkscrew esophagus: Diffuse esophageal spasm.
- Apple Core Sign (Barium meal): Carcinoma esophagus.
- Double Bubble Sign: Duodenal Atresia.
- Colon cut off sign: Acute Pancreatitis.
- Sentinel loop sign: Acute Pancreatitis.
- Mercedes Benz sign: Gallstones.
- Claw sign: Intussusception.
- Meniscus sign: Intussusception (Plain film).
- Target Sign: Intussusception (Plain film).
- Coiled Spring appearance: Intussusception (Barium study).
- Pseudokidney sign: Intussusception (Ultrasound sign).
- Coffee Bean sign: Sigmoid Volvulus.
- Bird of Prey sign: Sigmoid Volvulus.
- Rigler's sign/Inverted V sign/Cupola sign/Football sign: Pneumoperitoneum.
- String of Beads sign: Mechanical intestinal obstruction.

PUV/VUR/MCU is one of the most repeated hot areas across different entrance exams........So a bit more deeper..........

- An MCU or VCUG (Voiding Cystourethrogram) should be performed in suspected VUR after the 1st well-documented UTI.
- Grading of VUR:
    - Gr 1: reflux to only ureter
    - Gr 2: reflux to ureter, pelvis and calyces, but no dilatation
    - Gr 3: reflux to calyces with mild dilatation of calyces
    - Gr 4: reflux to calyces with moderate dilatation
    - Gr 5: gross dilatation of ureter/renal pelvis/calyces.
- Most common congenital obstructive lesion of the urethra: PUV.

- Most common type of PUV: Type 1 PUV. Least common Type 2. Three types in all.
- Congenital anomaly a/w PUV: Potter facies and Pulmonary Hypoplasia.(3P)/Prune Belly syndrome.
- Cobra Head Appearance on MCU: Ureterocele.
- Posterior urethral valves are vestiges of the Wolffian Duct.
- a/w "pear/keyhole" bladder.

SUBARACHNOID HEMORRHAGE

- Initial investigation in Acute SAH: Noncontrast CT.
- Gold standard investigation: cerebral 4 vessel angiography.
- Best investigation for subacute or chronic SAH: MRI.
- Best noninvasive investigation to investigate the etiology of SAH: MR Angiography.
- Most common cause of SAH: Aneurysm.
- Most common site of aneurysm: Anterior communicating artery.

HYDATID CYST

- Most pathognomonic finding: demonstration of daughter cysts within larger cyst.
- Egg shell calcification or Mural calcification on CT: Indicative of Echinococcus granulosus infection.
- Most specific investigation for Hydatid cyst: Immunoblotting – detection of antibodies to specific echinococcal antigens.
- Other ultrasonogram findings in Hydatid disease: cyst in cyst appearance/Honeycomb pattern/floating membrane sign/ultrasound water lilly sign.

THE WATER LILLIES.....

- Water Lilly sign in X-ray – Ruptured Pulmonary Hydatid cysts.
- Ultrasound Water Lilly sign – Hydatid cyst of liver.
- Drooping Water Lilly sign in IVU – Upper pole renal mass.

KERLEY B LINES (CHAPMAN 5TH ED.)

- Due to thickening of interlobular septa surrounding individual secondary pulmonary nodules.
- Interlobular septa contain lymphatics, venous radicals and interstitium.
- Any cause of lymphatic or venous obstruction or infiltrating/interstitial diseases cause Kerley B lines.

> Kerley B lines are best appreciated in costophrenic angles on X ray. Kerley B lines more clearly visible on CT.

Pulmonary venous pathology	Lymphatic pathology	Interstitial disease
LV failure	Lymphangitic spread of tumor	Pneumoconiosis
Mitral Stenosis	Diffuse pulmonary lymphangiomatosis	Erdheim Chester disease
Pulmonary Veno-occlusive disease	Congenital lymphangiectasia	Pulmonary hemorrhage
		Amyloidosis
		Alveolar Proteinosis

NUCHAL FOLD THICKNESS

> Nuchal fold is: the skin thickness at the posterior aspect of fetal neck.
> Definition of thickened nuchal fold: > or = to 6 mm between 18-24 weeks.
> Definition of thickened nuchal fold: > or = to 5 mm between 16-18 weeks.
> Nuchal fold thickness is NOT the same as Nuchal Translucency.
> Nuchal translucency is a specific measurement of fluid in the posterior aspect of neck at 11 to 14 weeks gestation.
> A thickened nuchal fold 6 mm or greater increases the risk of Down's syndrome 17 fold.
> Other DDs of thickened Nuchal fold: Turner's syndrome, Noonan syndrome, Multiple pterygium syndrome, skeletal dysplasia, congenital cardiac defects.
> Next investigation to be done in case of a thickened nuchal fold: Karyotyping.
> Nuchal fold index: Mean nuchal fold/mean biparietal diameter * 100.

EGG SHELL CALCIFICATION

Defined as

Shell like calcifications up to 2 mm thick in the Periphery of at least 2 lymph nodes

In at least 1 of which the ring of calcification must be complete

And 1 of the affected lymph nodes must be >1 cm in diameter. (Chapman's Aids to Radiological Differential Diagnosis, 5th ed.)

Silicosis (5%)

Coal Miner's Pneumoconiosis (1%)

Sarcoidosis (5%)

Lymphoma following Radiotherapy

EGG SHELL CALCIFICATION

- Hilar and Mediastinal nodal egg shell calcification is CHARACTERISTIC of SILICOSIS.
- Egg Shell Calcification is UNCOMMON in COAL WORKER'S PNEUMOCONIOSIS.
- Egg Shell Calcification in CT in HYDATID CYST.
- Egg On Side appearance in Transposition of Great Arteries. (TGA)